STATE OF THE ART IN QUANTITATIVE CORONARY
ARTERIOGRAPHY

DEVELOPMENTS IN
CARDIOVASCULAR MEDICINE

STATE OF THE ART IN QUANTITATIVE CORONARY ARTERIOGRAPHY

edited by

J.H.C. REIBER, PhD and P.W. SERRUYS, MD

Department of Cardiology, Thorax Center, Erasmus University
Rotterdam, The Netherlands

1986 **Springer-Science+Business Media, B.V.**

Library of Congress Cataloging in Publication Data

ISBN 978-94-010-8401-7   ISBN 978-94-009-4279-0 (eBook)
DOI 10.1007/978-94-009-4279-0

Table of contents

List of contributors

Amende I, MD, Abteilung Kardiologie, Medizinische Hochschule Hannover, Postfach 610180, D-3000 Hannover 61, Germany.

Blankenhorn DH, MD, University Southern California School of Medicine, 2025 Zonal Ave, Los Angeles, CA 90033, U.S.A.

Boer A den, BSc, Thoraxcenter, Erasmus University and University Hospital Dijkzigt, PO Box 1738, 3000 DR Rotterdam, the Netherlands.

Bove AA, MD, PhD, Division of Cardiovascular Diseases and Internal Medicine, Mayo Medical School, Rochester, Minnesota 55905, U.S.A.

Brand M van den, MD, Thoraxcenter, Erasmus University and University Hospital Dijkzigt, P.O. Box 1738, 3000 DR Rotterdam, the Netherlands.

Bürsch JH, MD, Abteilung Kinderkardiologie, Klinikum der Christian-Albrechts-Universität zu Kiel, Schwanenweg 20, 2300 Kiel 1, Germany.

Conti CR, MD, Department of Medicine, Division of Cardiovascular Medicine, University of Florida, College of Medicine, Box J-277, Gainesville, Florida 32601 and VA Medical Center, Gainesville, Florida 32601, U.S.A.

Feldman RL, MD, Department of Medicine, Division of Cardiovascular Medicine, University of Florida, College of Medicine, Box J-277, Gainesville, Florida 32601 and VA Medical Center, Gainesville, Florida 32601, U.S.A.

Feyter P de, MD, Thoraxcenter, Erasmus University and University Hospital Dijkzigt, P.O. Box 1738, 3000 DR Rotterdam, the Netherlands.

Geuskens R, MD, Thoraxcenter, Erasmus University and University Hospital Dijkzigt, P.O. Box 1738, 3000 DR Rotterdam, the Netherlands.

Gould KL, MD, Division of Cardiology, University of Texas, Medical School at Houston, P.O. Box 20708, Houston, Texas 77225, U.S.A.

Harrison DG, MD, Department of Internal Medicine and The Cardiovascular Center, University of Iowa, Iowa City, Iowa 52242, U.S.A.

Heethaar RM, PhD, Department of Cardiology and Department of Medical Physics, University Hospital, State University, Catharijnesingel 101, 3583 CP Utrecht, the Netherlands.

Heintzen PH, MD, Abteilung Kinderkardiologie, Klinikum der Christian-Albrechts-Universität zu Kiel, Schwanenweg 20, 2300 Kiel 1, Germany.

Hemphill L, MD, University of Southern California, School of Medicine, 2025 Zonal Ave, Los Angeles, California 90033, U.S.A.

Herrmann G, MD, Abteilung Kardiologie, Medizinische Hochschule Hannover, Postfach 610180, D-3000 Hannover 61, Germany.

Hiratzka LF, MD, Department of Internal Medicine and The Cardiovascular Center, University of Iowa, Iowa City, Iowa 52242, U.S.A.

Kirkeeide, RL, PhD, Division of Cardiology, University of Texas Medical School at Houston, P.O. Box 20708, Houston, Texas 77225, U.S.A.

Kooijman, CJ, MSc, Thoraxcenter, Erasmus University and University Hospital Dijkzigt, PO Box 1738, 3000 DR Rotterdam, the Netherlands.

Lee PL, PhD, Jet Propulsion Laboratory, California Institute of Technology, 4800 Oak Grove Drive, Pasadena, California 91109, U.S.A.

Leeuw, P de, MSc, Philips Medical Systems, Best, The Netherlands.

Lichtlen PR, MD, Abteilung Kardiologie, Medizinische Hochschule Hannover, Postfach 610180, D-3000 Hannover 61, Germany.

Lipton MJ, MD, Department of Radiology, University of California San Francisco, California 94143, U.S.A.

Macdonald RG, MD, Department of Medicine, Division of Cardiovascular Medicine, University of Florida, College of Medicine, Box J-277, Gainesville, Florida 32601 and VA Medical Center, Gainesville, Florida 32601, U.S.A.

Marcus, ML, MD, Department of Internal Medicine and the Cardiovascular Center, University of Iowa, Iowa City, Iowa 52242, U.S.A.

Moldenhauer K, MD, Abteilung Kinderkardiologie, Klinikum der Christian-Albrechts-Universität zu Kiel, Schwanenweg 20, 2300 Kiel 1, Germany.

Nichols WW, PhD, Department of Medicine, Division of Cardiovascular Medicine, University of Florida, College of Medicine, Box J-277, Gainesville, Florida 32601 and VA Medical Center, Gainesville, Florida 32601, U.S.A.

Pepine CJ, MD, Department of Medicine, Division of Cardiovascular Medicine, University of Florida, College of Medicine, Box J-277, Gainesville, Florida 32601 and VA Medical Center, Gainesville, Florida 32601, U.S.A.

Quante W, BSc, Abteilung Kardiologie, Medizinische Hochschule Hannover, Postfach 610180, D-3000 Hannover 61, Germany.

Reiber JHC, PhD, Thoraxcenter, Erasmus University and University Hospital Dijkzigt, PO Box 1738, 3000 DR Rotterdam, The Netherlands.

Ritman EL, MD, PhD, Department of Physiology and Biophysics, Mayo Medical School, Rochester, Minnesota 55905, U.S.A.

Sandor T, DP, Department of Radiology, Brigham and Women's Hospital, Harvard Medical School, Massachusetts 02215, U.S.A.

Schmiel FK, MD, Department of Cardiology, Medizinische Einrichtungen der Universität Düsseldorf, Medizinische Klinik und Poliklinik, Klinik B, Moorenstrasse 5, 4000 Düsseldorf 1, Germany.

Schuurbiers JCH, BSc, Thoraxcenter, Erasmus University and University Hospital Dijkzigt, PO Box 1738, 3000 DR Rotterdam, the Netherlands.

Serruys PW, MD, Thoraxcenter, Erasmus University and University Hospital Dijkzigt, P.O. Box 1738, 3000 DR Rotterdam, The Netherlands.

Selzer RH, MSc, Jet Propulsion Laboratory, California Institute of Technology, 4800 Oak Grove Drive, Pasadena, California 91109, U.S.A.

Shircore A, BSc, Informatics General Corp., 21050 Van Owen Street, Canoga Park, California 91304, U.S.A.

Simon R, MD, Abteilung Kardiologie, Medizinische Hochschule Hannover, Postfach 610180, D-3000 Hannover 61, Germany.

Slager CJ, MSc, Thoraxcenter, Erasmus University and University Hospital Dijkzigt, PO Box 1738, 3000 DR Rotterdam, the Netherlands.

Spears JR, MD, Beth Israel Hospital, Cardiovascular Division, 330 Brookline Avenue, Boston, Massachusetts 022150, U.S.A.

Spiller P, MD, Department of Cardiology, Medizinische Einrichtungen der Universität Düsseldorf, Medizinische Klinik und Poliklinik, Klinik B, Moorenstrasse 5, 4000 Düsseldorf 1, Germany.

Stegehuis H, MSc, Department of Cardiology and Department of Medical Physics, University Hospital, State University, Catharijnesingel 101, 3583 CP Utrecht, the Netherlands.

Vogel RA, MD, Department of Cardiology, Veterans Administration, 2215 Fuller Road, Ann Arbor, Michigan 48105, USA.

Werf T van der, MD, Department of Cardiology, St. Radboud Hospital, Catholic University, Geert Grooteplein Zuid 8, 6525 AG Nijmegen, the Netherlands.

Wijns WW, MD, Thoraxcenter, Erasmus University and University Hospital Dijkzigt P.O. Box 1738, 3000 DR, Rotterdam, the Netherlands.

White CW, MD, Department of Internal Medicine and the Cardiovascular Center, University of Iowa, Iowa City, Iowa 52242, U.S.A.

Introduction

Over the past twenty years, technical advances in coronary arteriography have contributed to our understanding of the pathophysiologic aspects and natural history of coronary artery disease. Probably more than 700.000 coronary arteriograms are performed annually throughout the world. Usually, these arteriograms are interpreted visually to determine the morphologic extent and severity of coronary artery disease. These subjective determinations, which are hampered .by relatively large intra- and interobserver variations, are used as a basis for critically important therapeutic decisions: Which arteries are to be revascularized, which lesions are suitable for coronary bypass surgery or for percutaneous coronary angioplasty? To improve on this clinical decision making, on the treatment and follow-up of such patients, new, objective and reproducible techniques for the assessment of the extent and severity of coronary artery disease, both in terms of anatomy and functional significance of the lesions, must be made widely available. With such new procedures and technologies the efficacy of new therapeutic procedures, the effects of vasodilating and constricting drugs, and the results of long-term studies on the regression and progression of atherosclerotic plaque can be determined in an objective and cost-effective manner.

In this book the state-of-the-art in quantitative coronary arteriography is reviewed, including the progress in *technical and clinical developments* in coronary arteriography (conventional cineangiography, digital cardiovascular imaging and X-ray tomography), the methodology and clinical applications of *quantitative coronary cineangiography* which allows the assessment of objective and reproducible measurements on arterial dimensions from 35 mm cinefilm, the measurement of *coronary blood flow* from contrast injections, and finally, the determination of the *physiologic significance* of coronary lesions and the relation to the morphologic abnormalities.

Each chapter has been authored by an expert from either Europe or the USA, who has contributed to the developments in his particular field. The basic principles of each technique, the results from validation studies and the clinical applications are described in detail. Guidelines are provided for standardized acquisition and analysis of angiographic studies to minimize the variations result-ing from the many potentially existent error sources.

We hope that this book will show the (clinical) cardiologist, radiologist, and physicist how and to which extent the present technological and clinical develop-ments in quantitative coronary arteriography may influence the clinical decision making in patients with coronary artery disease and in which way it may facilitate new clinical research studies.

Michel E. Bertrand, M.D.
Chairman, Working Group
'Coronary blood flow and mechanism
of angina pectoris' of the
European Society of Cardiology.

Part I: Technical developments in coronary angiography

Quality considerations on cine-imaging and PTCA-fluoroscopy anticipating a digital future

Paul de Leeuw

Summary

In a modern catheterization laboratory coronary cineangiography, PTCA procedures and digital radiography are performed with one and the same X-ray system. On the basis of an optimization analysis of the image quality using the concepts of window signal-to-noise ratio and equivalent blur, overall performance can roughly be estimated. Some important aspects of a realistic X-ray system design resulting from this analysis have been identified. Specifically, the X-ray loadability and its loading strategy play a crucial role with respect to signal detection sensitivity and the safe, efficient use of X-ray radiation. The analysis shows also that some basic limitations exist to the use of digital substraction techniques for moving objects. Last but not least, it shows that the video camera performance is critical with respect to the imaging tasks during PTCA and digital procedures.

Introduction

Although the technique of coronary cineangiography has been widely used for more than fifteen years, it still remains one of the most difficult radiographic procedures from a technical point of view. In recent years, digital imaging techniques have proven to be very useful especially in conjunction with Percutaneous Transluminal Coronary Angioplasty (PTCA). This combination has stimulated the discussions about quantitation of images both from the manufacturer's and the user's point of view. High quality images are a prerequisite for the successful application of quantitation techniques, reason to review briefly a number of requirements for high quality angiographic imaging.

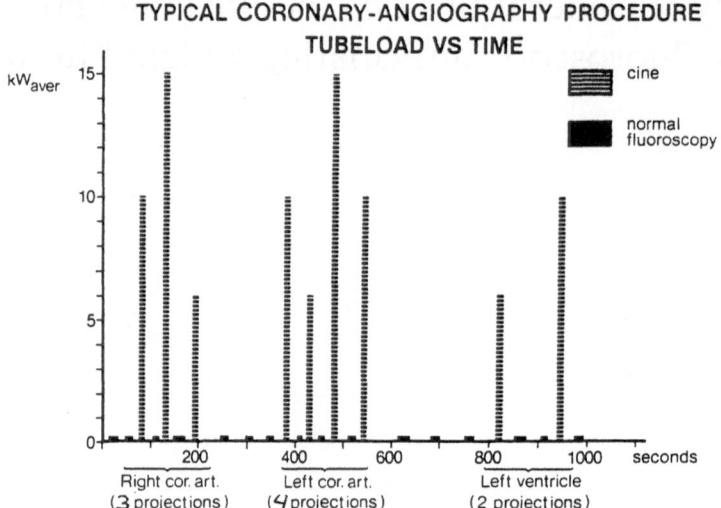

Figure 1. X-ray tube loading by fluoroscopy (average 200 W) and 8–12 cineruns (50 images/s, 10 sec. duration per cinerun). Peak and average power during cineruns are dependent upon the projection angles.

X-ray generation

Under the usual conditions for coronary procedures (Figure 1), today's X-ray tube technology is an important limiting factor in the quality of cineangiographic images. The large number of images (up to 4000) obtained during the 15–30 minutes of a typical coronary angiographic procedure, severely restricts the energy per image available. This limited energy per image determines on the one hand the flux of X-ray photons to the image intensifier and therefore the noise in the image, and on the other hand the average kilovolt (kV) level at which the X-rays can be generated and therefore, among others, the detail contrast in the image. The power applied to the tube requires a certain focal spot size, which also influences the image quality. (Table 1).

Table 1. The power that can be delivered by the X-ray tube depends on the selected focal spot size.

Focal spot	0,8	0,5	0,3	mm
Power	80	40	15	kW

However, with cineangiography and PTCA the energy per image is restricted to a larger extent by other parts of the X-ray tube; under these circumstances the focal spot size selected for a particular energy level is not a major contributor to the detoriation of the image in terms of sharpness and contrast (see also Tables IV

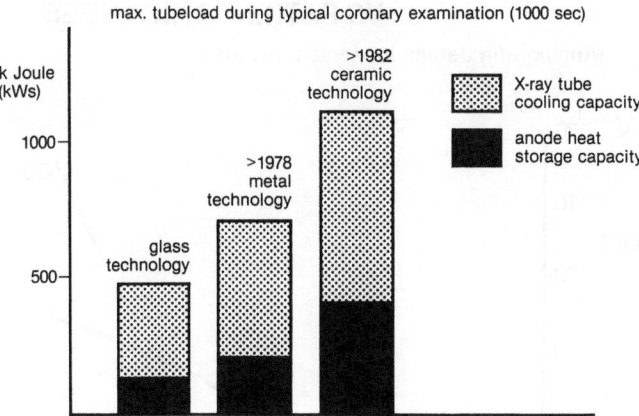

Figure 2. Medium term loadability of X-ray tubes. Cooling over a period of 1000 seconds and anode heat storage capacity determine maximum angiographic heat load.

and V). The X-ray dose levels at the maximum energy levels per image that can be achieved for cineangiography and PTCA with today's X-ray tube technology are generally found acceptable. Figure 2 shows the maximum energies that can be dissipated by X-ray tubes of different technologies. Critical temperatures in X-ray tubes are avoided by using the anode as a heat buffer and by constructions resulting in an increased cooling efficiency.

The resulting maximum heat load to the tube during the time of a short coronary procedure (duration approximately 1000 sec.) gives a much better impression of the capabilities of an X-ray tube than the anode heat storage capacity only. Especially a high cooling capacity of the X-ray tube guarantees a fast and uninterrupted procedure.

When the X-ray tube has been designed with emphasis only on the heat storage capacity of the anode, unacceptable waiting times may occur during the angiographic procedures at the moment that the anode is fully loaded. Comparison of the different tube technologies demonstrates clearly the superior performance of the ceramique X-ray tube over the conventional glass tube. This will be apparent in the image by a much better detail contrast relative to the noise.

Geometric versus motion unsharpness

From the overall energy limitations of e.g. a ceramique X-ray tube it can easily be derived that an average of 250 Joule is approximately available per cine-image.

The amount of X-ray absorption is very much dependent on the angiographic projection used, so that the energy per image should be made dependent on the specific absorption in a selected projection in order to achieve the optimum

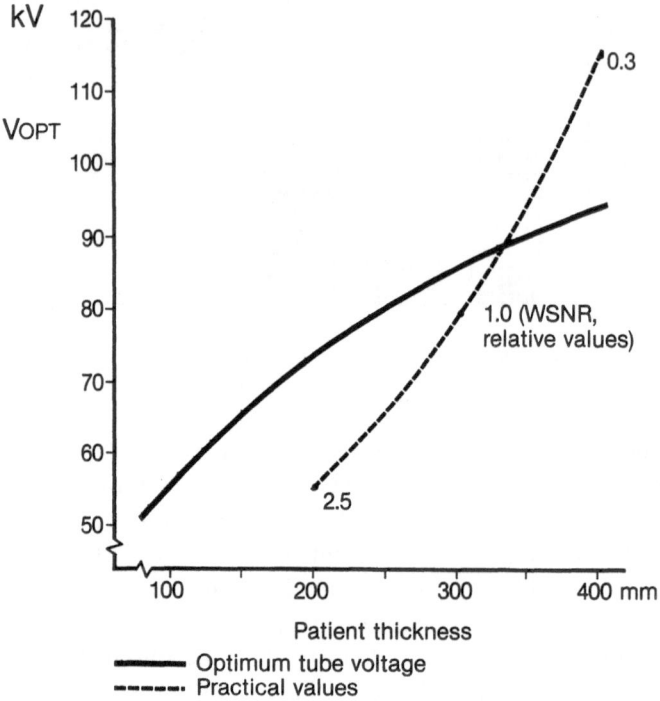

OPTIMUM X-RAY TUBE VOLTAGE
VS PATIENT THICKNESS

(Angiografin details immersed in water)

Figure 3. X-ray tube voltages for optimal window signal-to-noise ratio. (continuous curve). Values often found in practice; nonoptimal tube loading (dotted curve).

kV-levels (Figure 3). A suitable range of energy levels with an average value of 250 Joule is then 150 to 350 Joule/image.

The specific amount of energy available for one image can be obtained either from a low-power X-ray pulse with a rather long exposure time or from a high-power X-ray pulse with a short exposure time.

The exposure time and the focal spot size should be chosen such that a good balance is achieved between the motion unsharpness caused by the movement of the cardiac vessels and the geometric unsharpness caused by the finite focal spot size.

Taking into account the cardiac motion (Figure 4) and the geometric magnification factors which range from 1.3 to 1.5 depending on the angiographic projection used, a combination of a 0,8 mm focal spot with 4–5 ms exposure time has been found optimal for projections with large amounts of X-ray absorption (Figure 5, upper curve) and a 0,5 mm focal spot with 2,5–3 ms exposure time for projections with small amounts of absorption. (Figure 5, lower curve).

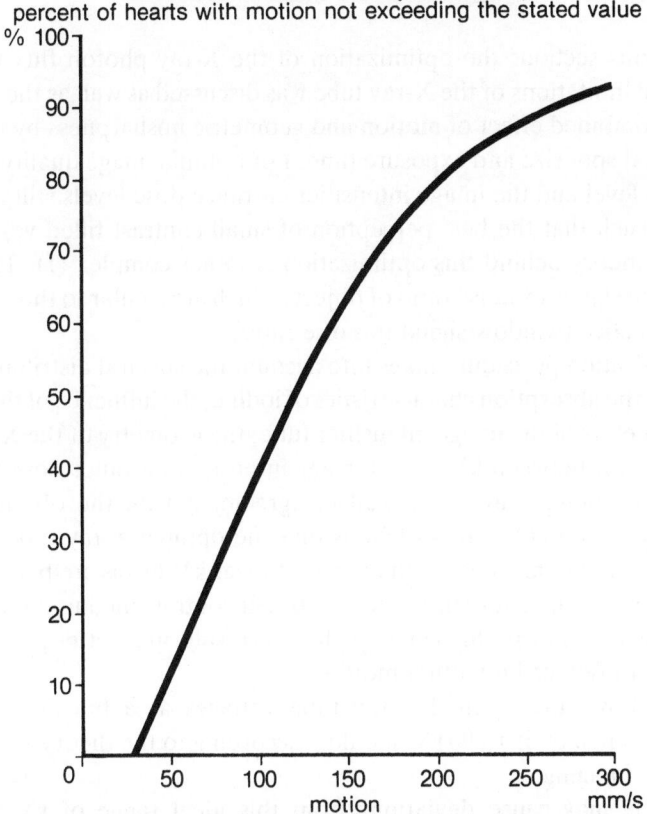

Figure 4. Cardiac motion; percentage of human hearts with motion not exceeding the stated value.

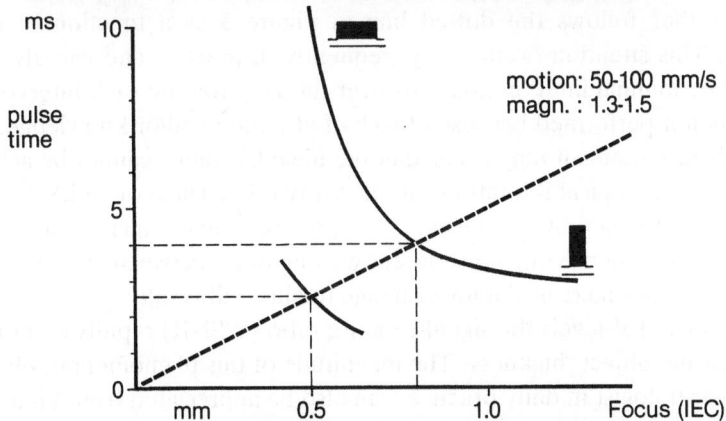

Figure 5. The combined effect of geometric and motion unsharpness is minimized for the pulse time and focal spot values as indicated. Energy per image is 350 J for the upper curve and 150 J for the lower curve.

Optimum X-ray tube voltage

In the previous sections the optimization of the X-ray photon flux within the technological limitations of the X-ray tube was discussed as well as the minimization of the combined effect of motion and geometric unsharpness by the proper choice of focal spot size and exposure time. For optimal image quality the X-ray tube voltage level and the image intensifier entrance dose levels still need to be determined such that the best perception of small contrast filled vessels is obtained. The theory behind this optimization is rather complex (1). This theory maximizes the signal-to-noise ratio of objects which are similar to those observed in clinical practice (window signal-to-noise ratio).

The optimization procedure takes into account the spectral distribution of the X-ray beam, the absorption characteristics of iodine, the influence of the grid, the design parameters of the image intensifier tube, the geometry of the X-ray beam and the trade-off between kV_{max} and image intensifier entrance dose.

The results obtained are very well in agreement with the observations in practical cineangiography. It is obvious that the optimal X-ray tube voltage is dependent upon the thickness of the object. Lower kV-levels are better adapted to the absorption characteristics of iodine-based contrast medium; on the other hand, an X-ray beam with high energy photons results in a better penetration of the object with reduced quantum mottle.

Figure 3 shows the optimal X-ray tube voltages as a function of patient thickness. A range of 65 to 90 kV should – according to the theory – be used for cinecoronary imaging.

Two effects may cause deviations from this ideal range of kV-levels. As described in the previous sections the energy per image should be dependent upon the amount of X-ray absorption in a selected projection. However, in many X-ray systems the loading strategy of the X-ray tube is not optimal; as a result, the kV-level rather follows the dotted line in Figure 3 as a function of object thickness. This situation occurs very frequently in practice and can always be corrected by manual intervention; however, in daily routine such interventions are usually not performed because of lack of attention and/or knowledge.

With obese patients it may occur that the ideal kV-range cannot be achieved within the technological limitations of the X-ray tube. The correct kV-level can then only be obtained by increasing the energy per image (increased exposure time); as a consequence one must accept waiting times between cineruns. If the energy level is not increased a lower image quality will result.

Even at ideal kV-levels the signal-to-noise ratio (WSNR) rapidly deteriorates with increasing object thickness. The magnitude of this phenomenon, observed by every cardiologist in daily practice, can also be appreciated from Figure 3. It can only be minimized by careful selection of the angiographic views and by using a good patient positioning technique. The image intensifier entrance doses are also determined by the preceding optimization process.

I.I. ENTRANCE DOSE

USA	: 30 - 35 uR/image 30 images/s	9" I.I. mode
Europe	: 15 - 20 uR/image 50 images/s	

Entrance dose/s :

USA	: 900 - 1050 uR/s
Europe	: 750 - 1000 uR/s

Table 2. Radiation doses at the entrance of the image intensifier commonly applied in the USA and Europe for cine-images.

The large differences in dose levels considered optimal in the USA and in Europe (Table 2) disappear when the different frame rates (30 images/s vs 50 images/s) are taken into account. The entrance doses/s, which really determine the kV-level, are roughly the same. Differences in image quality of the cinefilms from the USA and Europe (lower amounts of X-ray photons and thus noiser images in Europe), are hardly noticeable when the films are reviewed at reduced speed, because of the noise integration process in the perception apparatus of the human observer.

X-ray generators for cine-angiography

In the previous sections the requirements for the X-ray generators for cine-angiography have been determined. These requirements are summarized in Table 3.

Particular attention should be given to the loading strategy of the X-ray tube

X-RAY GENERATORS FOR CINE-ANGIOGRAPHY

Operational values

High tension range	50-120 kV
Maximum tube current	1200 mA
Maximum power output	120 kW
Exposure times	2-10 ms
Rise time of pulses	0.2 ms/100 KV
Framerates mono plane	10-100 im/s
bi plane	20-200 im/s

Optimal loading strategy of X-ray tube

Table 3. X-ray generator requirements for cardiac cine-angiography and PTCA.

avoiding the necessity of manual intervention when angiographic views are changed.

Modulation transfer functions

The spatial resolution of a cineangiographic system is basically limited by three factors: (1) the focal spot size of the X-ray tube in combination with the geometric magnification; (2) the motion of the heart; and (3) the image intensifier resolution. The overall performance of a system can be obtained by multiplication of the modulation transfer functions (MTF's) of the various subsystems involved. A less exact, but practical method is to derive from the MTF a single parameter δ, the equivalent blur diameter.

Comparison of the δ_i's of the various subsystems provides a good insight in the contribution of each of the subsystems to the degradation of the resolution. This method has been described in detail by Verhoeven (2).

Under the assumption that all MTF curves have roughly the same shape, the various δ_i's can be combined into the parameter δ_{tot}, which describes with reasonable accuracy the performance of the entire imaging chain, according to the following formula:

$$\delta_{tot} = (\delta_1^n + \delta_2^n + \delta_3^n + \ldots)^{1/n}$$

with $n = 1.5$.

δ_{tot} is roughly equal to the spatial distance between the points of 10% and 90% contrast of a step response function (edge transition). The situation for cine-

CINE CORONARY ANGIOGRAPHY

	δ-MOTION	δ-FOCUS	δ-I.I.	δ-TOTAL
M = 1.3	0.2-0.4 mm	0.23 mm	0.48 mm	0.71 mm
M = 1.5	0.2-0.4	0.4	0.42	0.78 mm

focus   : 0.8 mm (IEC)
pulsetime: 4 ms   high abs. projections

M = 1.3	0.1-0.2 mm	0.15 mm	0.48 mm	0.59 mm

focus   : 0.5 mm (IEC)
pulsetime: 2.5 ms   low abs. projections

M: geometric magnification – motion: 50-100 mm/s – I.I. mode: 9''

Table 4. Spatial resolution of a cine-angiographic system. Contribution by the various factors to the overall equivalent blur diameter.

angiography is summarized in Table 4. It is evident that the image intensifier resolution plays a major role in the overall performance. The geometric factor should be kept as small as possible for two reasons: (1) the resolution degrades with increasing magnification; (2) the signal-to-noise ratio decreases with increasing focus to image intensifier distance because of less favorable energy transfer conditions.

PTCA-procedures

From an imaging point of view the PTCA-procedures add several new elements to the conventional coronary cineangiography. High quality fluoroscopy is required during the critical phases of the angiographic procedure; in addition, short imaging runs are frequently made for review and documentation. In general, these runs are recorded simultaneously on cinefilm and on a videorecorder.

Figure 6 shows the timing of a typical PTCA-procedure. Since a complete coronary angiography is usually performed immediately prior to the PTCA, the X-ray tube load is increased considerably compared to the situation for normal coronary angiography.

The X-ray tube performance with respect to the quality of the fluoroscopic and fluorographic images should be considered in detail, when a tube is selected for PTCA-procedures.

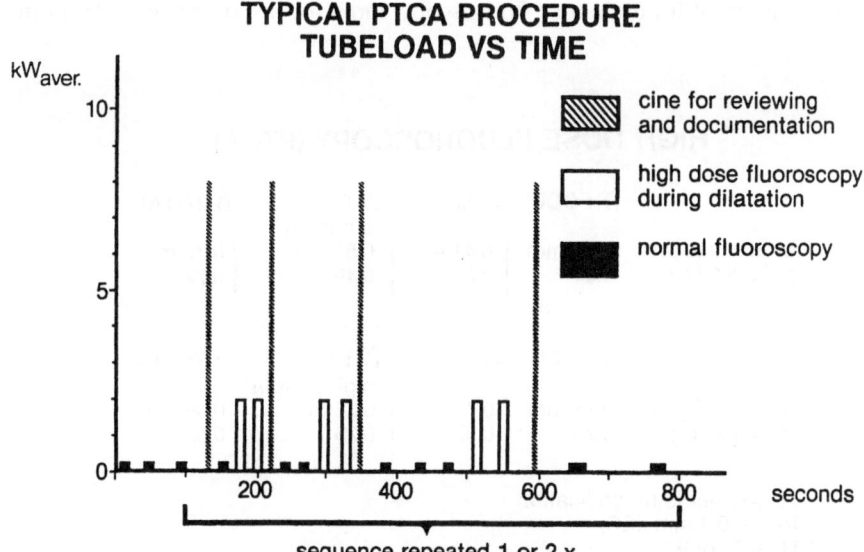

Figure 6. X-ray tube loading by standard fluoroscopy (average 200 W), high dose fluoroscopy (2 kW) and cineruns (50 images/s, 5 seconds duration).

The use of video recording and digital imaging are increasingly important for PTCA-procedures. Selection of roadmaps for catheter guidance, immediate review of the results of attempts to dilate the coronary vessels and the availability of images in a digital format for subsequent processing are so useful that electronic imaging becomes an indispensable part of an X-ray system for cardiac angiography. In such a system the T.V. camera is used for both fluoroscopy and fluorography, reason to include the T.V. camera in the assessment of the spatial resolution performance of the entire system.

Modulation transfer function with TV

High contrast fluoroscopy with increased X-ray dose is important to clearly visualize the catheter during the critical phases of the PTCA procedure. This high dose fluoroscopy can be achieved with a 0.3 mm focal spot resulting in a radiation dose of 300–400 µR/min. at the input of the image intensifier. The major factors determining the spatial resolution in such a system are the focal spot size and the resolution of the image intensifier and of the TV-camera. In Table 5 the contributions of the various components are shown for two imaging chains: (1) with a standard 1"-target TV camera; (2) with a high performance $1^{1}/_{4}$"-target TV camera.

Comparing the $\delta \cdot$ TV and resulting $\delta \cdot$ TOTAL values for the two camera systems illustrates the importance of TV camera selection, not only for reasons of image quality but also to ensure optimal conditions for quantification of e.g. vessel diameter. With high dose fluoroscopy and a focal spot size of 0.3 mm the

HIGH DOSE FLUOROSCOPY (PTCA)

	δ-FOCUS	δ-I.I.	δ-T.V. standard	δ-TOTAL
M = 1.3 (6.5")	0.11 mm	0.41 mm	0.51 mm	0.77 mm
M = 2.0 (9")	0.21	0.32	0.49	0.72

	δ-FOCUS	δ-I.I.	δ-T.V. high perform.	δ-TOTAL
M = 1.3 (6.5")	0.11 mm	0.41 mm	0.28 mm	0.59 mm
M = 2.0 (9")	0.21	0.32	0.26	0.55

M: geometric magnification
focus: 0.3 mm (IEC)
I.I.: 6.5" or 9"
radiation dose: 300-400 µR/min.

Table 5. As Table 4, but now for high dose fluoroscopy.

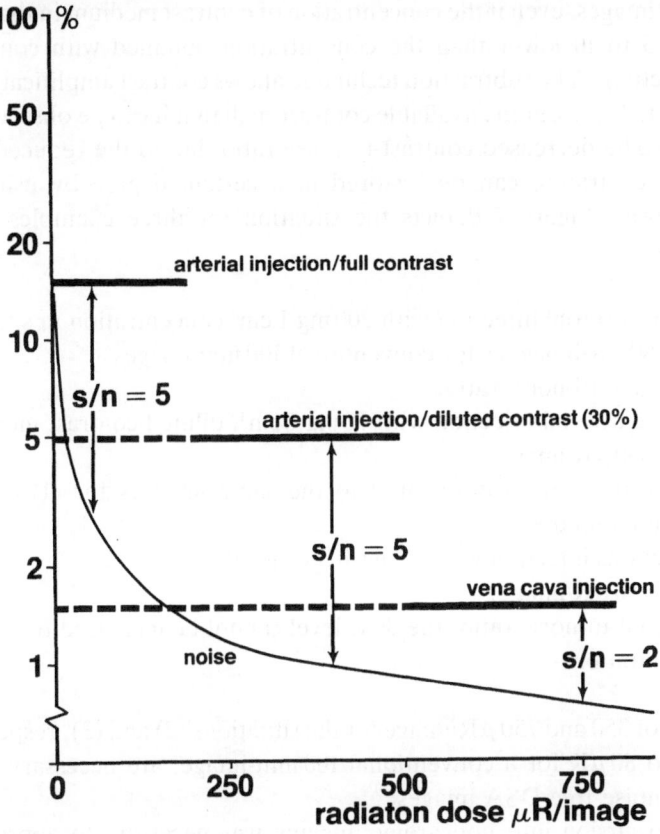

Figure 7. Image contrast versus quantum noise in digital images (512²) before subtraction. Angiographic details immersed in 20 cm water.

spatial resolution improves with geometric magnification, this in contrast with the situation for cine-angiography.

High performance TV does not necessarily imply the use of a 1249 line TV system or 1024² digitization matrices. The improvement is obtained to a large extent by using TV camera's with an improved MTF; the other parts of the chain may consist of standard video components and 512² matrices for digital imaging. However, it is beyond the scope of this paper to analyze the spatial resolution performance of digital imaging systems; for such information the reader is referred to other publications.

Digital imaging

Digital subtraction angiography (DSA) has proven to be very useful for the diagnosis of abnormalities in static vessels. The technique is capable of producing high quality images, even if the concentration of contrast medium in the vessels is a factor of 3 to 10 lower than the concentration obtained with conventional arterial injections. The subtraction technique allows contrast amplification which is necessary to bring out the available contrast such that it can be observed by the human eye. The decreased contrast-to-noise ratio due to the reduced contrast medium concentration can be restored to a certain degree by using higher radiation doses. Figure 7 depicts the situation for three examples of DSA-applications:

(1)   Selective arterial injection with 200 mg I/cm³ concentration in situ.
Dose level: 80 μR/image as for conventional 100 mm images.
Adequate signal-to-noise ratio.
(2)   Selective arterial injection with 70 mg I/cm³, diluted contrast medium.
Dose level: 350 μR/image.
The signal-to-noise ratio is restored to the same level as for (1) due to the increased radiation dose.
(3)   Intravenous injection with 20 mg I/cm³, in situ.
Dose level: 750 μR/image.
Reduced signal-to-noise ratio; the dose level cannot be increased further due to technical limitations.

Dose levels of 350 and 750 μR/image for the situations (2) and (3), respectively as compared to 80 μR for a conventional 100 mm-image, are necessary to obtain reasonably noise-free DSA images.
    A brief excursion into noncardiac imaging was necessary to appreciate the difficulties which occur when trying to apply the DSA-technique for moving vessels, while maintaining the high frame rates commonly used for cardiac imaging. The trade-off between the concentration of contrast injected and the applied radiation dose can be exploited only in a very restricted manner for cardiac applications. The X-ray tube limitations (see before) prohibit the use of higher radiation doses per image with high frame rates.
    An increased dose/image at a reduced frame rate, which is technically feasible, has the disadvantage of increased motion unsharpness due to long exposure times and loss of dynamic information (Figure 8):

(1)   Selective arterial injection with 200 mg I/cm³ in situ. Dose level: 20 μR/image as for conventional cine-images. The rather low signal-to-noise ratio is improved during dynamic review due to noise integration over several images. Motion unsharpness: 0,15–0,4 mm.

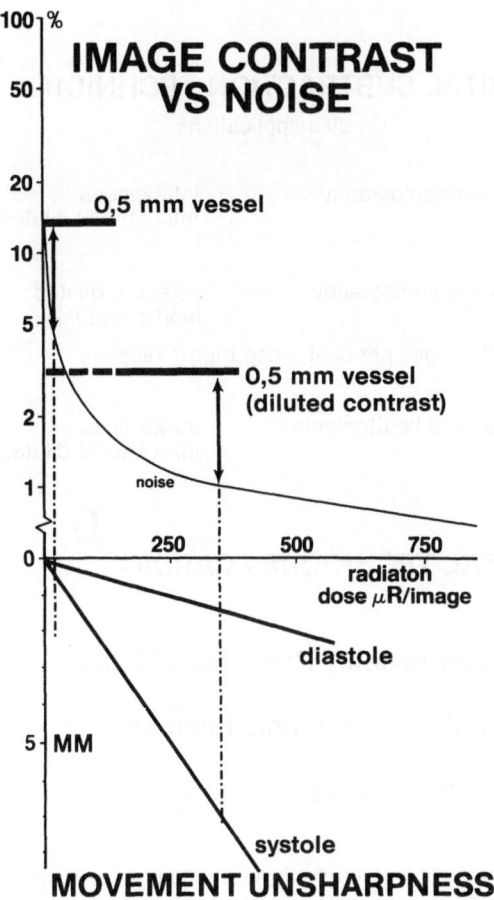

Figure 8. As Figure 7 for cardiac images; however, in this figure the motion unsharpness associated with the applied radiation doses is shown additionally.

(2)   Selective arterial injection with 40 mg I/cm³, diluted contrast. Dose levels necessary for an acceptable noise-free image cause motion unsharpness up to several millimeters.

The use of the DSA-technique with reduced concentration of the contrast medium – by diluted arterial or intravenous injection – is therefore restricted to those cases, where either sufficient object contrast is available and moderate spatial resolution is required, or reduced frame rates during the heart phase are adequate, or the object that needs to be visualized has a low X-ray absorption.
Table 6a lists some examples of cardiac applications with DSA. Although cardiac digital imaging most probably will not bring any dramatic changes in the injection technique, the advantages of the features mentioned earlier for PTCA and listed in Table 6b are so great, that digital imaging will rapidly penetrate further into the

a

DIGITAL SUBTRACTION TECHNIQUE

Cardiac applications

● Left ventriculography   intravenous
                                           intra-arterial diluted

● Coronary angiography   selective diluted
                                           (aortic root inj.)

  1 or 2 images per beat / ecg trigg / diastole

● Congenital heartdefects   intravenous
                                           intra-arterial diluted

b

DIGITAL TECHNIQUE · CARDIO

● Instant review / Roadmap (PTCA)

● Real time image enhancement

● Analytical data processing

Table 6. Cardiac applications of digital technology. a) subtraction technique; b) others.

cardiac field. With the progress of further developments, especially in archiving large number of images, a full transition from film-based imaging to digital imaging may be expected.

References

1. Boer JA den: Image formation in diagnostic X-ray equipment. Ph. D. thesis, Delft 1983.
2. Verhoeven LAJ: Digital subtraction angiography; the technique and an analysis of the physical factors influencing the image quality. Ph.D. thesis, Delft 1985.

Digital coronary arteriography

Robert A. Vogel

Summary

Digital angiography combined with image enhancement techniques such as inter-frame subtraction has proven clinically useful for intravenous and low-dose direct ventriculography. Considerable further interest is now directed toward imaging the coronary arteries and bypass grafts, determining lesional geometry and assessing blood flow parameters. Although intravenous contrast administration has not proven acceptable for these purposes, aortic root and selective arteriographic approaches are quite promising. Currently digital aortography is considered to be the most accurate means for determining bypass graft patency, but does not provide adequate visualization of either the distal portions of the grafts or of the coronary arteries.

Digital selective coronary arteriography provides slightly less spatial resolution, but considerably greater density resolution than conventional arteriography, and enables direct stenosis geometry and blood flow measurements. We have recently implemented an automated edge-detection method which analyses both geometric (absolute diameter) and videodensitometric (relative area) parameters of digitally acquired and stored coronary arteriograms (512×512 or 1024×1024 pixels with 8-bit grey levels). In addition, a digital radiographic technique which uses ECG-gated mask-mode subtraction of selectively injected coronary arteriograms to generate color and intensity coded parametric images, has been developed. These images depict the timing and density of the contrast medium bolus as it traverses the coronary circulation. Regional coronary flow reserve data are obtained by this technique through analysis of baseline and hyperemic parametric studies. Animal validation studies suggest that this approach is reasonably accurate. Application of this technique to patients with and without coronary artery disease confirms the difficulty with using percent diameter stenosis to predict the physiological significance of intermediate coronary stenoses. A close correlation between regional coronary flow reserve and the results of exercise scintigraphy seems to exist.

Combined with its ventriculographic applications, digital radiographic techniques clearly offer great promise in developing a fuller comprehension of the complexities of human coronary artery disease. It is likely in the near future that with improvements in data storage, digital coronary arteriography will largely replace film-based catheterization procedures.

Introduction

During the last decade, digital computer techniques have been widely applied to several areas of medical imaging, including computer tomography, cardiac scintigraphy, and digital radiography. Recently implemented digital acquisition and enhancement methods have supplanted long existent film-based analog image subtraction approaches. These technological developments pioneered at the Universities of Wisconsin, Arizona, and Kiel and at the Mayo Clinic (1–4), have now been embodied in commercial systems which are being applied and tested in numerous medical centers. Digital angiography was first introduced as a technique for enabling the visualization of peripheral arterial structures using intravenous contrast administration. Soon after its introduction, right and left ventricular imaging was reported using this technique (5). Whereas the ventricles have sufficient volume to be imaged in this manner, saphenous vein bypass grafts and coronary arteries have, in general, been visualized by aortic root injection and selective arteriography (6, 7). This trend toward intra-arterial contrast administration has paralleled a similar shift for the digital radiographic field, in general. Unlike peripheral arteriography, cardiac applications have often involved quantitative measurements and functional imaging which take greater advantage of the numerical nature of the images involved (8, 9). The recent cardiac applications of digital angiography, namely image enhancement and immediate review, quantitative stenosis determinations, and assessment of coronary blood flow and flow reserve, are summarized in this paper.

Digital instrumentation

The digital radiographic process uses conversions of fluoroscopic or radiographic images into digital format for subsequent image enhancement and storage. Important technical features of this process include: radiographic technique, image matrix size and framing rate, and storage medium. Unlike standard catheterization imaging techniques, which usually use floating radiographic parameters which adapt to image intensifier output, all digital radiographic techniques require constant parameters (10–12). This has required some modifications of existing radiographic equipment as many catheterization facilities have used 'add-on' digital equipment. Unlike digital ventriculography which requires only 256 × 256 8-bit pixel matrix resolution, but mandates 30 frames per second temporal sampling, coronary artery and saphenous vein bypass graft imaging requires much greater spatial, but less temporal image resolution. Pixel matrices of 512 × 512 or 1024 × 1024 dimension have been used with radiographic exposure of about 25 μR per frame. This radiographic exposure level coupled to the rapid translational velocity of coronary arteries (up to 10 cm per second) necessitates the use of radiographic X-ray pulsing with pulse width between 3 and 10 ms. Also, unlike the digital radiographic technique originally described, current coronary artery imaging uses progressive plumbicon readout rather than standard interlaced video, and direct digital disk, rather than analog image storage (13). Although coronary artery imaging requires very high spatial resolution, initial trials of framing rates of 2–8 frames per second have been reported to give equivalent clinical information to standard 30 frames per second cineradiography (7). Current commercial hardware allows 512 × 512 matrix acquisitions at 30 frames per second and 1024 × 1024 matrix acquisitions at 7 frames per second. Array processors allow for rapid image enhancement and analysis but, digital tape storage methods remain slow and cumbersome. Clinical archiving is often accomplished on photographic hard copy or analog video tape.

Digital coronary arteriography

Although selective coronary arteriography has remained the most important standard for the assessment of coronary artery disease, recent data and developments have pointed out several important limitations of this film-based method. Moreover, with the introduction of angioplasty and thrombolytic interventions, immediate review capabilities having excellent spatial resolution have become necessary. These new requirements cannot be met with film storage technology. Intra- and interobserver variability in visual assessment of stenosis severity remains substantial, and major inaccuracies using postmortem comparisons have been reported (14–16). Lastly, difficulty with the use of the clinically widely used percent stenosis criteria for the prediction of the physiological significance of individual coronary lesions has been reported (17).

Three applications of digital coronary arteriography are currently under investigation as solutions to these problems: (1) image manipulation and archiving, (2) quantitative stenosis determinations, and (3) assessments of coronary flow and flow reserve. Most current investigations of digital coronary arteriography use selective contrast injection. Efforts to implement intravenous coronary imaging using automated adaptive attenuation filters have not resulted in clinically usable data (18), and studies of intra-aortic contrast injection have demonstrated significant errors in evaluating coronary anatomy (19). The latter technique, however, has been useful for evaluating saphenous vein bypass graft patency.

The specific value of digital subtraction as compared with viewing and analyzing unsubtracted images is still to be defined, although the portions of arteries which overlie the diaphragm tends to be better visualized using subtraction. Clearly, a significant advantage of using the digital format for either subtracted or unsubtracted arteriograms is the ability to immediately review previous acquisitions during interventional studies. Live fluoroscopy can be superimposed or viewed adjacent to previously acquired arteriograms providing the operator with a 'roadmap' of the anatomy. Magnification of areas of interest and filtering algorithms which reduce quantum mottle and/or enhance edges may also prove helpful.

Quantitative stenosis measurements

In an attempt to increase the visual assessment of lesional severity, several quantitative methods have been applied to standard arteriography with reductions in interpretational variability (20–22). These techniques tend to be time consuming and may not take into consideration the distortion of spatial dimensions caused by pincushion and differential magnification effects. Brown *et al.* initially described a cinefilm based method which embodies pincushion and magnification distortion correction, but uses operator-defined contours (23). This geometric approach can be applied to orthogonal views of a single lesion. The resultant analysis of absolute minimal cross-sectional area of the lesion has been reported to be both reproducible and accurate. True digital radiographic methods are not employed by this approach which is, to date, fairly time consuming.

Spears *et al.* have pointed out that errors in analyzing elliptical stenoses can occur even using geometric analysis of orthogonal views (24). An alternate approach to geometric analysis is that of videodensitometry for either relative or absolute measurements. This method also has limitations. It can be affected by contrast streaming, and absolute videodensitometric determinations require corrections for multiple radiographic factors such as veiling glare, system nonlinearity, and beam hardening. The videodensitometric approaches described by several groups may be better suited to digital coronary arteriography because of the greater density resolution of the digital compared with the film-based technique (8, 25–29).

With advances in computer hardware and edge-detection algorithms, automated approaches to quantitative geometric and densitometric coronary artery stenosis assessment have been reported (30). Technical and biological variability even in automated edge-detection approaches clearly exists, but not to the extent of visual assessment. Correlations of absolute dimensions with physiological assessments of lesional severity are closer than with visual estimation of percent stenosis. Moreover, these methods finally offer the degree of precision and reproducibility necessary to investigate lesion progression and regression.

Our laboratory has recently implemented an automated edge-detection method which analyzes both geometric (absolute diameter) and videodensitometric (relative area) parameters, of digitally acquired and stored selective coronary arteriograms. This method can be used to evaluate coronary stenoses during interventional procedures as it requires neither film development nor subjective operator edge tracing. Pincushion distortion is corrected on the original arteriogram using a vectorial pixel shifting algorithm. Regional vectors are determined using data derived from imaging an orthogonal BB (ball bearings) phantom. Image matrices of either 512 × 512 or 1024 × 1024 pixels with 8-bit grey levels can be analyzed using this program which requires minimal operator interaction and about 20 seconds running time.

The digital arteriographic frames are stored with the ECG-signal facilitating selection of end-diastolic images. The initial step is magnification calibration which uses the catheter as a reference. The operator identifies the catheter using a light-pen, following which the computer magnifies that region of the arteriogram fourfold for 512 × 512 images and twofold for 1024 × 1024 images. The operator then identifies an acceptable point along the catheter. An automated edge detection algorithm identical to that used for the stenosis quantification (see below) determines the catheter diameter over a length of about 1 cm. With knowledge of the catheter size the image magnification is then calibrated (Figure 1a).

The operator then identifies the stenosis under investigation, which is magnified, and subjected to an automated analysis by the following scheme. A polar coordinate search algorithm is used to identify the centerline of the artery following operator assignment of the approximate center of the lesion and the length of artery to be evaluated. Orthogonal lines at closely spaced intervals are then identified which lie perpendicular to the arterial centerline. The first and second derivatives of the contrast medium density are analyzed along these lines. The arterial 'edge' is determined at an arbitrary spacing between these derivatives, and the arterial density is determined at its edge. Using continuity criteria, a threshold based contour is determined which best passes through these derivative determined 'edges'. Finally, the cumulative arterial contrast density is summed between the opposite edges of each perpendicular segment (Figure 1b).

Color coded data are presented superimposed on both the original and schematized arterial segment including: absolute diameter, percent diameter narrowing, and relative cross-sectional (densitometric) area. This technique has been validated in arterial phantoms from 0.5 to 5.0 mm diameter with excellent reproducibility and accuracy being found. Some overestimation of absolute dimensions of those less than 0.7 mm is observed. This is not found using densitometric assessments although the latter underestimates diameters greater than 4 mm. We have compared application of this automated approach using 512 × 512 and 1024 × 1024 digital images to film-based studies digitized in 2000 × 2000 matrices. The most accurate approach was that using 1024 × 1024 direct digital acquisition.

Although 2000 × 2000 film images possessed similar resolution of small diameters (less than 1 mm), they contained significantly greater noise and, therefore, less precision. Thus, it appears that digital coronary arteriography with automated analysis provides the most accurate means for quantitating coronary stenoses.

Coronary flow techniques

Although better predictions of the hemodynamic significance of individual coronary stenoses has been reported using quantitative coronary stenosis determinations, poor correlations between percent stenosis and coronary flow reserve measured intraoperatively and at the time of angioplasty have been reported (17,

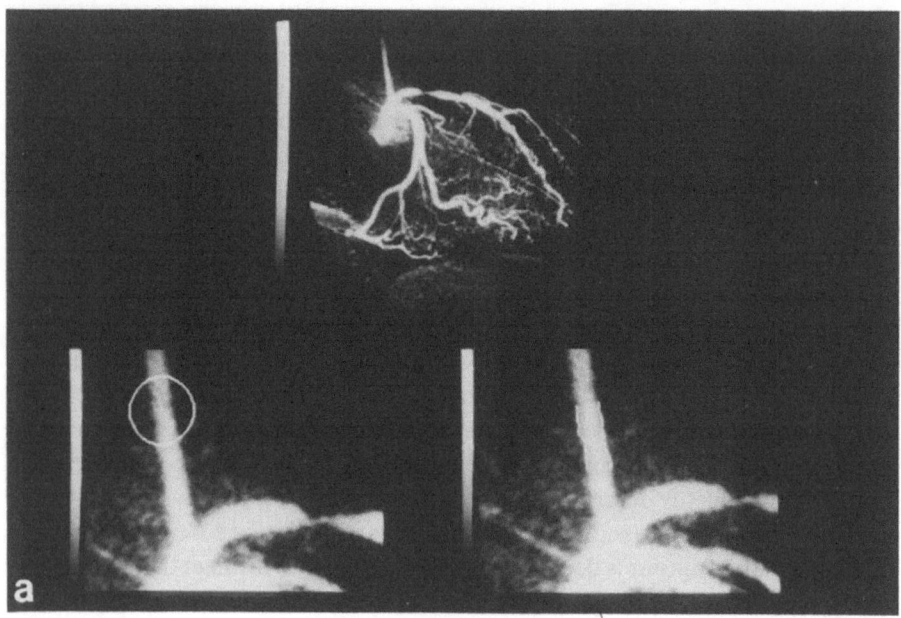

Figure 1a. Calibration of a digital coronary arteriogram is accomplished by identification of the catheter and automated edge-detection of its diameter.

Figure 1b. A coronary stenosis acquired using digital arteriography is quantitated by operator identification of the stenosis and automated edge-detection. Geometric coronary diameter (absolute and relative) and densitometric relative area stenosis are also calculated automatically in about 20 seconds.

Figure 2. Parametric digital coronary arteriograms under baseline (left) and hyperemic (right) conditions are depicted for a normal right coronary artery in the RAO projection.

ARTERY DIAMETER (MM) 0.64
X-SECT AREA (RELATIVE) 1.48
P
D
3.04
% STEN
DIAM.
79.6%
0

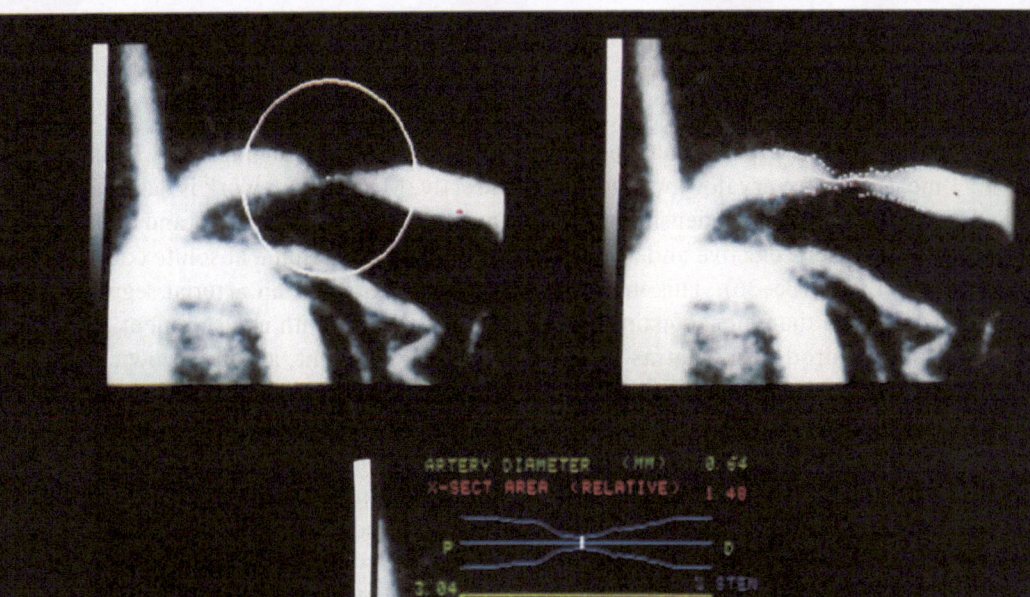

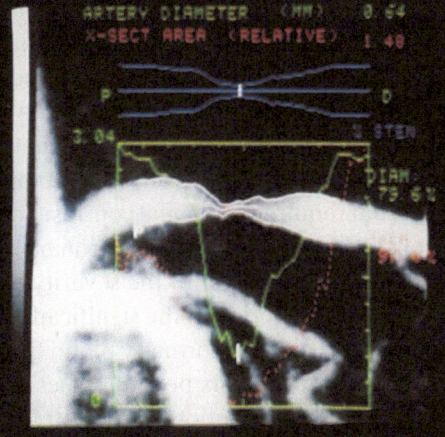

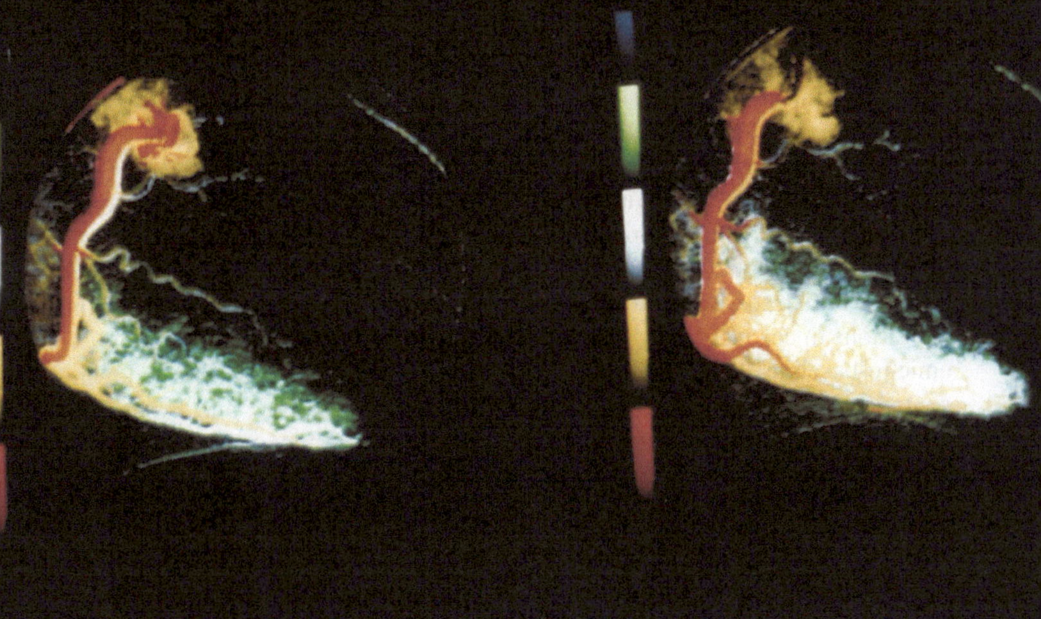

31, 32). This problem has lead to interest in using the digital arteriogram to measure coronary flow or flow reserve directly. Much recent work is based upon the film-based videodensitometric approaches of Rutishauser *et al.* and Smith *et al.* who used selective and aortic root injections to determine absolute coronary blood flow (33–36). This method uses determinations of an arterial segment's length and diameter to estimate its volume. Together with measurement of the time required for a contrast bolus to transit the segment, absolute flow can be calculated. This method has been recently shown to be accurate and capable of assessing phasic flow (37). This approach is generally limited to proximal predivisional coronary arterial segments whose courses need to be relatively perpendicular to the X-ray beam. Additionally, precise determinations of vessel diameter are mandatory. In an attempt to reduce some of these problems, Foerster *et al.* developed a method for measuring relative coronary flow. Flows are assessed by ratios comparing the videodensitometric areas under the baseline and hyperemic condition transit curves (38). This can be accomplished in more distal and circuitous arteries, but requires that equal contrast boluses be administered under the two conditions. The resultant index, coronary flow reserve (39, 40), is an important hemodynamic parameter of the severity of coronary stenoses. It is by this index that the clinical criterion of the significance of coronary artery stenoses was established. Measurement of coronary blood flow or flow reserve, however, is complicated by numerous factors beyond issues of arterial geometry.

In opposition to tracer, dye dilution, and electromagnetic methods for assessing blood flow, all contrast media substantially affect blood flow itself, vascular volume, and ventricular function, although nonionic media may do so less than ionic agents. The effects of a 3 ml bolus of ionic contrast medium on coronary blood flow, as measured by electromagnetic flowmeter in a canine model, has been studied in our laboratory (41). Both baseline flow and initially hyperemic flow induced by a 10-second prior injection of the same contrast medium bolus are affected in three phases. Initially, during the interval of contrast medium injection, a small increase, of usually <10% of initial flow, is observed despite free reflux of contrast into the sinus of Valsalva. After this period of minor flow increment, a 30–70% decrease in flow ensures, which is likely caused by the combined effects of the contrast medium hyperosmolality and high viscosity on the microcirculation. The widely recognized third phase of reactive hyperemia then follows. Baseline flow increases approximately threefold and already hyperemic flow by about 20%. Both curves peak at approximately 10 seconds, which occurs whether or not coronary stenosis is present. Despite the substantial alterations in coronary flow induced by the contrast medium the ratio of hyperemic-to-baseline flow remains uniform during the first five seconds following contrast injection. These findings suggest that absolute flow and hyperemic-to-baseline flow ratios should be measured during the first 1.5 and 5 seconds following contrast injection, respectively.

Problems in addition to alterations in blood flow exist with using contrast medium to measure coronary blood flow. For application of the dilutional principle, an indicator must be administered in known or fixed amount, remain wholly intravascular and be detectable quantitatively downstream. Without sub-selective (direct intra-arterial) injection at low flow rates to prevent reflux, it is difficult to administer contrast medium in known or fixed amounts. Furthermore, under conditions of slow administration, substantial streaming usually occurs. Contrast agents also increase intravascular volume affecting downstream detection by increasing the volume-of-interest under study. It is for these reasons of blood flow variation and capillary vasodilation that transit-time approaches have been the most frequently employed.

Parametric imaging

During development of the Dynamic Spatial Reconstructor, Robb and colleagues first proposed the use of ECG-synchronized mask-mode subtraction for the purpose of measuring regional blood flow (42). These investigators demonstrated that digital subtraction resulted in a significant increase in the ability to visualize contrast medium in its myocardial or microcirculation phases. Our laboratory has combined this digital approach with the transit-time analysis of Rutishauser and Smith. We use dual parameter functional images to depict the timing and density of a selectively injected contrast medium bolus as it traverses the coronary circulation (9, 13, 43). Coronary flow reserve is estimated in myocardial regions-of-interest by quantitatively comparing data encoded in baseline and hyperemic condition parametric or functional images. This technique was first implemented using cinefilm image storage with subsequent analog-to-digital conversion, but currently uses direct digital disk image storage, which allows rapid application during routine cardiac catheterization. Other subsequent methodological changes include the use of mask-mode subtraction rather than time interval differencing, atrial pacing, and power contrast injection.

Following the initial methods, the parametric imaging method estimates regional flow using the vascular volume/transit-time principle. It differs from previous methods by measuring data over myocardial rather than arterial regions-of-interest. The parametric imaging technique uses atrial pacing to regularize cycle length to provide optimal interframe registration and selective, ECG-synchronized, power contrast medium injection to standardize the timing and flow rates of the contrast bolus. As mentioned above, in addition to increasing coronary flow, contrast agents increase vascular volume. Thus, both transit-time and vascular volume need to be measured to determine even parameters of relative flow. This was not understood when this method was first described, at which time vascular volume was assumed to remain constant following hyperemic stimulus (9). Subsequent studies, however, have demonstrated that use of an assumed fixed vascular volume results in underestimation of flow reserve (13).

Mean mask-mode subtracted radiographic density, as a function of time, over myocardial regions-of-interest, are used to assess both appearance times and vascular volumes. Wavefront appearance-time analysis is accomplished using a threshold criterion of approximately one-third maximal density. This approach results in the determination of appearance-time during the first four to five seconds after contrast administration. This is the period in which flow ratios remain approximately constant. Under the assumption that the vascular space contains full-strength contrast media, vascular volume is approximated by the product of a radiographic system transfer function constant and the region-of-interest density. Under equivalent radiographic conditions, vascular volume is proportional to mean density, assuming that the vascular space has been filled with contrast medium. This assumed that additional vasodilitation has not yet occurred at the time of the measurement. Using density measurements at a time thought to meet these requirements, the hyperemic-to-baseline flow ratio (coronary flow reserve (CFR)) is calculated by the following equation:

$$CFR = \frac{\text{vascular volume}_h}{\text{appearance-time}_h} \div \frac{\text{vascular volume}_b}{\text{appearance-time}_b}$$

where h = hyperemia and b = baseline. Despite the many assumptions and the difficulties associated with use of contrast media, a good correlation between electromagnetic flowmeter and digital radiographic determinations of relative regional coronary blood flow was found in a canine model using this method of analysis (13).

This volumetric approach to measuring relative flow can be implemented on a pixel-by-pixel basis using parametric images in which individual pixel color and intensity are modulated according to the transit-time and density values calculated for each pixel. These parametric images differ from those used previously in that each pixel contains information on two different parameters. In contrast to single region-of-interest techniques, parametric images have the advantages of providing simultaneous visualization of the entire coronary circulation and allow recognition of contrast medium injection problems, such as streaming. A clinical example of functional images obtained under baseline and contrast-induced hyperemic conditions is shown in Figure 2. The color of each pixel is coded according to the number of cardiac cycles required for contrast medium appearance determined by threshold criterion: red, yellow, white, green and blue denote appearance within the first through the fifth cardiac cycles, respectively. The intensity of each pixel is coded according to contrast medium density data. Figure 2 depicts a normal right coronary artery circulation and visually demonstrates significantly reduced transit-time and increased vascular volume in the hyperemic study by earlier colors and greater intensity of the pixels within the myocardial region perfused by this artery.

Clinical applications and limitations

Several centers are beginning clinical experience with this technique for measuring relative blood flow. Parametric images can be generated rapidly during cardiac catheterization although atrial pacing, ECG-synchronized power contrast medium injection, digital equipment capable of direct digital storage, and fixed patient positioning need to be added to the routine technique of selective arteriography. No substantial problems have arisen yet with the use of either atrial pacing or power contrast injection. Routine contrast medium volumes are employed (approximately 5 and 7 ml administered over 2 cardiac cycles for the right and left coronary arteries, respectively). Patient motion, which causes registration artifacts on the functional images, has proven to be the most persistent problem, necessitating the repetition of many studies.

From a pathophysiological viewpoint, it needs to be emphasized that coronary flow reserve is affected by numerous factors other than epicardial stenosis, including myocardial hypertrophy, arterial hypertension, prior myocardial infarction, vessel collateralization, coronary spasm, syndrome X, prolonged ischemia, acute endothelial injury (e.g. angioplasty), and vasoactive drugs. The additional factors of arterial blood pressure, ventricular end-diastolic, and intrathoracic pressure (e.g. Valsalva maneuver), which can vary during arteriography can also affect flow reserve. Lastly, as a parameter of relative flow, coronary flow reserve determinations are altered by variations in baseline flow.

Higher levels of hyperemic flow can be achieved with the use of agents other than contrast media. Especially promising is intracoronary papaverine which increases blood flow about fourfold. Use of either contrast agents or papavarine appear to be quite safe. Clearly, however, even with maximal stimulation, flow reserve, as a physiological parameter, has significant limitations which must be considered during individual coronary artery assessment. It is hoped that radiographic methods capable of measuring absolute coronary flow during routine catheterization may be developed. This would prove useful for differentiating epicardial arterial stenosis from the many other causes of abnormal flow reserve.

Within these limitations, our laboratory has found the parametric imaging approach to measuring flow reserve helpful for the assessment of: individual coronary artery disease severity, the efficacy of coronary angioplasty and bypass surgery, and ischemia in patients without coronary artery disease. Figure 3 depicts the coronary flow reserve values in 92 individual coronary arterial distributions in two groups of patients, the first having entirely normal coronary arteriograms, and the second having coronary artery disease, but without prior myocardial infarction or visible collaterals. The presence of collaterals has been found to be associated with reduced flow reserve, even in normal arteries supplying collaterals to other vessels (44). This effect on normal arteries is not associated with abnormal stress perfusion of ventricular function and disappears promptly following angioplasty which eliminates collateral flow. Both groups of patients in

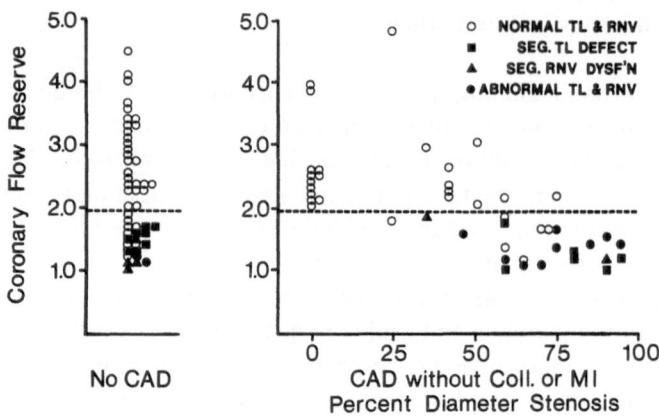

Figure 3. Coronary flow reserve, percent arterial stenosis and stress scintigraphic results are shown for patients without (left) and with (right) coronary artery disease.

Figure 3 were investigated because of chest pain syndromes and had stress thallium-201 scintigraphy and radionuclide ventriculography within two days of their coronary arteriography. Seven of 18 individuals with entirely normal coronary arteries were found to have abnormal stress perfusion and/or ventricular function results (45). Low coronary flow reserve was observed in arterial distributions in all of the patients within this group, but in only 2 of 11 patients without abnormal stress test results. Abnormal segmental stress perfusion and/or wall motion was observed only in arterial distributions with low flow reserve. A history of hypertension was commonly found in both subgroups. These data support the presence of true myocardial ischemia in some patients with chest pain and normal coronary arteries and suggest that differences between the findings of coronary arteriography and stress scintigraphy should not be attributed wholly to false scintigraphic results.

Figure 3 also depicts the coronary flow reserve and stress scintigraphic data obtained in 19 patients with coronary artery disease without prior infarction or visible collaterals (46). Data are presented using percent arterial stenosis determined by caliper measurements in the individual arterial distributions studied. Similar to the data from patients without coronary artery disease, abnormal stress test results were found only in distributions with low coronary flow reserve. Similar close correlations between coronary flow reserve measured by xenon-133 washout and stress scintigraphy have also been reported (4). A slightly better correlation was found between percent arterial stenosis and segmental coronary flow reserve in this study ($r = -.61$) than that described using other methodologies. Examination of the current data, however, shows that only stenoses <25% or >75% provide assurance that an individual lesion is either physiologically insignificant or significant, respectively. Although a 50% criterion appears to optimally separate lesions into these categories, about one-quarter of intermediate lesions between 25% and 75% stenosis will be incorrectly assessed using this standard. Clearly, not all of the distributions studied had concordance of flow reserve and stress scintigraphic data. Five of the six distributions in this intermediate category with low flow reserve values and normal stress test results occurred in patients with multivessel disease and had abnormal scintigraphic results in other arterial distributions with lower flow reserve values. This points out a limitation of stress scintigraphy in that patients cannot always exercise to the level at which ischemia is produced in each distribution in which coronary disease is present. Stress scintigraphy and flow reserve results were usually concurrent in patients with only single vessel disease.

The ability to evaluate relative coronary flow in the catheterization laboratory now provides a means of evaluating coronary blood flow as well as anatomy. Combined with its ventriculographic applications, clearly digital radiographic techniques offer great promise in developing a fuller comprehension of the complexities of human coronary artery disease.

References

1. Wood EH, Sturm RE, Sanders JJ: Data processing in cardiovascular physiology with particular reference to roentgen videodensitometry. Mayo Clin Proc 39, 1964: 849–865.
2. Heintzen PH, Brennecke R, Bürsch JH, Lange P, Malerczyk V, Moldenhauer K, Onnasch D: Automated videoangiocardiographic image analysis. IEEE Computer 8, 1975: 55–64.
3. Frost MM, Fisher HD, Nudelman S, Roehrig H: A digital video acquisition system for extraction of subvisual information in diagnostic medical imaging. In: Optical Instrumentation in Medicine VI, SPIE 127, 1977: 208–215.
4. Kruger RA, Mistretta CA, Houk TL, Riederer SJ, Shaw CG, Goodsitt MM, Crummy AB, Zwiebel W, Lancaster JC, Rowe GG, Flemming D: Computerized fluoroscopy in real time for noninvasive visualization of the cardiovascular system. Radiology 130, 1979: 49–57.
5. Kruger RA, Mistretta CA, Houk TL, Kubal W, Riederer SJ, Ergun DL, Shaw CG, Lancaster JC, Rowe GG: Computerized fluoroscopy techniques for intravenous study of cardiac chamber dynamics. Invest Radiol 14, 1979: 279–287.
6. Drury JK, Gray R, Diamond GA, Whiting J, Pfaff M, Vas R, Wheeler W, Nathan M, Forrester JS, Swan HJC, Nivatpumin T: Computer enhanced digital angiography visualizes coronary bypass grafts without need for selective injection. Circulation 66 (Suppl II), 1982: II-229. (Abstract)
7. Tobis J, Nalcioglu O, Iseri L, Johnston WD, Roeck W, Castleman E, Bauer B, Montelli S, Henry WL: Detection and quantitation of coronary artery stenoses from digital subtraction angiograms compared with 35-millimeter film cineangiograms. Am J Cardiol 54, 1984: 489–496.
8. Kruger RA: Estimation of the diameter of and iodine concentration within blood vessels using digital radiography devices. Med Phys 8, 1981: 652–658.
9. Vogel R, LeFree M, Bates E, O'Neill W, Foster R, Kirlin P, Smith D, Pitt B: Application of digital techniques to selective coronary arteriography: Use of myocardial contrast appearance time to measure coronary flow reserve. Am Heart J 107, 1984: 153–164.
10. Bailey NA: Video techniques for x-ray imaging and data extraction from roentgenographic and fluoroscopic presentations. Med Phys 7, 1980: 472–491.
11. Kruger RA: Basic physics of computerized fluoroscopy difference imaging. In: Digital Subtraction Arteriography: an Application of Computerized Fluoroscopy. Mistrette CA, Crummy AB,

Strother CM, *et al.* (Eds), Yearbook Medical Publishers, Inc., Chicago, 1982: 16–22.

12. Ovitt TW, Fisher III DH: Ideal configuration for intravenous digital subtraction angiography machine. Cardiovasc Intervent Radiol 6, 1983: 300–302.

13. Hodgson JMcB, LeGrand V, Bates ER, Mancini GBJ, Aueron FM, O'Neill WW, Simon SB, Beauman GJ, LeFree MT, Vogel RA: Validation in dogs of a rapid digital angiographic technique to measure relative coronary blood flow during routine cardiac catheterization. Am J Cardiol 55, 1985: 188–193.

14. Grondin CM, Dyrda I, Paternac A, Campeau L, Bourassa MG, Lespérance J: Discrepancies between cineangiographic and postmortem findings in patients with coronary artery disease and recent myocardial revascularization. Circulation 49, 1974: 703–708.

15. Zir LM, Miller SW, Dinsmore RE, Gilbert JP, Harthorne JW: Interobserver variability in coronary angiography. Circulation 53, 1976: 627–632.

16. Fisher LD, Judkins MP, Lespérance J, Cameron A, Swaye P, Ryan T, Maynard C. Bourassa M, Kennedy JW, Gosselin A, Kemp H, Faxon D, Wexler L, Davis KB: Reproducibility of coronary arteriographic reading in the Coronary Artery Study (CASS). Cath Cardiovasc Diagn 8, 1982: 565–575.

17. White CW, Wright CB, Doty DB, Hiratza LF, Eastham CL, Harrison DG, Marcus ML: Does visual interpretation of the coronary arteriogram predict the physiologic importance of a coronary stenosis? N Engl J Med 310, 1984: 819–824.

18. Peppler WW, Kudva B, Dobbins III TJ, Lee CS, Lysel MS van, Hasegawa BH, Mistretta CA: Digitally controlled beam attenuator. In: Application of Optical Instrumentation in Medicine X, SPIE, 347: 106–111.

19. Ross AM, Johnson RA, Katz RJ, Varghese PJ, Leiboff RH, Bren GB, Schwartz H, Wasserman AG: Diagnosis of coronary disease by aortic digital subtraction angiography. Circulation 68 (Suppl III), 1983: III–43. (Abstract)

20. Gensini GG, Kelly AE, Da Costa BCB, Huntington PP: Quantitative angiography: the measurement of coronary vasomobility in the intact animal and man. Chest 60, 1971: 522–530.

21. Feldman RL, Pepine CJ, Curry RC, Conti CR: Quantitative coronary arteriography using 105–mm photospot angiography and an optical magnifying device. Cathet Cardiovasc Diagn 5, 1979: 195–201.

22. Rafflenbeul W, Smith LR, Rogers WJ, Mantle JA, Rackley CE, Russell Jr RO: Quantitative coronary arteriography: Coronary anatomy of patients with unstable angina pectoris reexamined 1 year after optimal medical therapy. Am J Cardiol 43, 1979: 699–707.

23. Brown BG, Bolson E, Frimer M, Dodge HT: Quantitative coronary arteriography: Estimation of dimensions, hemodynamic resistance, and atheroma mass of coronary artery lesions using the arteriogram and digital computation. Circulation 55, 1977: 329–337.

24. Spears JR, Sandor T, Baim DS, Paulin S: The minimum error in estimating coronary luminal cross-sectional area from cineangiographic diameter measurements. Cathet Cardiovasc Diagn 9, 1983: 119–128.

25. Sandor T, Als AV, Paulin S: Cine-densitometric measurement of coronary arterial stenoses. Cathet Cardiovasc Diagn 5, 1979: 299–245.

26. Crawford DW, Brooks SH, Barndt Jr R, Blankenhorn DH: Measurement of atherosclerotic luminal irregularity and obstruction by radiographic densitometry. Invest Radiol 12, 1977: 307–313.

27. Kishon Y, Yerushalmi S, Deutsch V, Neufeld HN: Measurement of coronary arterial lumen by densitometric analysis of angiograms. Angiology 39, 1979: 304–312.

28. Hoornstra K, Hanselman JMH, Holland WPJ, Wey Peters GW de, Zwamborn AW: Videodensitometry for measuring blood vessel diameter. Acta Radiol Diagn 21, 1980: 155–164.

29. Nichols AB, Gabrieli CFO, Fenoglio JJ, Esser PD: Quantification of relative coronary arterial stenosis by cinevideodensitometric analysis of coronary arteriograms. Circulation 69, 1984: 512–522.

30. Reiber JHC, Serruys PW, Kooijman CJ, Wijns W, Slager CJ, Gerbrands JJ, Schuurbiers JCH,

Boer A den, Hugenholtz PG: Assesment of short-, medium- and long-term variations in arterial dimensions from computer-assisted quantitation of coronary cineangiograms. Circulation 71, 1985: 280–288.

31. Harrison DG, White CW, Hiratzka LF, Doty DB, Barnes DH, Eastham CL, Marcus ML: The value of lesion cross-sectinal area determined by quantitative coronary angiography in assessing the physiologic significance of proximal left anterior descending coronary arterial stenoses. Circulation 69, 1984: 1111–1119.

32. Banka VS, Argarwal JB, Bodenheimer MM, Wertheimer JH, Gessman LJ, Weintraub WS, Helfant RH: Determination of the severity of coronary stenoses in man: correlation of angiography and hemodynamics. Circulations 64 (Suppl IV), 1981: IV–108 (Abstract).

33. Rutishauser W, Bussmann W-D, Noseda G, Meier W, Wellauer J: Blood flow measurement through single coronary arteries by roentgen densitometry. Part I. A comparison of flow measured by a radiologic technique applicable in the intact organism and by electromagnetic flow meter. Am J Roentgenol, Rad Therapy and Nucl Med 109, 1970: 12–20.

34. Rutishauser W, Noseda G, Bussmann W-D, Preter B: Blood flow measurement through single coronary arteries by roentgen densitometry. Part II. Right coronary artery flow in conscious man. Am J Roentgenol, Rad Therapy and Nucl Med 109, 1970: 21–24.

35. Smith HC, Frye RL, Donald DE, Davis GD, Pluth JR, Sturm RE, Wood EH: Roentgen videodensitometric measure of coronary blood flow. Determination from simultaneous indicator – dilution curves at selected sites in the coronary circulation and in coronary artery-saphenous vein grafts. Mayo Clin Proc 46, 1971: 800–806.

36. Smith HC, Sturm RE, Wood EH: Videodensitometric system for measurement of vessel blood flow, particularly in the coronary arteries, in man. Am J Cardiol 32, 1973: 144–150.

37. Spiller P, Schmiel FK, Pölitz B, Block M, Fermer U, Hackbarth W, Jehle J, Körfer R, Pannek H: Measurement of systolic or diastolic flow rates in the coronary artery system by X-ray densitometry. Circulation 68, 1983: 337–347.

38. Foerster JM, Link DP, Lantz BMT, Lee G, Holcroft JW, Mason DT: Measurement of coronary reactive hyperemia during clinical angiography by video dilution technique. Acta Radiol 22, 1981: 209–216.

39. Gould KL, Lipscomb K, Hamilton GW: Physiologic basis for assessing critical coronary stenosis. Instantaneous flow response and regional distribution during coronary hyperemia as measures of coronary flow reserve. Am J Cardiol 33, 1974: 87–94.

40. Gould KL, Lipscomb K: Effects of coronary stenoses on coronary flow reserve and resistance. Am J Cardiol 34, 1974: 48–55.

41. Hodgson JMcB, Mancini GBJ, Vogel RA: Characterization of changes in coronary blood flow during the first six seconds after contrast injection. JACC 3, 1984: 589 (Abstract).

42. Robb RA, Wood EH, Ritman EL, Johnson SA, Sturm RE, Greenleaf JF, Gilbert BK, Chevalier PA: Three-dimensional reconstruction and display of the working canine heart and lungs by multiplanar X-ray scanning videodensitometry. Comput Cardiol 1974: 151–163.

43. Vogel RA, Bates ER, O'Neill WW: Coronary flow reserve measured during cardiac catheterization. Arch Int Med (in press).

44. LeGrand V, Aueron FM, Bates ER, O'Neill WW, Hodgson JMcB, Mancini GBJ, Vogel RA: Reversibility of coronary collaterals and alteration in regional coronary flow reserve after successful angioplasty. Am J Cardiol 54, 1984: 453–454.

45. LeGrand V, Hodgson JMcB, Aueron FM, Bates ER, Mancini GBJ, Smith JS, Vogel RA: Abnormal coronary flow reserve and abnormal radionuclide exercise tests in patients with normal coronary angiograms. JACC 5, 1985: 531 (Abstract).

46. LeGrand V, Hodgson JMcB, Aueron FM, Mancini GBJ, Bates ER, Smith JS, LeFree MT, Vogel RA: The correlation of percent diameter coronary stenosis with the functional significance of individual coronary artery stenoses. JACC 5, 1985: 475 (Abstract).

47. Port SC, Lassar TA, Schmidt DH: Coronary flow reserve after dipyridamole predicts adequacy of ventricular function during exercise. Circulation 70 (supp II), 1984: II–22 (Abstract).

Digital imaging modalities for coronary and myocardial wall studies

Joachim H. Bürsch, P.H. Heintzen and K. Moldenhauer

Summary

The continued development of digital imaging techniques has resulted in advanced diagnostic capabilities for the assessment of coronary artery disease and myocardial ischemia. Enhancement of vascular and tissue opacification, as well as the extraction of perfusion parameters are the basic procedures in digital coronary angiography. In this survey different acquisition and processing modes are discussed within the limitations of the spatial and temporal resolution of current imaging systems.

Coronary artery studies involve morphologic and flow analysis. The use of a 1024×1024 matrix reveales comparable spatial resolution as the conventional cinefilm; however, at this resolution the temporal resolution is limited to rates of 8 images/sec. The 512×512 image matrix allows real-time acquisition with a rate of 30 images/sec and is practical for most of the diagnostically relevant problems. Temporal aspects of vascular contrast flow have even been assessed with a 256×256 matrix, specifically taken advantage of the improved signal-to-noise ratio per picture element.

Myocardial imaging is another important application that provides dimensional measurements of the left ventricular wall, as well as detection of regional perfusion annomalies. ECG-gated image integration and subtraction are the basic processing steps. Finally, digital densitometry has been developed to assess myocardial flow and flow reserve quantitatively.

This chapter ends with a discussion of an economical solution for digital storage requirements of coronary angiograms.

Introduction

The development of digital imaging techniques for studies of the coronary circulation has been a diagnostic challenge because of its potential clinical value and particular qualities of this vasculature. Technical limitations were mostly related to the small size and significant motion of coronary arteries as well as their low contrast opacification and that of the myocardium. Interestingly, it was the latter aspect that stimulated the application of digital enhancement techniques for studies of myocardial opacification and flow distribution (12, 20).

A variety of diagnostic approaches have been proposed that will be outlined in this survey which covers both coronary vascular examinations and myocardial perfusion studies.

Image acquisition considerations

Digital equipment for high resolution real-time acquisition of cardiovascular angiograms has been improved during the past decade. A characteristic feature of present systems is the video data scanning rate of 7.5 million samples per second, digital conversion (8–10 bit resolution) and subsequent storage in digital memory. This acquisition rate is equivalent to the product of spatial and temporal resolution, i.e. low imaging rates correspond to high spatial matrix resolution and vice versa (Figure 1). For example, the use of a 1024×1024 matrix allows for detailed morphologic analysis, but is limited to a temporal resolution of 7 images per second. A 256×256 matrix facilitates acquisition rates of more than 60 images per second and provides temporal resolution of at least 20 msec. Consequently, the latter system seems more appropriate for dynamic cardiovascular studies, despite its rather limited spatial resolution.

Another aspect concerns the signal-to-noise ratio (SNR) as a function of spatial resolution. If the number of raster lines in the video camera is doubled, the spot size decreases by a factor of four and the signal-to-noise ratio is reduced. To compensate for high image noise levels an increase in X-ray dose is necessary, which may in turn become a limiting factor. Low spatial resolution corresponds to low quantum noise per picture element (pixel) favoring densitometric parameter extraction. A 512×512 matrix comprises a good compromise between resolution and SNR, and is preferable for quantitative evaluation of coronary angiograms. Finally, pulsing of the X-ray generator as well as progressive line scanning of the video camera are important requirements to minimize misregistration by vascular motion.

With the development of improved instrumentation the interest in functional studies have steadily increased (10, 11). The present generation of digital systems allows the definition of regions of interest (ROI's) for measurement of temporal variation in contrast absorption. Moreover, the extraction of functional data on a picture element basis has become technically feasible. Densitometric analysis can be used to measure a value that is proportional to the total amount of contrast medium in areas of the vasculature. In order to account for the exponential relationship between the amount of contrast medium and the X-ray absorption,

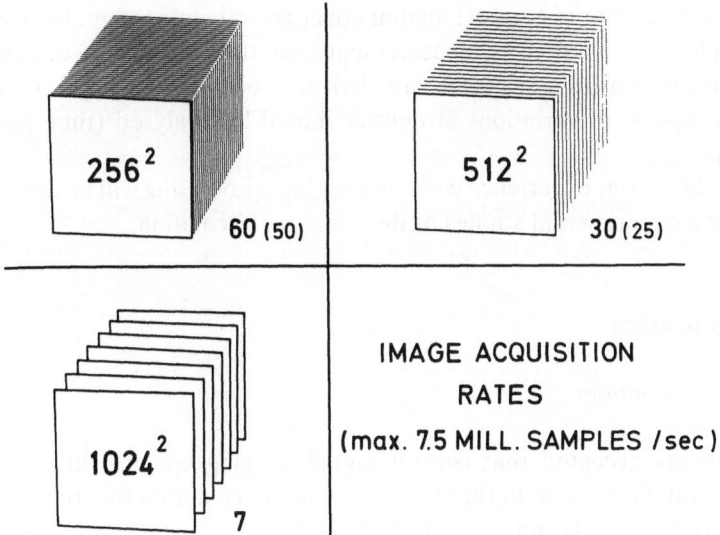

Figure 1. Acquisition modalities of digital systems relating the matrix format to frame rates per second (numbers in the lower right corner of each panel). A rate of 7.5×10^6 samples/sec was assumed.

the detected intensity is logarithmically converted. Several factors have been discussed as fundamental constraints governing the performance of densitometry for quantitative studies (2), such as X-ray scattering and veiling glare of the image intensifier. However, integrated measurements of X-ray absorption over relatively large ROI's (2% of the projection area or more), lead to linear measure-

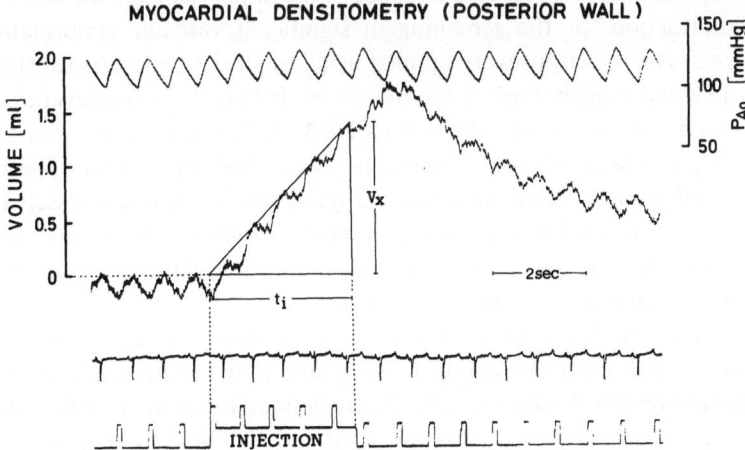

Figure 2. Densogram in an animal study after selective contrast injection of 3 ml of contrast medium (constant infusion rate) into the left circumflex coronary artery. ti = injection duration; Vx = contrast material volume that had entered the coronary vasculature.

ments of the amount of contrast medium over an adequate range. Figure 2 gives an example of such a density measurement from the posterior myocardial wall. Contrarily, if densitometric data are derived from individual pixels only the temporal aspects of variations in density should be analyzed (time parameter imaging).

On this basis, our experience with digital image processing will be discussed for clinical and experimental studies of the coronary circulation.

Coronary imaging

Vascular morphology

It is generally accepted that current digital imaging systems do not provide diagnostic qualities equal to that from conventional cinefilm for studies of coronary artery lesions. Technical limitations in digital imaging result from limited resolution and noise (4). Accurate measurements of coronary stenoses with sizes on the order of 1 mm would require a matrix of 1024×1024 picture elements in the standard viewing field. As already noted, this limits the frame rate to seven images per second. Furthermore, a large focal spot in the X-ray tube is required to facilitate an adequate X-ray dose and to keep quantum noise per picture element reasonably low. The use of a large focal spot size in turn degrades the spatial resolution of radiographic images. Therefore, current studies using digital subtraction angiography (DSA) have been based on a 512×512 image matrix with a rate of 30 frames per second. It has been demonstrated that these systems allow for the detection of significant lesions, especially in the major coronary arteries.

Clinical applications have taken advantage of the improved contrast sensitivity of image subtraction for the screening of significant vascular abnormalities. Hence, intra-aortic injections were applied using small size catheters for studies of the patency and morphology of the main vessels (24). Less invasiveness has been the important aspect for intravenous DSA-studies in patients with saphenous vein bypass grafts. These examinations yielded high success rates, particularly because of the large diameters and negligible motion of these vessels (15). Another application of DSA in coronary angiography has been the use of algorithms for edge enhancement and densitometric analysis for percentage cross-sectional narrowing measurements (1, 19).

Two acquisition modes are preferred for coronary studies. Selection of a single contrast image and a corresponding mask image is the method of choice to achieve optimal results. Unfortunately, this technique has some practical drawbacks as far as real-time imaging is concerned and also in the event of cardiac arrhythmia. Therefore, another approach has been developed, namely averaging mask images over a period of one or more cardiac cycles. The socalled 'blurred' mask mode is illustrated in Figure 3. It facilitates real-time subtraction of contrast

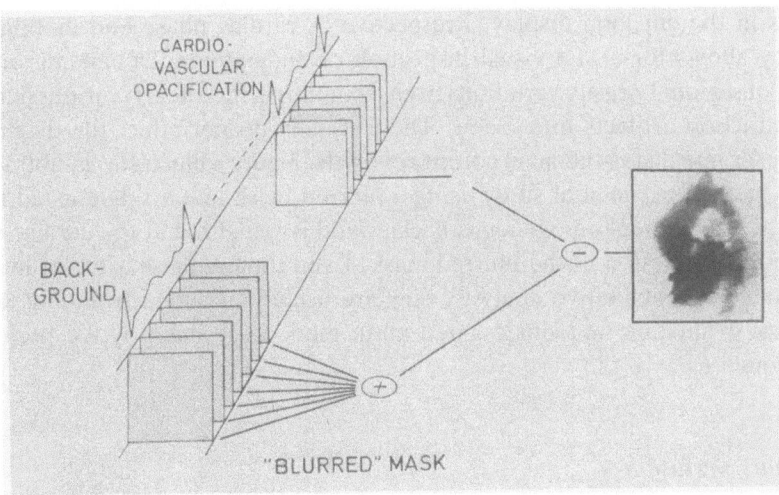

Figure 3. Diagram of the 'blurred mask' subtraction mode for cardiac studies.

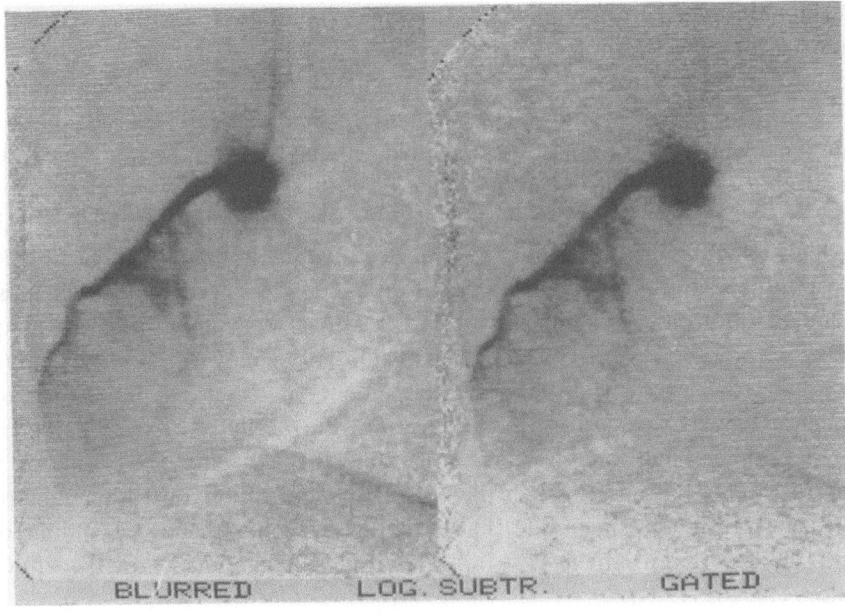

Figure 4. Use of two imaging modes in an experimental study for imaging the left anterior descending coronary artery (256 × 256 image matrix). Left: Subtraction image formed by integration of a blurred mask and a single contrast image. Right: Same study (as left) using a single mask and a single contrast image from identical cardiac phases. The blurred mask study reveales background inhomogeneities, especially at the posterior wall; this is not the case with the optimal ECG-gated mask image.

images in the cineloop display, irrespective of cardiac phase and motion and thereby allows for a fast visual inspection of angiograms. Depending on the extent of regional density variations from the nonopacified heart, various degrees of subtraction artifacts may occur. These usually do not affect the diagnostic quality for imaging of the main coronary vessels. Figure 4 illustrates a subtraction image in an experimental study using a blurred mask and a single gated mask image. Usually, nonhomogeneous background is visualized at the cardiac walls due to phasic motion in the blurred mask. Even though these artifacts may be acceptable for qualitative analysis, they are usually excluded from any densitometric evaluation and single gated mask mode subtraction is the preferred technique.

Coronary perfusion

Temporal aspects of the passage of contrast material through the arterial vasculature can be assessed in two different ways. The first principle utilizes image subtraction and the second is based on the processing of density-time curves detected at each picture element.

The difference between images of the angiographic contrast phase over one or more cardiac cycles indicates the regional change of contrast medium. This acquisition mode is called gated-interval difference imaging. Gating from the ECG corrects for phasic motion of the regularly beating heart and is the basis for minimizing misregistration of the opacified vessels. Because the spatial positions of coronary arteries will not remain identical over several cardiac cycles, some blurring of the vasculature may be observed. Consequently, high resolution imaging systems will not result in any improvement in this field of application and most of the studies have been successful with 256×256 matrices. The diagnostic value of difference imaging is to compare the propagation of radio-opaque indicator along different vessels; as an example, this may be used to document any delayed washout from poststenotic segments of vessels. Usually aortic root injections are performed in this application. Furthermore, a sequence of difference images may be processed for studies of the temporal course of the contrast bolus passage through the coronaries and the myocardium. Figure 5 illustrates this processing mode. The resulting set of images may be combined to one single temporal image that indicates the propagation of flow by different colors (14, 16, 17, 21).

The other approach utilizes the processing of temporal variations in X-ray opacity at each of the picture elements and is called time parameter extraction (3, 7, 13). A set of coronary densograms is depicted in Figure 6. ECG-gated image acquisition of the entire angiogram is necessary to establish regional density-time curves. A low resolution image matrix (256×256) in these studies is preferred to improve the SNR. Several algorithms are in use for the calculation of representa-

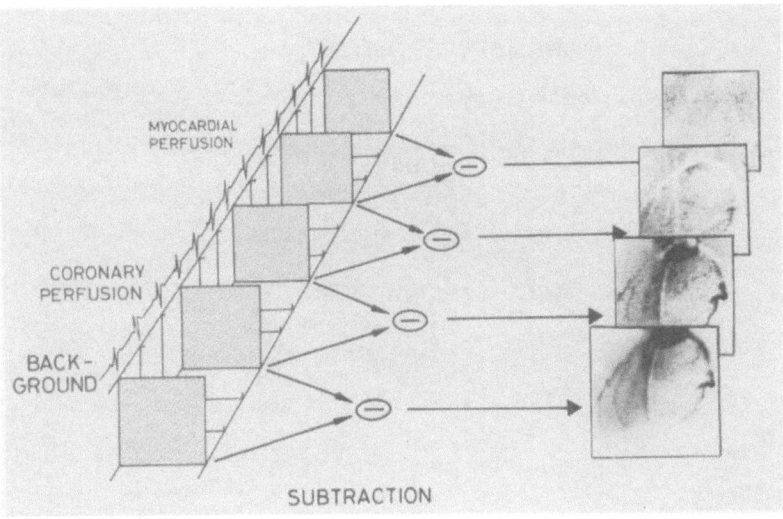

Figure 5. Diagram of the gated-interval difference mode.

tive time data from the contrast dilution curves (pixel densograms). Typical parameters are the timing of the line of gravity of the curve and, more suitably, the mean appearance time as derived from the bolus front (initial curve section ending at the peak amplitude). The calculated parameters are displayed as a parameter image in a color coded format. This type of parameter image provides temporal information similar to that of the described gated-interval difference technique; however it has the advantage that segments based on any desired time interval may be defined interactively, irrespective of heart rate. This approach is advantageous for interindividual studies. Examples are illustrated in Figures 7 and 8.

Temporal imaging of the coronary vasculature provides a good predictive value of myocardial perfusion in hearts with stenosed coronary vessels. Vogel, LeFree and coworkers (23) have clearly demonstrated the utility of this technique for estimating the coronary flow reserve (9). Experimental infarction studies in our laboratory, however, did not show good results as compared with densitometric measurements of the amount of contrast medium from the myocardial perfusion phase. It is our impression that the specificity of flow velocities in native vessels is not a reliable reflection of quantitative changes in volume flow. Nevertheless, visualization of the time of contrast flow and its spatial distribution definitely has gained diagnostic significance for the evaluation of coronary artery disease. The different methods described may be applied as complementary diagnostic approaches.

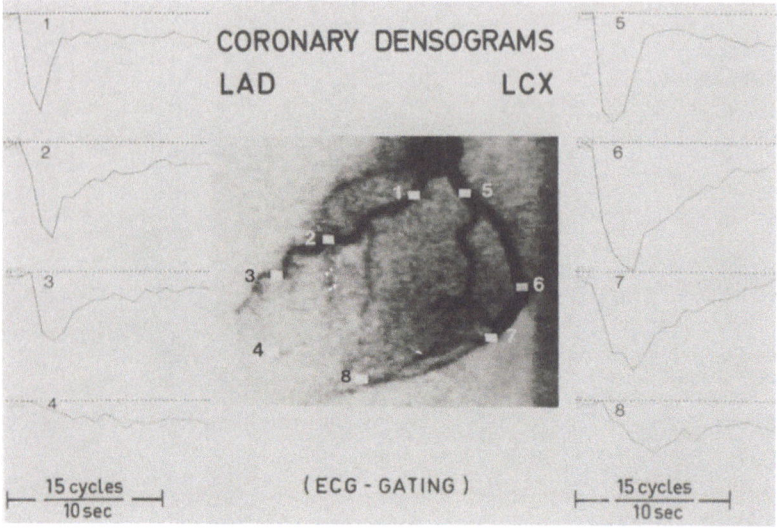

Figure 6. Illustration of regional density-time curves as detected from 4 ROI's (white rectangles) from each of the two coronary arteries. Curves have been established by interpolation of density data obtained from sequential ECG-gated images. Time parameters are preferably calculated from the initial curve sections (early slope of curves).

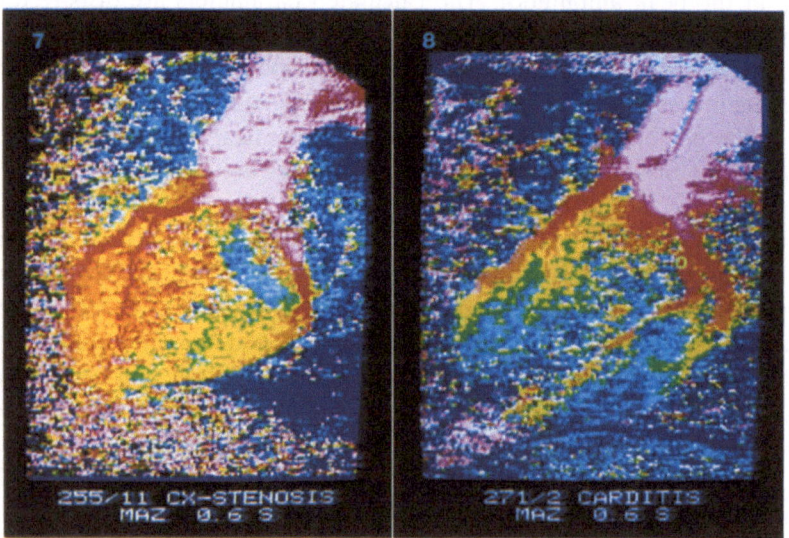

Figure 7. Time parameter image of left coronary arteries in an experimental infarction study (proximal LCX-stenosis) indicating delayed contrast flow to the posterior left ventricular wall.

Figure 8. Time parameter image of left coronary arteries in an animal showing vascular segments that indicate flow propagation within 0.6 sec. ECG-gated image acquisition was utilized.

Myocardial imaging

Visualization of LV wall

Different aspects of myocardial imaging by digital subtraction techniques have been discussed previously. Visualization of the opacified myocardium facilitates both the detection of nonperfused myocardial regions and the dimensional measurements of the ventricular wall. Digital subtraction of ECG-gated images from the pre-injection period and from the time of microvascular contrast perfusion is the basic subtraction mode. The success of myocardial imaging is highly dependent on the suppression of background structures. Thus, ECG-gating as well as suspended respiration are the basic requirements. As a result, the myocardial shell can be adequately visualized, especially, if selective coronary injections are performed. Myocardial imaging quality can be improved by contrast enhancement, although is limited by the effects of increased image noise. Consequently, integration of images from the pre-injection period and from the contrast phase has been found important in enhancing myocardial images.

Numerous studies have demonstrated that averaging of four ECG-gated images from each of the two contrast phases provides a compromise between the practical feasibility and optimal contrast enhancement in coronary angiography. Image integration and subtraction are schematically depicted in Figure 9. Corresponding to the relationship between signal-to-noise ratio and roentgen dose (D): SNR ~ $\sqrt{D}$, SNR doubles as a result of the integration of 4 images. The sequence of gated contrast images usually begins with the onset of contrast washout from the main coronary arteries and ends before venous runoff has occurred. It may be

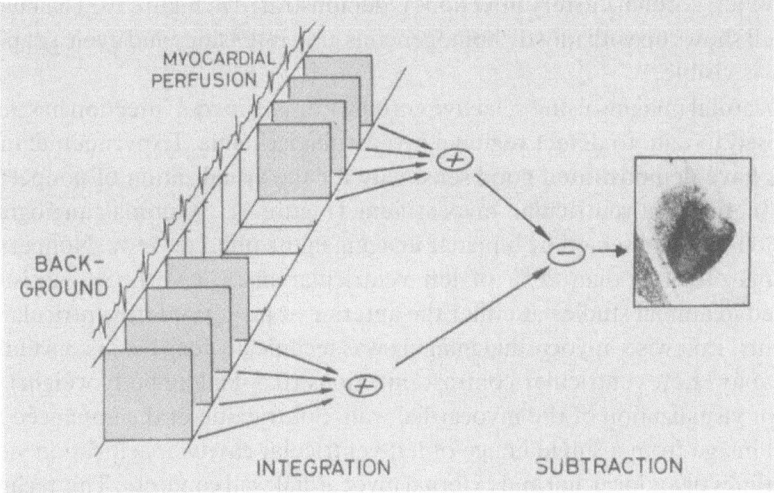

Figure 9. Diagram of integration of images to improve signal-to-noise ratio.

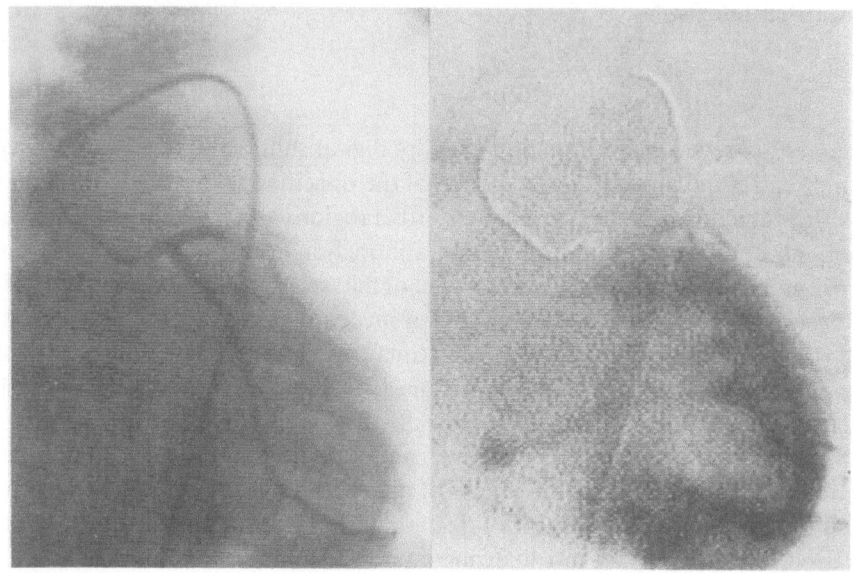

Figure 10. Myocardial image in a patient study using selective left coronary artery injection. Left: Original coronary angiogram. Right: Visualization of the left ventricular wall using image integration and subtraction.

emphasized, that the resulting subtracted image cannot represent a strictly defined time of regional contrast opacification. However, this fact is not necessarily negative, because unforeseen flow abnormalities with different times of opacification are thereby encountered. A typical example of a clinical study with selective left coronary artery injections is demonstrated in Figure 10. The myocardial shell shows up with mostly homogeneous gray intensities and even a papillary muscle is visible.

Myocardial imaging using selective coronary or aortic root injection has mainly been used to date to detect regional myocardial ischemia. Experimental infarct studies have demonstrated good sensitivity for the visualization of nonperfused zones in the left ventricular myocardium (Figure 11). Optimal angiographic conditions were obtained by biplanar imaging in the oblique views. Nonperfused segments of more than 20% of left ventricular mass have been consistently detected in animal studies at either the anterior or posterior left ventricular wall segments. Likewise, myocardial imaging was technically feasible in conventional levography. Left ventricular contrast injections (0.5–1 ml/kg body weight) were used for visualization of the myocardial wall. Subtraction of the enhanced myocardial image from a single image of left ventricular cavity opacification yielded the outlines of endocardial and external myocardial wall contours. This technique has been found to be less reliable for the detection of myocardial ischemia because only the most peripheral wall shell is visible. Other parts of the myocar-

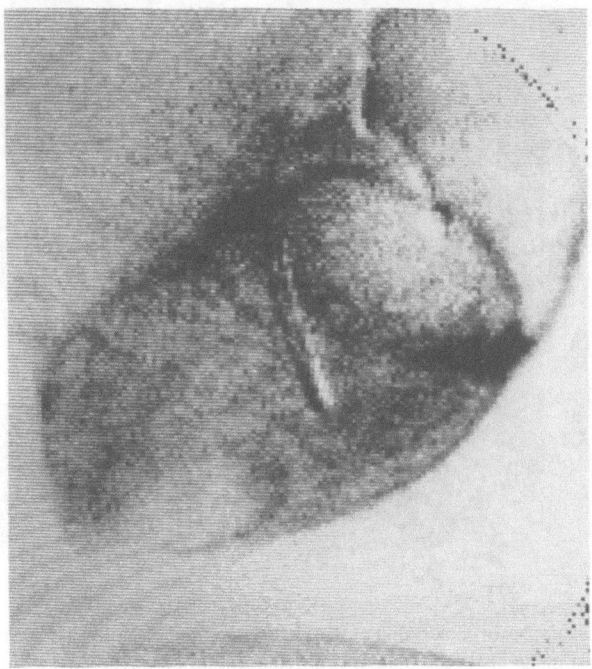

Figure 11. Myocardial image from an experimental infarct study demonstrating a nonperfused zone at the apico-posterior wall of the left ventricle.

dium are superimposed by the opacified cavity. Nevertheless, estimation of the infarct size with this technique has proven successful when compared to postmortem measurements.

Relevant diagnostic information was also obtained from measurements of left ventricular myocardial volume using videometry (18), as well as from regional wall thickening studies (6, 21), both of which may be regarded as a diagnostic adjunct to conventional angiocardiographic examinations. An example from a patient study is illustrated in Figure 12.

Perfusion studies

In order to assess myocardial perfusion in a quantitative manner densitometric analysis was combined with the digital subtraction technique. The basic idea of this analytic procedure was to measure the total amount of radio-opaque indicator from the myocardial regions that are supplied by each of the three main coronary arteries (8). Preliminary studies indicated that oblique projections of the heart were adequate to separate the perfusion regions of the LCX and the LAD coronary arteries without significant overlap. RCA studies were easiest to

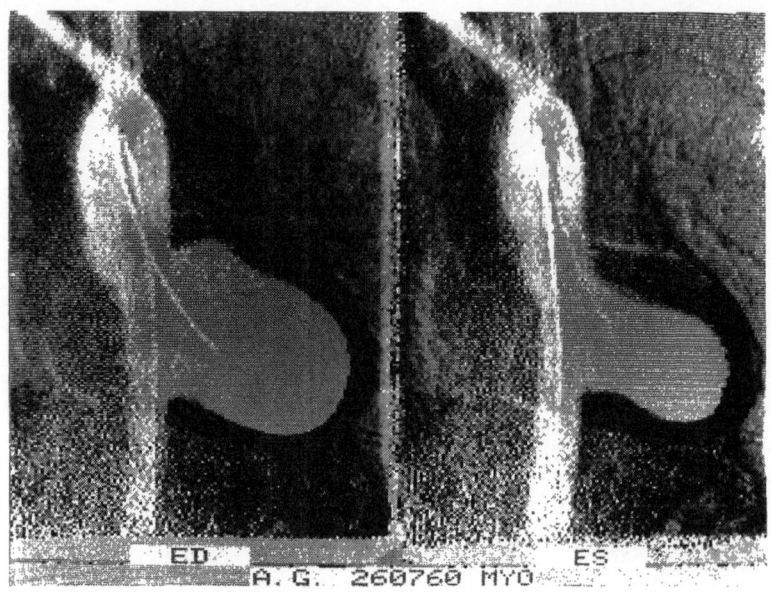

Figure 12. Clinical example for illustration of myocardial wall imaging after left ventricular contrast injection. A contrast image from the time of ventricular filling was subtracted from the myocardial perfusion image for visualization of the internal and external wall contours. Left: End-diastolic phase. Right: End- systolic phase.

assess because they were not accompanied by left coronary artery opacification. Thus, it was possible to analyze densitometrically the three main wall regions separately and for comparison with each other.

In these studies processing of images differed somewhat from the imaging modes described. Usually a single contrast image was selected as defined by a characteristic event during the course of angiography (e.g. end of injection). Subsequently, a single mask image was selected from the corresponding cardiac phase. In order to assure optimal registration several consecutive mask images from the corresponding cardiac phases were tested. This practice became an important feature in order to derive high quality density data from hypoperfused myocardial regions. Logarithmic conversion of image data was necessary to account for the exponential relationship between fractional X-ray absorption and the amount of contrast medium transradiated. An illustration of this processing mode is depicted in Figure 13.

Regional measurements of contrast accumulation in the myocardium were established by manual outlining of the different wall segments. An example from selective left coronary artery injections is given in Figure 14. Densitometric analyses was usually applied to images corresponding to the end of contrast injection. A special power syringe was used to provide accurate and constant injection flow rates on the order of 3–4 ml/sec. Significant backflow of contrast

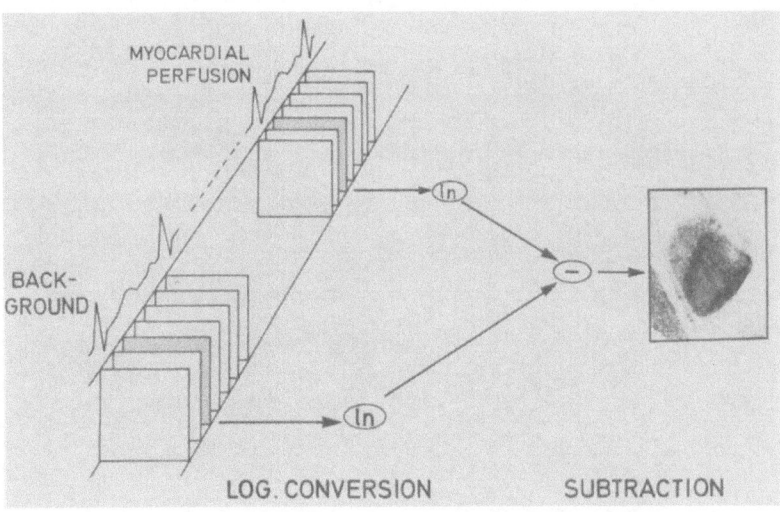

Figure 13. Diagram of mask mode subtraction using a single pre-injection image and a contrast image. Image data must be converted logarithmically for subsequent densitometric analysis.

medium into the ascending aorta was a regular finding. Consequently, regional density data indicated the amount of contrast medium that had entered the myocardial wall segment by antegrade flow. These data were used as relative measures of coronary blood flow for comparison in the different regions.

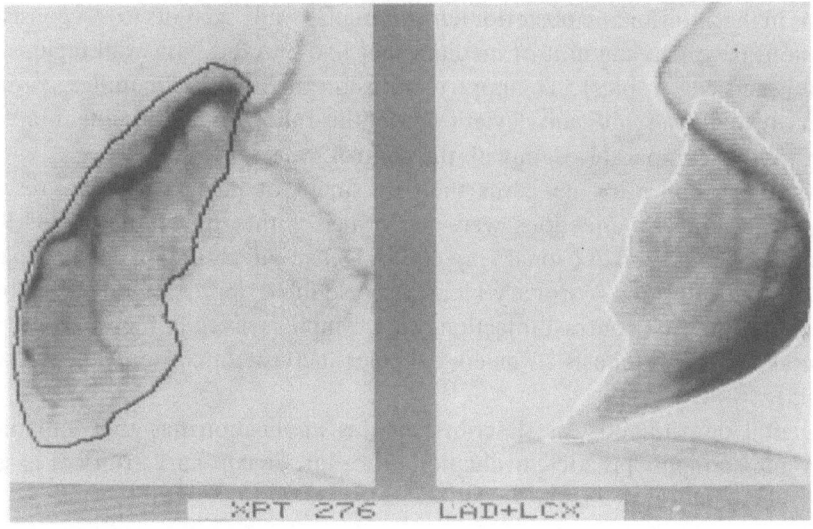

Figure 14. Myocardial contrast images in an experimental study after selective injection into the LAD (left) and LCX (right) coronary arteries.

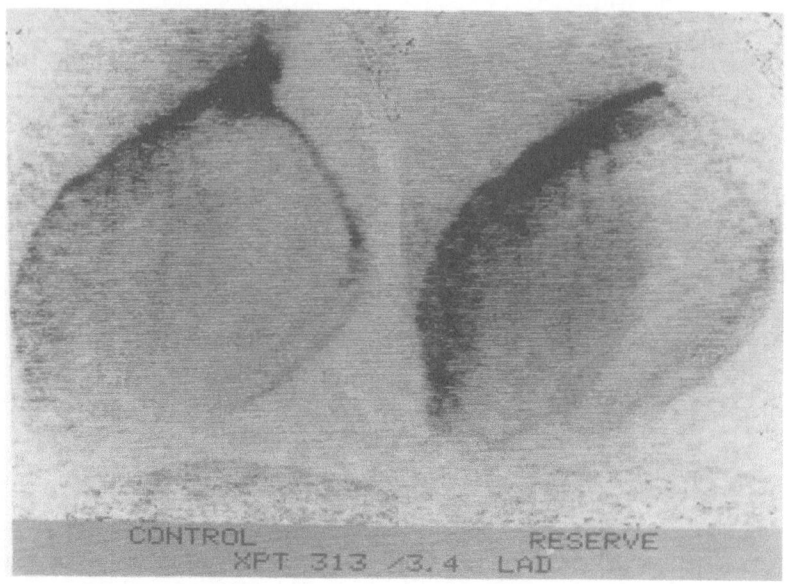

Figure 15. Myocardial contrast images from an experimental study using duplicate contrast injections into the LAD coronary artery (each 3 ml/sec) for study of coronary flow reserve. Left: Mask mode image of first contrast injection. Right: Mask mode image of second contrast injection obtained 15 seconds after the first injection. Significantly increased contrast accumulation in the myocardium is visualized. Densitometric analysis revealed an increase of contrast flow by a factor of two.

Similarly, injection into the main left coronary artery was used to estimate flow ratios in the anterior and posterior left ventricular wall segments (5). A consistent relationship of the amount of medium that had entered both wall regions was established (1:1 in pigs). Temporary occlusion of the left circumflex coronary artery revealed a significant deviation from this ratio, while subsequent reperfusion yielded comparable data with the control state.

Another application concerns the assessment of myocardial flow reserve. Duplicate contrast injections were performed within time intervals of 10–15 seconds using selective coronary injections. Densitometry of the regional opacifications indicated that coronary blood flow doubled approximately as a consequence of the first contrast injection. An example is given in Figure 15. Experimental coronary stenosis revealed a smaller increase in coronary flow reserve (<1.5).

Digital densitometry as described in this application has the potential of becoming a highly practicle evaluation procedure in coronary artery disease.

Digital storage requirements

Many of the described imaging modalities are essentially based on ECG-gating and only a small number of angiographic images is actually needed for the specific problem under study. However, the use of optional imaging modes and supplementary information from the entire image sequence necessitates the acquisition and storage of the complete angiographic sequence in real time. As stated before, current roentgen-video systems are capable of producing a practical data rate of 7.5 million samples per second. Presently, an economical solution to these high-speed storage needs is a real-time digital disk subsystem. High data rates of more than 9 Mbytes/s are accomplished by the use of special interfaces connected to Winchester disks or with real-time data reduction.

The minimum requirement needed for clinical examinations is the real-time storage capability of at least 1 angiographic sequence. For 10 seconds of imaging a storage capacity of 75 Mbyte is needed. Even more flexibility is provided by real-time storage of the total number of studies for each patient. Assuming 8 angiographic scenes with a duration of 10 sec each, 2400 images per patient are obtained, leading to a total data volume of 600 MByte per patient without data reduction.

Subsequent processing and retrieval requires an additional removable long-term backup medium for archival storage. The traditional way of storing such large data volumes is the use of digital magnetic tapes which have a relatively low cost per Mbyte of storage. Access time, shelf life (about 3 years), reliability and durability of magnetic tapes however are not satisfactory. Archiving with optical laser disks with direct access to single images will be advantageous. At present the access-time is not as high as that of Winchester disks. However, the capacity of about 2 Gigabyte/disk allows storage of more than 8000 images ($512 \times 512 \times 8$ bits). The permanence of this medium is an additional benefit for this application and provides high data safety. The price per Mbyte of the laser disk medium will be comparable to that of magnetic tapes and the lifetime of the optical disks is considerably longer (more than 10 years) than that of magnetic tapes.

References

1. Alderman EL, Berte LE, Harrison DC, Sanders W: Quantitation of coronary artery dimensions using digital image processing. In: Digital Radiography, WR Brody (Ed.). SPIE 314, 1981: 273–278.
2. Brennecke R, Hahne HJ, Bürsch JH, Heintzen PH: Digital videodensitometry: Some approaches to radiographic image restoration and analysis. In: Radiological functional analysis of the vascular system, F. Heuck (Ed.), Springer, Berlin Heidelberg New York, 1983: 79–88.
3. Brennecke R, Bürsch JH, Heintzen PH: Functional analysis by digital angiography: basic physics and technology. In: Contrast media in digital radiography, R. Felix, W Frommhold, J Lissner, TH Meaney, HP Niendorf, E Zeitler (Eds.). Exerpta Medica, Amsterdam, 1983: 37–50.

4. Brody WR: Digital Radiography. Proc SPIE 314, 1981.

5. Bürsch JH, Hahne HJ, Beyer C, Seemann S, Meissner L, Brennecke R, Heintzen PH: Myocardial perfusion studies by digital angiography. Comp Cardiol, 1983: 343–346.

6. Bürsch JH, Radtke W, Rünger T, Moldenhauer K, Hoffmann B, Heintzen PH: Endocardial and epicardial contour detection of the left ventricle by digital angiocardiography. In: Ventricular Wall Motion, U Sigwart, PH Heintzen (Eds.), Georg Thieme Verlag, New York, Stuttgart, 1984: 49–57.

7. Bürsch JH, Heintzen PH: Parametric imaging. Radiologic Clinics of North America, 1985: 321–333.

8. Bürsch JH: Densitometric studies in digital subtraction angiographie: Assessment of pulmonary and myocardial perfusion. Herz, 1985 (in press).

9. Gould KL, Lipscomb K, Hamilton GW: Physiologic basis for assessing critical coronary stenosis. Instantaneous flow response and regional distribution during coronary hyperemia as measures of coronary flow reserve. Am J Cardiol 33, 1974: 87–94.

10. Heintzen PH, Brennecke R, Bürsch JH, Hahne HJ, Lange PE, Moldenhauer K, Onnasch D, Radtke W: Quantitative analysis of structure and function of the cardiovascular system by roentgen-video-computer techniques. Mayo Clin Proc 57, 1982: 78–91.

11. Digital Imaging in Cardiovascular Radiology. Heintzen PH, Brennecke R (Eds): Georg Thieme Verlag, Stuttgart, New York, 1983.

12. Heintzen PH, Brennecke R, Bürsch JH: Computerized videoangiocardiography. In: Coronary Heart Disease, M Kaltenback, P Lichtlen, R Balcon, W-D Bussmann (Eds.). Georg Thieme Verlag, Stuttgart, New York, 1978: 116–121.

13. Höhne KH, Obermöller U, Riemer M, Witte G: Advanced techniques for digital angiography of the heart. In: Digitale Radiographie, HE Riemann, J Kollath (Eds.). Schnetztor, Konstanz, 1984: 146–154.

14. LeFree MT, Vogel RA, O'Neill WW, Bates ER, Smith DN, Pitt B: A digital radiographic technique for visualization and quantitation of regional myocardial perfusion. Comp Cardiol 1982: 153–156.

15. Luska G, Hendrickx Ph, Kuhl A, Lichtlen P: Peripher venöse digitale Subtraktionsangiographie (DSA) zur Kontrolle von aortokoronaren Venenbypassgrafts (ACVB). Fortschr Röntgenstr 142, 1985: 35–40.

16. O'Neill WW, Vogel RA, LeFree M, Bates E, Kirlin P. Beaumon G, Pitt B: Digital coronary radiographic assessment of relative regional coronary blood flow. Circulation 66, 1982: II–229 (Abstract).

17. Ratib O, Chappuis F, Rutishauser W: Digital angiographic technique for the quantitative assessment of myocardial perfusion. Ann Radiol 28, 1985: 193–197.

18. Radtke W, Bürsch JH, Brennecke R, Hahne HJ, Heintzen PH: Assessment of left ventricular muscle volume by digital angiocardiography. Invest Radiol 18, 1983: 149–154.

19. Reiber JHC, Slager CJ, Schuurbiers JCH, Boer A den, Gerbrands JJ, Troost GJ, Scholts B, Kooijman CJ, Serruys PW: Transfer functions of the X-ray-cine-video chain applied to digital processing of coronary cineangiograms. In: Digital Imaging in Cardiovascular Radiology. PH Heintzen, R Brennecke (Eds.). Georg Thieme Verlag, Stuttgart, New York, 1983: 89–104.

20. Robb RA, Wood EH, Ritman EL, Johnson SA, Sturm RE, Greenleaf JF, Gilbert BK, Chevalier PA: Three-dimensional reconstruction and display of the working canine heart and lungs by multiplanar X-ray scanning videodensitometry. Comp Cardiol. 1974: 151–163.

21. Rünger T: Die Messung der linksventrikulären systolische Myokardzunahme mit Hilfe der digitalen Subtraktionsangiographie. Ein Vergleich gesunder und experimentell infarzierter Herzen. Thesis, Kiel 1985.

22. Spiller P, Jehle J, Pölitz B, Schmiel FK: A digital X-ray image processing system for measurement of phasic blood flow in coronary arteries. Comp Cardiol 1982: 223–226.

23. Vogel R, LeFree M, Bates E, O'Neill W, Foster R, Kirlin P, Smith D, Pitt B: Application of

digital techniques to selective coronary arteriography: use of myocardial contrast appearence time to measure coronary flow reserve. Am Heart J 107, 1984: 153–164.

24. Whiting JS, Nivatpumin TH, Pfaff M, Vas R, Drury K, Diamond G, Swan HJC, Forrester JS: Assessing the coronary circulation by digital angiography: bypass graft and myocardial perfusion imaging. In: Digital Imaging in Cardiovascular Radiology, H. Heintzen, R, Brennecke (Eds.), Georg Thieme Verlag, Stuttgart, New York, 1983: 205–211.

Myocardial densograms from digital subtraction angiography with apparent cardiac arrest

Tjeerd van der Werf, H. Stegehuis and R.M. Heethaar

Summary

To study the perfusion of the myocardium, digitally subtracted coronary arteriograms were analyzed densitometrically. Since coronary arteries are in continuous motion, the conventional subtraction technique cannot be used in coronary arteriography without taking certain precautions. To prevent variations in cardiac contractions due to varying RR-intervals, heart rate was controlled by regular right atrial stimulation. Moreover, both the stimulation rate and cine frequency were brought into synchrony by triggering on the frequency of the electrical main current (50 cycles/s). In this way each cardiac cycle contained exactly the same number of frames and these were acquired at corresponding moments in the cardiac cycle. These two measures together were called: apparent cardiac arrest. Digital subtraction with the application of the concept of apparent cardiac arrest enables one to obtain good quality images of the coronary arterial tree, capillary filling, myocardial staining and wash-out of contrast material.

To test the method eleven candidates for percutaneous transluminal coronary angioplasty (PTCA) were studied. Following injection of 8 ml Ioxaglate in 2 s. into the left main stem (LMS) mean pixel grayness was determined in regions of interest over the LMS, over the myocardium supplied by the stenosed vessel (path. area) and over the normal vessel (control area) in end-diastolic frames acquired over a period of 15 s. From the grayness versus time curves appearance time (t_{ap}) and peak concentration time (t_{max}) were assessed. From these values the difference in build-up time between myocardium and LMS ($\triangle t_{bu}$) was calculated. Results (mean ± s.d.):

	path. area		control area	
	pre PTCA	post PTCA	pre PTCA	post PTCA
t_{ap}	1.1 ± 0.5	0.7 ± 0.5	0.7 ± 0.4	0.8 ± 0.5
t_{max}	7.1 ± 1.8	4.4 ± 0.8*	4.6 ± 0.9	4.4 ± 0.8
$\triangle t_{bu}$	3.9 ± 2.6	2.0 ± 1.1**	1.7 ± 1.2	2.0 ± 1.2

$* = p<0.01; ** = p<0.05$.

The parameters peak concentration time t_{max} and difference in build-up time $\triangle t_{bu}$ between myocardium and injection site demonstrate the expected improvement in myocardial perfusion by PTCA to values similar to those in control areas. This is in contrast to the parameter appearance time t_{ap}.

From our results it may be concluded that densitometry of digitally subtracted coronary arteriograms facilitates the quantitative analysis of parameters related to myocardial perfusion.

Introduction

Conventional coronary arteriography provides detailed information about the patho-anatomy of the coronary vessels during life. The quality of the angiographic images has considerably increased during the last decade by the development of more powerful X-ray generators, better X-ray tubes with increased heat capacity, and improved image intensifiers with cesium iodide input screens. Insight into the three-dimensional coronary anatomy has initiated the wide spread application of cranial and caudal angulations in order to be able to visualize narrowings and occlusions in vessels running anteriorly or posteriorly.

On the other hand, it should be realized that a number of problems in coronary arteriography still exist and probably will persist. These problems can be divided into three categories: 1) fundamental and structural problems related to the use of X-rays for image acquisition; 2) unsolvable situations in coronary anatomy; and 3) shortcomings of the human eye and brain.

The finite dimensions of the focus of the X-ray tube, being of the same order as the objects to be visualized, namely narrowed coronary arteries, is one example of a fundamental problem related to the use of X-rays for image acquisition. Another example is the noise, caused by quantum mottle that could be solved by employing higher doses, which are, however, undesired for the safety of patient and personnel. Unsolvable situations in coronary anatomy are suspected narrowings in kinks and curls of vessels, which cannot be adequately visualized in any projection. As to the third point, mentioned above, inter- and intraobserver variabilities have been described frequently. From the rheology's point of view, it is obvious that the impact of an increasing degree of narrowing on flow and on flow reserve is far from proportional, which necessitates more accurate assessments of the degree of narrowing with increasing degree of stenosis.

Ziedses des Plantes introduced over 40 years ago the idea of image subtraction into radiologic practice with the purpose to enhance image quality of films with poor definition. In recent years essentially the same principle has been applied to various fields of radiology by computer handling of X-ray images. Thanks to the large capabilities of such systems, it was not only possible to enhance image quality of poorly defined structures, but it also became possible to extend the objectives to comprise goals such as reducing contrast medium volume, reducing radiation dose and – most importantly – administering the contrast material for imaging of arteries intravenously, thus obviating selective arterial catheterization.

In relation to coronary arteriography it seems very questionable whether intravenous injection will become a real option. After intravenous injection the passage of the latter part of the contrast material through the left atrium and the left ventricle will degrade the coronary artery image quality to a level that diagnostic decision making will become very difficult. Fluoroscopy combined with video techniques open indeed possibilities to reduce radiation dose to the patients and personnel. In a previous study, we demonstrated that digital coronary subtraction angiography after selective intracoronary contrast administration is possible provided a good triggering method is applied (1). This triggering procedure was called: 'apparent cardiac arrest', essentially based on two requirements: 1) stimulating the heart at a strictly regular rate; and 2) synchronizing heart rate and cinepulses to the main's frequency. In applying this method we could demonstrate, firstly, an enhancement of conspicuousness of the larger coronary arteries and their pathological changes and, secondly, an intensification of myocardial filling, allowing a better appreciation of this phenomenon. It seemed important to us to continue the study of the second mentioned result, intensification of myocardial filling, since this phenomenon is related to myocardial flow. Study of this phenomenon could possibly open up possibilities to extract pathophysiological information, up till now hidden in the coronary arteriogram. In this context it is important to notice that our patients suffered from myocardial ischemia that, apart from other causes, indeed was caused by coronary narrowings, occlusions and insufficient collateral circulation, but that represents a far more intricate pathophysiological phenomenon in which the key word is myocardial flow (perfusion) or flow reserve.

Methods and patients

Basic principle underlying the concept of apparent cardiac arrest

The causes of motion of an object and changes in background can be divided into evitable and inevitable causes (Table 1). Table motion (known as 'panning') is evitable. The patient can be instructed not to move and can be trained to hold his or her breath at a constant level during the cinerun. The automatic brightness control unit of the X-ray equipment can be locked; otherwise, changes in radiation dose will occur after the injection of contrast agent. On the other hand, cardiac contractions causing motion of the object (the coronary arteries) and changes in background (the volume of the cardiac cavities and the ventricular myocardium) are inevitable and complicate the application of subtraction techniques. To cope with these problems, we developed the concept of apparent cardiac arrest in which contrast and non-contrast images are subtracted only if they have been obtained at comparable moments in the cardiac cycle, as if the heart was arrested. This approach requires a regular heart rate and synchrony between heart rate and cine frequency.

Practical realization of the concept of apparent cardiac arrest

A regular heart rate was obtained by stimulating the heart at a frequency slightly above the sinus rhythm by means of an externally triggered stimulator with a pacing catheter positioned against the right atrial wall. The reason for the use of the external trigger is explained later. With the X-ray equipment 25 cineframes/s are obtained in synchrony with the frequency of the electric main alternating current (50 cycles/s in Europe). To achieve synchrony between X-ray film frames and heart rate, the stimulator is also triggered at the frequency of the alternating electric current. Thereto, the main current's signal is fed into an electronic circuit that delivers a short pulse each time the main voltage exceeds a certain value, resulting in a pulse sequence with 20 ms between subsequent pulses. Adequate selection (by division) of these pulses results in a pulse train that is fed into the

Table 1. Causes of motion of the object and changes in background in coronary angiography.

Evitable
    Table motion ('panning')
    Patient motion
    Respiration
    Automatic brightness control
Inevitable
    Cardiac contractions

---

external input of the stimulator leading to intervals that are multiples of 40 ms. Optical insulation units prevent the occurrence of leakage currents in accordance with international safety standards.

Catheterization procedure

One dog and ten patients were studied. The dog was anaesthetized with methadon (Symoron®) and dehydrobenzoperidol (Droperidol®) and artificially ventilated with oxygen and nitrous oxide. A pacing catheter was advanced through a femoral vein to the right atrium. Coronary injections were performed through a size 7 left Judkins catheter using 8 ml metrizoate (Isopaque coronar®) with a power injector at a flowrate of 4 ml/s. The heart was stimulated just above its own frequency and at a considerably higher rate. Furthermore, a measurement was performed 20 s after intracoronary injection of 0,5 mg of nitroglycerin with the heartrate just above its own frequency.

Ten patients, scheduled for left side percutaneous transluminal coronary angioplasty (PTCA) were studied, all but one having a single stenosis in the left anterior descending artery and a normal circumflex artery. One patient had two stenoses, one in the left anterior descending artery and one in a large diagonal branch; this patient is counted twice as patient 10a and 10b (Tables 3 and 4). In the first four patients the contrast medium was injected manually into the left main stem through a size 9 guiding catheter for PTCA. Thereafter, this policy was changed in two ways. Contrast was injected with a power injector with a flowrate of 4 ml/s and a volume of 8 ml in order to standardize the injection technique. Furthermore, an especially for this purpose introduced size 8 Judkins catheter was used; it had been observed that a size 9 catheter could occlude the left main stem as was seen in two patients (not included in this paper) blocking contrast run-off. Natrium-meglumine ioxaglate (Hexabrix®) was used as contrast medium.

The cineangiographic investigations were performed before as well as after the PTCA procedure. Heart rate was controlled by right atrial stimulation with a frequency slightly above the basic rhythm and synchronized together with the cinepulse rate to the main's frequency, as pointed out before. In most patients the same rate could be used in the cineruns before and after the PTCA procedure. In 4 patients the rate after the PTCA procedure had to be set slightly higher. At the start of the dilatation procedure nifedipine (Adalat®) was routinely administered sublingually. In some patients intracoronary nitroglycerine was given in case of a difficult crossing of the narrowing with the dilatation catheter. The cinerun after the PTCA procedure was always performed at least 10 minutes following the last contrast administration, obviating the vascular dilating effect of the contrast medium.

In all but one case the left anterior oblique projection (usually 50–60°) was chosen with a slight cranial angulation (about 20°). In one case a 30° right anterior oblique projection was chosen. The angiographic projections before and after PTCA were always identical. The angiographic investigations were performed with Siemens X-ray equipment using a focal spot size of 0.6 mm at about 70 KVp and a tube current of about 100 mA. The automatic brightness control was turned off. During the cinerun the ECG and the cinepulse signal were recorded. The Kodak film (2496 RAR) was developed with a gradient of about 1.65. The films used for subtraction were obtained during the routine procedure with informed consent of the patient.

Subtraction procedure

In the laboratory, the film was analyzed in an off-line mode. It was placed on a spooler, equipped with a microprocessor controlled drivemotor. Following identification of the first frame, the desired frame number was touched in and the film automatically advanced to this particular frame. The video signals, obtained with a Vidicon high resolution camera with locked automatic light compensation, were connected to an image analysis system (VICOM). After analog-to-digital conversion, comparable noncontrast and contrast images were stored into memories I and II, respectively, with a spatial resolution of 512 × 512 pixels and 128 gray levels. Subtraction was performed and the results stored in memory III. For better visual inspection, the gray levels of the resulting images were amplified by a factor 4 or 8. After digital-to-analog conversion, the results could be displayed on a video monitor and stored on a video disk. Regions of interest were placed in subtracted images in which the mean pixel grayness was computed. For this study only end-diastolic frames were analyzed. The regions of interest were positioned over the left main stem, over a myocardial area of about 12 × 16 pixels in the region supplied by the narrowed and subsequently dilated vessel, the socalled, schemic area and over an area supplied by the normal circumflex actery, the control area. In a number of cases regions of interest were also placed over the coronary sinus. With respect to the coronary sinus it is important to realize that this vessel, contrary to the left main stem, is usually projected over the myocardium so that interpretation of grayness-versus-time curves from the coronary sinus will be hampered by myocardial filling.

Analysis of grayness-time curves

Mean pixel grayness values in the selected regions of interest for each end-diastolic frame were determined. From the heart rate the time interval was calculated. The moment of injection of contrast medium could be assessed from the film with the frame-counter. From the curves the appearance time, the build-up time, the maximal concentration time and – where possible – the mean circulation time and the recirculation time were calculated. Appearance time was defined as the period of time at which the curve reached 5% of its maximal value after the start of contrast medium injection. The maximal concentration time was defined as the time period where the curve reached its maximum after the start of contrast medium injection. The build-up time is the difference between the maximal concentration time and the appearance time. Mean circulation time was defined according to classical mathematics of dilution curves as indicated by Zierler (2). To calculate this value it is necessary to separate the first circulation peak from the recirculation. In other words, there must be a sufficiently long descending limb to determine a linear regression between time and the logarithmic value of the grayness. If that is the case the recirculation time could be determined as well. It is important to realize that all these variables are related to flow, but also to vascular volume between injection site and measuring site. Zierler stated the fundamental fact that flow equals volume divided by mean circulation time. Thus, mean circulation time is a parameter that may be compared from one situation to another only if vascular volume is constant.

Statistical analysis was performed by calculating mean and standard deviation of the results obtained during certain conditions. It is questionable whether the observation in areas supplied by stenosed vessels may be considered as samples taken from a normally distributed population. Therefore statistical analysis aimed at the comparison of certain conditions was performed with the Wilcoxon rank test for paired observations.

Results

Results in the dog

Figure 1 shows a total of nine curves obtained in the dog with regions of interest over the left stem (figures in left column), over the myocardium supplied by the left anterior descending artery (center column) and over the coronary sinus (right column), respectively. Measurements were also performed over a part of the myocardium supplied by the circumflex artery (not shown). The curves were obtained from cinefilms taken during a driven heart rate of 115 beats/min (figures in top row), a rate of 187 beats/min (center row) and again at a rate of 115 beats/min, but now 20 seconds after an intracoronary injection of 0.5 mg nitroglycerin (bottom row). In Table 2 the appearance time, the maximal concentration time, the build-up time and, where possible, the mean circulation time and the recirculation time have been summarized for these three conditions. The difference in mean circulation time between the myocardial area supplied by the left anterior descending artery and the left main stem decreases with increased oxygen demand imposed by the high heart rate from 4.9 s to 2.2 s. Interpretation of the results obtained after the administration of nitroglycerin is more difficult because it is probable that nitroglycerin influences vascular volume between injection and measuring site to a considerable degree. If vascular volume increased by the nitroglycerin administration, flow increases more than the decrease in the difference in mean circulation time between left anterior descending artery and the left main stem regions (from 4.9 to 3.3 s) suggests.

The curves over the coronary sinus are not suitable for straightforward analysis because of considerable baseline offset caused by filling of the overprojected myocardium supplied by the circumflex artery. The appearance time is subjectively defined at the sudden bend in the curve.

Table 2. Circulation times in a dog.

		t_{app}	t_{max}	t_{bu}	t	t_{rec}
	LMC	–	1.7	1.7	2.3	4.5
f = 115	LAD	1.2	6.3	5.1	7.2	9.2
	RCX	0.8	6.5	5.7	–	–
	CS	4.8	8.1	3.3	–	–
	LMC	–	2.0	2.0	2.9	5.4
f = 187	LAD	0.5	4.8	4.3	5.1	8.7
	RCX	2.0	7.1	5.1	–	–
	CS	4.3	8.0	3.7	–	–
f = 115+						
NITRO	LMC	–	1.9	1.9	3.7	6.1
	LAD	1.1	7.0	5.9	7.0	9.8
	RCX	1.9	7.3	5.4	–	–
	CS	4.0	9.2	5.2	–	–

Abbreviations:
f = heart rate, LMC = left main coronary artery, LAD = left anterior descending artery, RCX = circumflex artery, Cs = coronary sinus, t_{app} = appearance time, t_{max} = maximal circulation time, t_{bu} = build-up time, t = mean circulation time and t_{rec} = recirculation time. Circulation times are indicated in seconds.

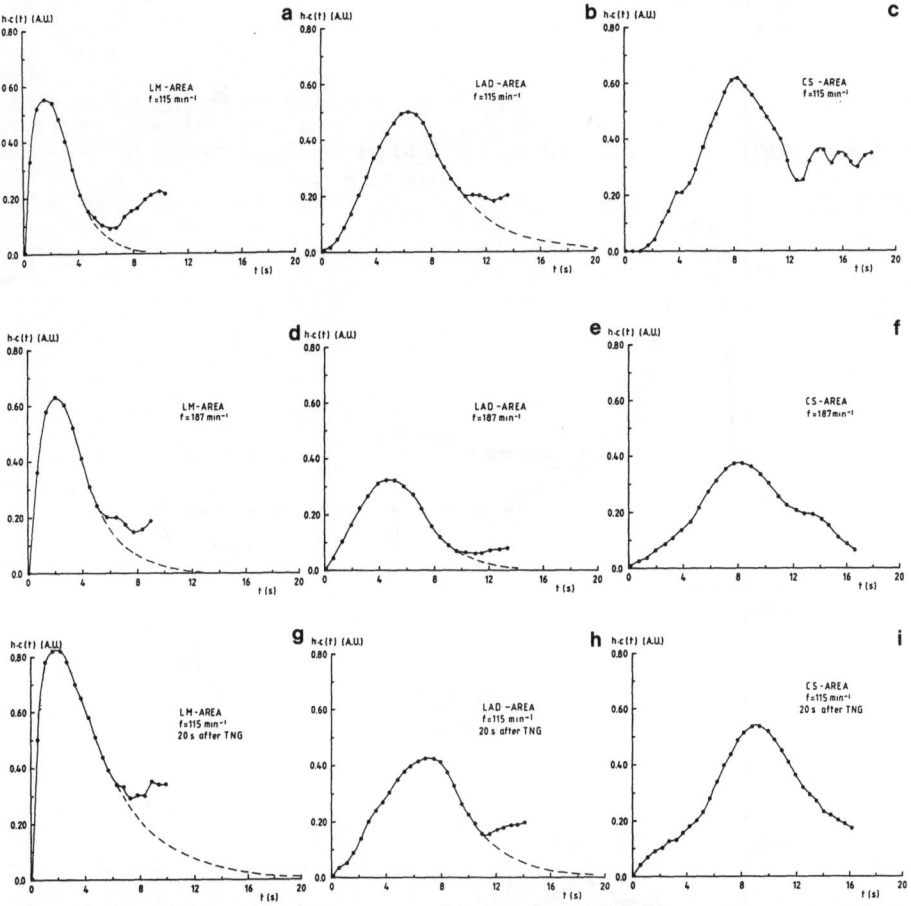

Figure 1. Grayness-time curves in a dog. Along the vertical axis grayness is plotted as the product of wall thickness (h) and iodine concentration (c(t)) in arbitrary units. Along the horizontal axis time (t) is plotted in seconds. Each dot represents an end-diastolic frame analyzed. The figures in the left column show the results obtained over the left main stem. The center vertical column those over the myocardium supplied by the left anterior descending artery, whereas the right column shows three evaluations of the coronary sinus area. The upper row measurements were obtained at a heart rate of 115 beats/min, the center row at a heart rate of 187/min and the lower row again at 115 beats/min, but now about 20 seconds after an intracoronary injection of 0.5 mg nitroglycerin (TNG). The broken lines in the left and middle column indicate the separation of the first circulation from the recirculation, achieved by replotting the extrapolated part of the curve from semilogarithmic graph paper. The calculated time parameters are presented in Table 2 and discussed in the text.

Results in the patients

Figure 2 shows a good example of the curves obtained over the left main stem (upper figure) and over a myocardial region supplied by the left anterior descending artery (lower figure) in a 63 year old woman before (dots) and after (squares)

60

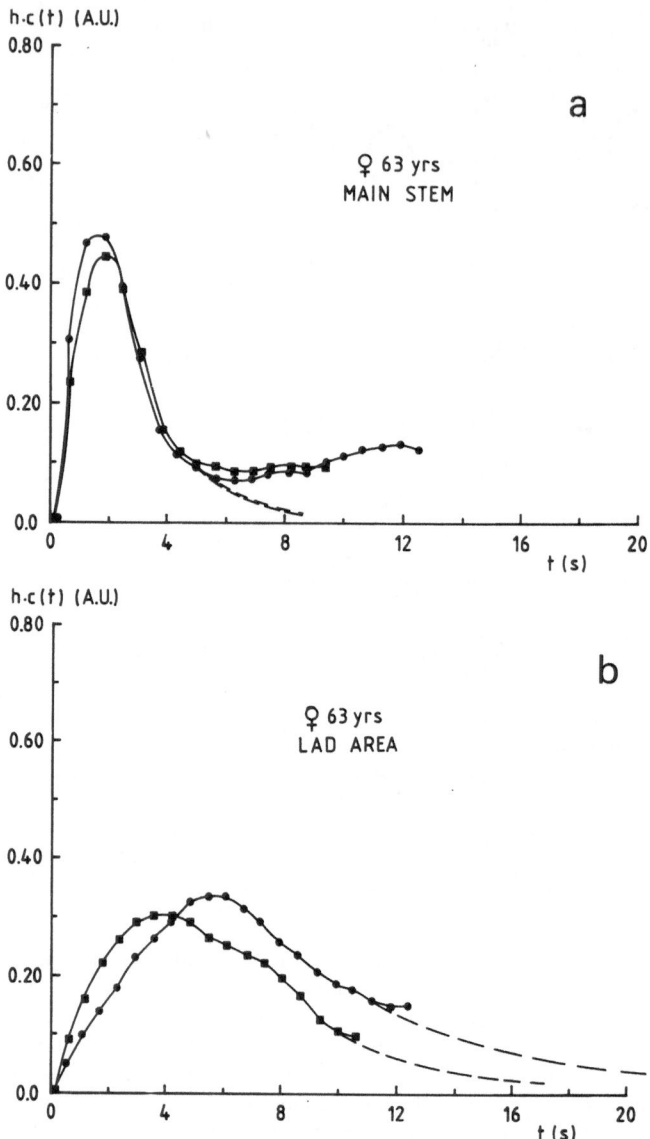

Figure 2. Grayness-time curves in a patient. In a 63 year old lady grayness-time curves were obtained over the left main stem (upper panel) and over the myocardium supplied by the left anterior descending artery (lower panel) before PTCA (dots) and after PTCA (squares). The parameters along the axes and the symbols used are the same as those of Figure 1. The calculated time parameters are included in Tables 3 and 4 under patient number 1. For further details see text.

PTCA. The descending limb has been extrapolated in a manner known from dye dilution theory. The mean circulation time in the left main stem region before and after PTCA equals 1.4 and 1.8 s, respectively. Over the myocardium supplied by the left anterior descending artery circulation times of 6.4 and 5.3 s are found, respectively. The difference in circulation times over the myocardium and over the left main stem decreases from 5.0 s before PTCA to 3.5 s after PTCA, suggesting an amelioration of local perfusion by more than 40%, provided vascular volume between injection and measuring site remained unchanged.

The results in the patients are summarized in Table 3.

Appearance time

The appearance time in the left main stem is always zero because the start of the contrast injection (with the catheter filled) was observed by the appearance of contrast in the left main stem. Furthermore, contrast concentration increased so rapidly that it was impossible to determine the moment in time that 5% of peak concentration was reached. Therefore, the maximal concentration time equals the build-up time. The appearance time in the control area before and after PTCA equaled 0.7 ± 0.4 s (mean $\pm$ standard deviation) and 0.8 ± 0.5 s, respectively. The appearance time in the 'ischemic' area after successful PTCA (0.7 ± 0.5 s) does not differ significantly from these values. Before PTCA, the appearance time in the 'ischemic' area was 1.1 ± 0.5 s, not differing significantly from the other observations.

Maximal concentration time

In the control area values of 4.6 ± 0.9 s and 4.4 ± 0.8 s were found before and after PTCA, respectively. Taking the control area values observed before and after PTCA together, maximal concentration time values of 4.5 ± 0.9 s were found. In the 'ischemic' area a significantly ($p < .01$) prolonged maximal concentration time (7.1 ± 1.8 s) was encountered before PTCA. After the successful procedure a value of 4.4 ± 0.8 s was found, which does not differ significantly from the values found in the control area. The differences in maximal concentration times in the left main stem before and after PTCA were not statistically significant.

Build-up time

As could be expected from the fact that build-up time is calculated from maximal concentration time and appearance time the same observations mentioned above hold also for this parameter. In the control area build-up time values of 3.9 ± 1.0 and 3.7 ± 0.9 s were found before and after PTCA, respectively; these values do not differ significantly from those found in the 'ischemic' area after successful dilatation of the supplying vessel: 3.8 ± 0.7 s. On the other hand, the values found for the 'ischemic' area before the procedure were again significantly higher: 6.0 ± 2.2 s ($p < .1$).

As can be seen from Table 3 it was not possible to calculate the mean circulation time in a number of cases. The best discrimination between the curves obtained before and after PTCA is given by the maximal concentration time. As

62

Table 3. Circulation times in patients.

f			Left main		'Ischemic' area				Control area			
			t_{bu}	t	t_{ap}	t_{max}	t_{bu}	t	t_{ap}	t_{max}	t_{bu}	t
1	pre	95	1.9	1.4	1.4	6.4	5.0	6.4	1.0	3.8	2.8	4.0
	post	95	1.9	1.8	1.6	5.8	4.2	5.3	0.8	5.0	4.2	5.1
2	pre	75	2.4	2.1	1.0	8.0	7.0	–	0.4	5.6	5.2	5.6
	post	83	1.8	2.1	0.6	5.5	4.9	4.7	0.5	6.2	5.7	7.0
3	pre	75	1.3	1.0	0.3	10.0	9.7	–	0.3	4.8	4.5	6.1
	post	83	1.1	1.0	0.3	5.4	5.1	–	0.3	4.0	3.7	5.1
4	pre	75	2.4	1.8	2.0	5.6	3.6	7.0	1.0	4.0	3.0	4.7
	post	83	1.8	1.5	0.2	3.8	3.6	3.3	1.5	3.8	2.3	3.8
5	pre	71	1.7	–	1.2	7.7	6.5	–	1.1	4.3	3.2	–
	post	71	2.6	–	1.3	4.3	3.0	–	1.8	5.1	3.3	–
6	pre	100	1.8	–	0.6	6.0	5.4	–	0.3	3.6	3.3	–
	post	100	1.2	–	0.4	3.6	3.2	–	0.6	4.2	3.6	–
7	pre	79	3.6	3.3	0.8	5.8	5.0	6.4	0.3	4.3	4.0	5.2
	post	79	2.7	3.6	0.8	4.9	4.1	4.1	0.6	4.9	4.3	5.8
8	pre	75	3.2	2.6	1.6	7.6	6.0	–	1.3	4.0	2.7	–
	post	88	2.7	2.3	1.0	4.1	3.1	7.5	1.4	4.1	2.7	4.4
9	pre	83	1.1	1.3	0.4	10.2	9.8	–	0.8	4.0	3.2	–
	post	83	1.1	0.9	0.3	3.2	2.9	–	0.3	3.2	2.9	–
10a	pre	88	2.0	1.3	1.2	4.8	3.6	5.4	0.8	6.1	5.3	5.2
	post	88	1.4	1.3	0.4	4.1	3.7	–	0.4	4.1	3.7	–
10b	pre	88	2.0	1.3	1.2	5.4	4.2	5.0	0.8	6.1	5.3	5.2
	post	88	1.4	1.3	0.4	4.1	3.7	–	0.4	4.1	3.7	–
mean pre			2.1±0.8		1.1±0.5	7.1±1.8	6.0±2.2		0.7±0.4	4.6±0.9	3.9±1.0	
mean post			1.8±0.6		0.7±0.5	4.4±0.8	3.8±0.7		0.8±0.5	4.4±0.8	3.7±0.9	
pre + post			2.0±0.7			p<.01	p<.1		0.8±0.4	4.5±0.9	3.8±1.0	

Abbreviations:
pre = before PTCA, post = after PTCA. All other abbreviations are the same as in Table 2.

suggested by Bürsch *et al.* the difference in build-up time over a vascular bed is related to flow (3, 4). Therefore, we calculated the differences of the build-up times for the 'ischemic' area and for the left main stem, as well as the differences for the control areas and the left main stem before and after PTCA. The results are presented in Table 4. If all control area values are taken together the mean and standard deviation equals 1.8 ± 1.2 s; therefore, a measurement exceding the value of $1.8 + (2 \times 1.2) = 4,2$ s is pathological. In the pre-PTCA 'ischemic' observations 4 patients have values above 4.2 s, indicated with an asterix. After PTCA all values are within normal limits.

Table 4. Differences in build-up times between myocardium and left main stem in patients

	'Ischemic' area		Control area	
	pre	post	pre	post
1	$5.0 - 1.9 = 3.1$	$4.2 - 1.9 = 2.3$	$2.8 - 1.9 = 0.9$	$4.2 - 1.9 = 2.3$
2	$7.0 - 2.4 = 4.6^*$	$4.9 - 1.8 = 3.1$	$5.2 - 2.4 = 2.8$	$5.7 - 1.8 = 3.9$
3	$9.7 - 1.3 = 8.4^*$	$5.1 - 1.1 = 4.0$	$4.5 - 2.4 = 2.1$	$3.7 - 1.1 = 2.6$
4	$3.6 - 2.4 = 1.2$	$3.6 - 1.8 = 1.8$	$3.0 - 2.4 = 0.6$	$2.3 - 1.8 = 0.5$
5	$6.5 - 1.7 = 4.8^*$	$3.0 - 2.6 = 0.4$	$3.2 - 1.7 = 1.5$	$3.3 - 2.6 = 0.7$
6	$5.4 - 1.8 = 3.6$	$3.2 - 1.2 = 2.0$	$3.3 - 1.8 = 1.5$	$3.6 - 1.2 = 2.4$
7	$5.0 - 3.6 = 1.4$	$4.1 - 2.7 = 1.4$	$4.0 - 3.6 = 0.4$	$4.3 - 1.2 = 3.1$
8	$6.0 - 3.2 = 2.8$	$3.1 - 2.7 = 0.4$	$2.7 - 3.2 = -0.5$	$2.7 - 2.7 = 0$
9	$9.8 - 1.1 = 8.7^*$	$2.9 - 1.1 = 1.8$	$3.2 - 1.1 = 2.2$	$2.9 - 1.1 = 1.8$
10a	$3.6 - 2.0 = 1.6$	$3.7 - 1.4 = 2.3$	$5.3 - 2.0 = 3.3$	$3.7 - 1.4 = 2.3$
10b	$4.2 - 2.0 = 2.2$	$3.7 - 1.4 = 2.3$	$5.3 - 2.0 = 3.3$	$3.7 - 1.4 = 2.3$
mean	3.9 ± 2.6	2.0 ± 1.1	1.7 ± 1.2	2.0 ± 1.2
			1.8 ± 1.2	

Abbreviations:
same as for Tables 2 and 3.
* abnormal values (see text)

Discussion

Sandor *et al.* studied myocardial contrast accumulation following the administration of contrast material into the left main stem in two patients (5). They found that only an increase in contrast concentration could be observed (observation period 8 heart beats). Therefore, we decided to take cineruns of about 20 seconds duration, the first three seconds being reserved for the acquisition of noncontrast images. Als and coworkers (6) suggested that the contrast medium not only passes through the capillaries, but also invades the surrounding perivascular space so that the passage of the contrast cannot simply be considered as the normal dye washin and washout. In a number of patients we could observe a grayness-time curve with a shape not different from a typical dye dilution curve. Plotted on semilogarithmic paper the descending limb appeared to be a straight line for a considerable portion. In a number of patients it was impossible to perform this procedure because of a very slowly descending limb. In all patients, however, there was a top followed by a descending limb. It is uncertain whether the observed differences in washout behavior are based on technical difficulties or on different contrast dynamics in certain patients.

The grayness-time curves obtained in the way described above are not calibrated in terms of iodine concentration. Therefore no attention was paid to the absolute amplitude of the curves. Most time parameters are very sensitive to errors due to irregularities in the curves. The parameter that does not have this disadvantage, mean circulation time however, is not only influenced by flow, but also by vascular volume between injection site and measuring site. This implies the risk of drawing incorrect conclusions about flow if, in between, pharmacological interventions have been applied that possibly change vascular tone. It is therefore important to emphasize the fact that we waited for about 10 minutes after the end of the dilatation procedure to perform the post-PTCA cinerun. It is reassuring that all time parameters derived from curves obtained over the control region before and after PTCA do not differ significantly, suggesting that the effects of medication have already subsided at the time the post-PTCA film was taken. This gives more weight to the significant differences observed in the films over the 'ischemic' area before and after the dilatation.

This study was undertaken to perform a preliminary test of the method described. PTCA patients were chosen for the study because in at least a part of this population changes between the measuring results before and after the dilatation were to be expected. To that end the study can be considered successful: in a number of patients delayed filling of the myocardium supplied by the stenosed vessel was demonstrated, and furthermore restoration of filling to values within normal limits after the procedure could also be proven.

In our opinion this method holds great promises for the future. It will be possible to develop a system with which only one cinepulse can be delivered at each end-diastolic moment, observing the rules of the concept of apparent cardiac arrest. This cinepulse can be given with a higher dose than normal reducing quantum mottle, because the other pulses during the cardiac cycle can be spared. The image can be transferred directly to a video disk obviating the cine-video conversion with inherent losses. By increasing right atrial driving rate, more insight into flow reserve can be acquired.

Conclusions

From this study we may draw the following conclusions:
1. with careful triggering, observing the rules of the socalled apparent cardiac arrest principle, using digital videosubtraction grayness-time curves of good quality can be obtained.
2. In the majority of the patients myocardial grayness-time curves, obtained after injection of contrast material, obey the laws of dye dilution curves.
3. In a number of patients the washout of contrast material cannot be treated in a manner known from dye dilution practice, either caused by divergent contrast dynamics or by technical imperfections.
4. Peak concentration of contrast in the myocardium occurs 4.5 ± 0.9 seconds after the start of the injection into the left main stem with a build-up time of 3.8 ± 1.0 seconds.

5.   In a number of PTCA patients maximal concentration time and build-up time are prolonged and after a successful dilatation restored to normal.

6.   A number of patients in whom a PTCA procedure was indicated had, during a (nearly) normal heart rate and consequently normal oxygen demand, normal time parameters although they suffered from disabling angina.

Acknowledgements

The authors wish to express their gratitude to Ans Maandag for her secretarial assistance. This study was supported by the Interuniversity Cardiology Institute (ICI), Utrecht and by The Netherlands Organization for the Advancement of Pure Research (ZWO), The Hague.

References

1. Werf T van der, Heethaar RM, Stegehuis H, Meijler FL: The concept of apparent cardiac arrest as a prerequisite for coronary digital subtraction angiography. JACC 4, 1984: 239–244.
2. Zierler KL: Circulation times and the theory of indicator-dilution methods for determining blood flow and volume. In: Handbook of Physiology, section 2: Circulation 1: American Physological Society, Washington DC 1962: 585–615.
3. Bürsch JH: Use of digitized functional angiography to evaluate arterial blood flow. Cardiovasc Intervent Radiol 6, 1983: 303–310.
4. Bürsch JH, Hahne H-J, Brennecke R, Heintzen PH: Digitale Funktionsangiographie: Eine Methode zur arteriellen Durchblutungsmessung. Radiologe 23, 1983: 202–207.
5. Sandor T, Paulin S, Sridhar B: Densitometric evaluation of myocardial contrast accumulation. In: Optical Instrumentation in Medicine VI. SPIE 127, 1977: 349–352.
6. Als AV, Paulin S, Serrur J, Sandor T: Evaluation of myocardial blush. Abstracts of the 15th International Congress of Radiology. Brussels 1981: 98.

A tomographic approach to intravenous coronary arteriography

Erik L. Ritman and A.A. Bove

Summary

Coronary artery anatomy can be visualized using high speed, volume scanning X-ray CT. A single scan during a bolus injection of contrast medium provides image data for display of all angles of view of the opacified coronary arterial tree. Due to the tomographic nature of volume image data the superposition of contrast filled cardiac chambers, such as would occur in the levophase of an intravenous injection of contrast agent, can be eliminated. Data are presented which support these statements.

The Dynamic Spatial Reconstructor (DSR) was used to scan a life-like radiologic phantom of an adult human thorax in which the left atrial and ventricular chambers and the major epicardial coronary arteries were opacified so as to simulate the levophase of an intravenous injection of contrast agent. A catheter filled with diluted contrast agent and with regions of luminal narrowing (i.e. 'stenoses') was advanced along a tract equivalent to a right ventricular catheterization. Ease of visualization of the catheter 'stenoses' and the accuracy with which they can be measured are presented.

Introduction

Evaluation of pathological alterations in coronary artery anatomy is likely to continue to provide an important index of the jeopardy of the blood supply to the myocardium. The gold standard for evaluation of coronary anatomy is selective coronary arteriography. Although this method involves little risk in capable hands there is sufficient morbidity to restrict its use to symptomatic patients. Generally this examination requires overnight hospitalization. These restrictions curtail use of coronary arteriography as a method for evaluating presymptomatic patients or for repeated follow-up of patients undergoing medical treatment or surgery.

On the assumption that it would be advantageous to perform coronary angiography in just those patients for whom the benefit to risk ratio of selective coronary arteriography is questionable, a method needs to be developed to reduce the risk to the patient. In order of increasing importance these risks are caused by:

a. need for multiple contrast injections to obtain multiple views.
b. entry into arterial system.
c. cannulation of the coronary orifices.

We are developing a computed-tomography based method for overcoming all three causes of risk. To demonstrate the feasibility of the proposed approach we use the Dynamic Spatial Reconstructor (DSR), a fast, volume imaging X-ray scanner which operates on the computed tomography principle (1). Although this current device is not yet optimal for routine clinical use in coronary arteriography, it is well suited to demonstrate the power of the method and the important technical features a clinically useable system should possess.

The important features of the current DSR (2) that are relevant to coronary arteriography can be summarized as follows:

1. *It scans a volume.* This cylindrically shaped volume, which is 21.5 cm in axial height and 21.5 cm in transaxial diameter, is large enough to contain all but the very largest hearts. The entire coronary arterial tree must be scanned if false negative readings, due to inability to visualize all parts of the coronary arterial tree, are to be avoided.

2. *It scans this volume synchronously.* If the volume were to be scanned in time-sequential portions, the resulting image of the entire coronary arterial tree may be an incorrect representation of the tree, even though each section scanned could be accurately imaged.

3. The entire *volume is scanned within a brief aperture time.* The coronary arteries, and the contrast medium within the coronary arteries, move rapidly. Consequently, scan aperture duration should be small relative to the distance the coronary arteries (or contrast agent) move in that period of time. In the slow filling phase of the cardiac cycle a scan aperture of 50 msec would generally be quite satisfactory. This aperture time is achieved in the DSR by using the scan data recorded during three time-sequential electronic scans, each of which is repeated at 16.7 msec intervals.

4. The *timing of the scan aperture can be retrospectively selected* to occur within 16.7 msec of the most desirable phase of the cardiac cycle and can be of any retrospectively selected duration commensurate with the duration of end diastole (or any other phase of the cardiac cycle). This operational flexibility allows for individualized optimization of the trade-off between scan aperture duration (the longer the scan the higher the quality of the reconstructed tomographic images) (3) and the loss of image sharpness due to cardiogenic motion.

5. The *scans can be repeated continuously* for up to 20 seconds. This allows for retrospective selection of those cardiac cycles which show optimal opacification of the epicardial coronary arteries or myocardium.

Demonstration of 3-D coronary arteriography

To illustrate how these capabilities of the DSR enable us to overcome the risks of selective coronary arteriography, we had the Humanoid Company* manufacture a realistic chest phantom. It consists of the rib cage and spinal column of a 175 cm tall, 73.5 kg weight male with chest wall and diaphragm and liver made of 'dry' water, a tissue equivalent material (Figure 1). The thoracic cavity is occupied by an animal's fixed lungs. A porcine heart with the left atrial and ventricular chambers, the aorta and coronary arteries filled with approximately 1:8 diluted contrast agent is suspended in its appropriate anatomic location (Figure 2). A 3 mm diameter tract was left within the phantom so as to provide a path via a brachial entry to the superior vena cava, right atrium, right ventricle and right ventricular outflow tract. This tract permits us to insert a catheter with a 2 mm diameter lumen. We modified the lumen of the catheter with different severity

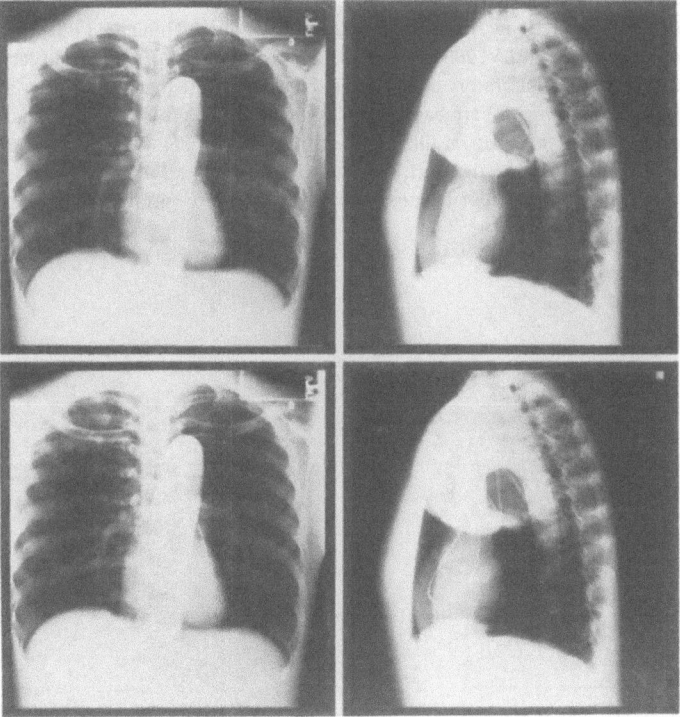

Figure 1. Upper Panels – AP and lateral chest X-rays of the radiological test phantom used in these studies. Note the contrast medium opacifying the left cardiac chambers and intrathoracic aorta. The coronary arteries also contain contrast medium and are best seen in the lateral views. *Lower Panels* – Same views as in upper panel but with a 2 mm diameter catheter in place within the tract (see text).

* Humanoid Systems, 17022 Montanero Street, Carson, CA 90746

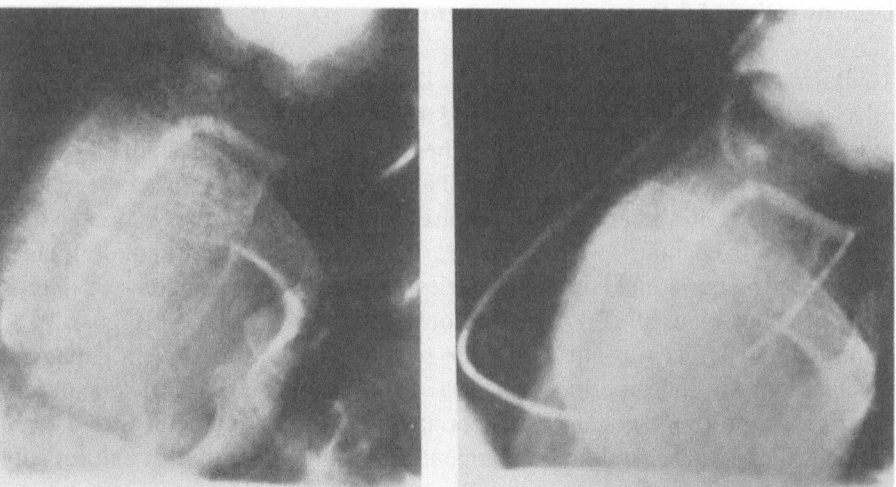

Figure 2. Left Panel – Cineframe, from RAO angle of view, of the Humanoid Phantom. The 35 mm cineframe was obtained at 110 kV, 200 mA and 60 frames/seconds using a General Electric System at the cardiac catheterization laboratory of an affiliated hospital. Note that the coronary arteries (filled with ~1:8 diluted contrast agent) are barely visible when the background is lung and difficult to see when the background is the contrast-filled left ventricular chamber or aortic root. *Right Panel* – Cineframe of phantom after a catheter (1.8 mm lumen filled with 1:2 diluted contrast medium with multiple 50% stenoses of different lengths) was advanced up to intrathoracic tract (see text for details).

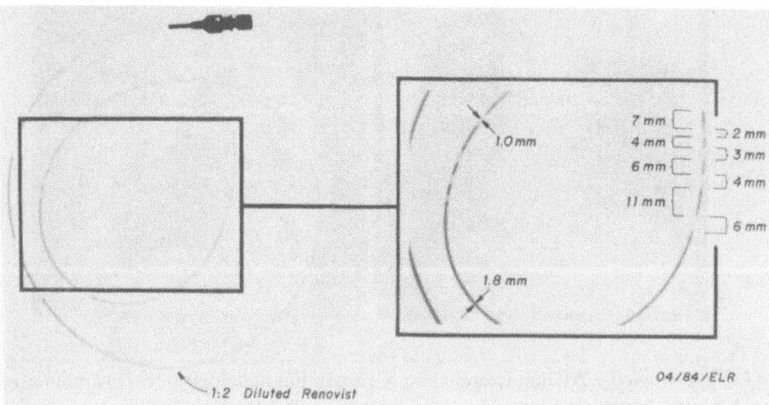

Figure 3. X-ray of 1.8 mm lumen, 2.5 mm outside diameter, plastic catheter filled with 1:2 diluted roentgen contrast medium. The lumen has been 'narrowed' at various locations as indicated. This catheter is advanced up the tract inside the radiologic phantom so as to simulate a stenosed opacified coronary artery.

and length 'stenoses' and filled the lumen with different concentrations of contrast agent. An example of such a catheter is shown in Figure 3. The removable catheter allows for quantitation of stenoses under conditions mimicking either selective or right sided angiography.

The dilution of contrast agent to be expected in the root of the aorta following contrast injection into the right side of the circulation is of the order of 1:8 (Figure 4). This means that a main stem coronary artery of 4 mm diameter results in a change in the X-ray transmission which, through the average adult's chest, is within the range of most X-ray imaging systems and of the current DSR. For a 1 mm diameter vessel, however, this results in a change in the X-ray transmission that is generally not reproducibly detectable with conventional electro-optical X-ray imaging systems.

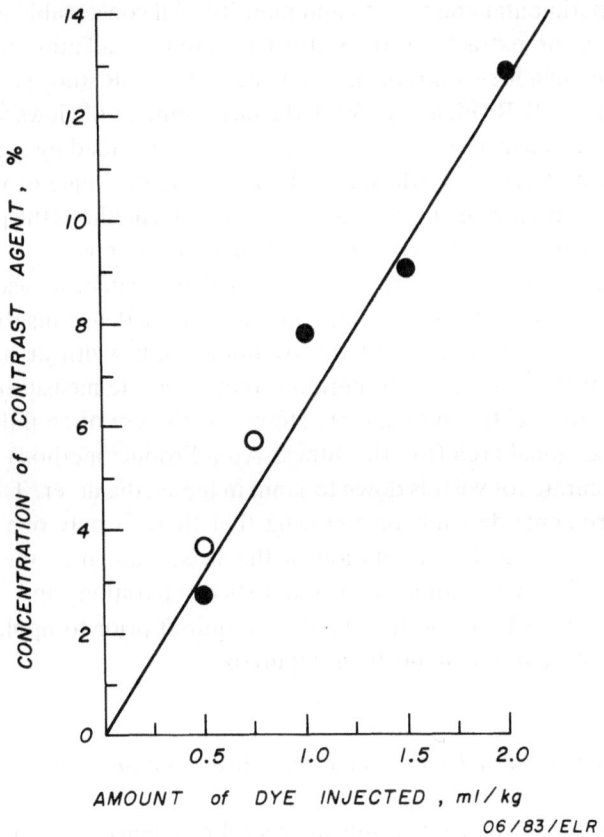

Figure 4. The concentration of diluted contrast agent in root of aorta, following injection of a bolus of contrast agent into the right ventricular outflow tract, increases linearly with volume of the bolus. Concentration was measured by continuous sampling of blood from the root of the aorta of two anesthetized dogs (one dog open circles, other dog closed circles). A concentration of 10% represents 32 mg Iodine/ml of blood.

The following discussion uses data obtained with the radiological phantom to demonstrate how each of the three major risks of coronary arteriography can be diminished by the functional features of the DSR.

(a) Reduction of number of angiographic injections

Because a volume is imaged in a single DSR scan sequence all angles of view can be displayed on completion of the scan. This capability involves computer-generated projection, dissolution, selective dissection (or erasure) and rotation of the volume image prior to its display (4). In brief, this method allows one to compute angiographic views identical to those generated by rotating the patient (and/or the X-ray system) in conventional angiography. This has been demonstrated in experimental animals (5) and man (6). All conceivable angles of view are available at no extra 'cost' of contrast injected or radiation exposure. The X-ray exposure of a 10 second coronary angiographic DSR study is expected to be approximately 10–12 R (Figure 5). With the large number of views available from a single scan, the chances of missing the presence or misreading the severity of a stenosis should be reduced. Moreover, by adjusting the angle of view to match previous studies performed by conventional (or DSR) methods the progression of a lesion can be followed more conveniently and accurately.

The accuracy with which vessel cross-sectional area can be measured using the DSR has been demonstrated (5, 7). The present DSR has insufficient spatial resolution (expressed in terms of the traditional full width at half maximum deflection (FWHM) criterion) to permit direct, accurate measurement of coronary arterial cross-sectional diameter. However, the use of an indirect index of vessel cross-sectional area (the Brightness Area Product method) permits measurements accurate for vessels down to 1 mm in lumen diameter. The accuracy of these measurements depends on knowing that there is only one vessel in the region of interest, on the orientation of the vessel lumen to the scan planes, scanned slice thickness, adjacent scanned slice separation, and scan aperture duration (2). The 3-D image reformatting required prior to application of the method is illustrated schematically in Figure 6.

(b) Replacement of selective coronary with aortic root injection

Injection into the aortic root results in several problems. First of all, it is often difficult to ensure that an adequate amount of contrast medium enters the coronary arteries due to complex streaming within the aortic root and because those very vessels with stenoses and reduced coronary flow will tend to receive a smaller fraction of the injected bolus. A second problem is that if both coronary arteries are well filled the mutual superposition of the right and left coronary

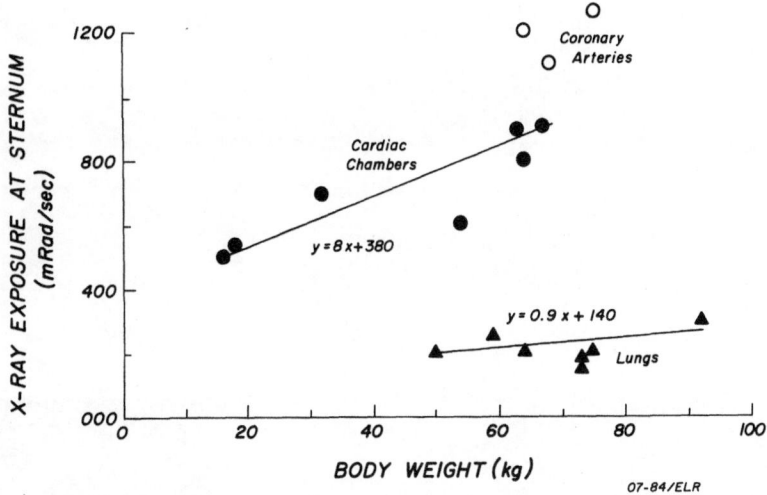

Figure 5. X-ray exposure of patients scanned in the DSR. Exposure was measured with thermolucent detectors (TLDs) on the sternum. Exposures to the thyroid was less than 10% of the sternal exposure and to the eyes and gonads was less than 1% of the sternal exposure. As indicated, X-ray exposures for coronary angiography would generally be expected to be higher than for ventricular angiography. Based on the ventricular angiography studies, the exposure in coronary angiography is expected to be linearly proportional to the weight of the subject.

trees, and of the proximal main stem artery on the contrast filled, aortic root, may result in obscuration of significant lesions. Using the DSR, the latter problem is overcome by the ability to rotate the image of the coronary tree until the superposition is eliminated. The first problem is one of injection technique but also of scanner density resolution. In our hands the roentgen opacity of the coronary arteries, following aortic root injection, is comparable to that achieved by a right-sided injection of contrast agent and presents little advantage. Indeed, left ventricular angiography often results in better opacification of the coronary arteries.

(c) Replacement of intra-arterial with right-sided injection of contrast

Intravenous injection of contrast agent has the advantage of reduced morbidity but creates two major problems. One is that the concentration of contrast agent is reduced by the time the bolus passes through the coronary arteries. The other, more serious problem, is that the pulmonary veins and left cardiac chambers are also filled with contrast agent so that superposition obscures the coronary arterial tree. This superposition is such that often no single angle of view can be found to overcome it completely.

The fundamental power of volume images is that it eliminates superposition.

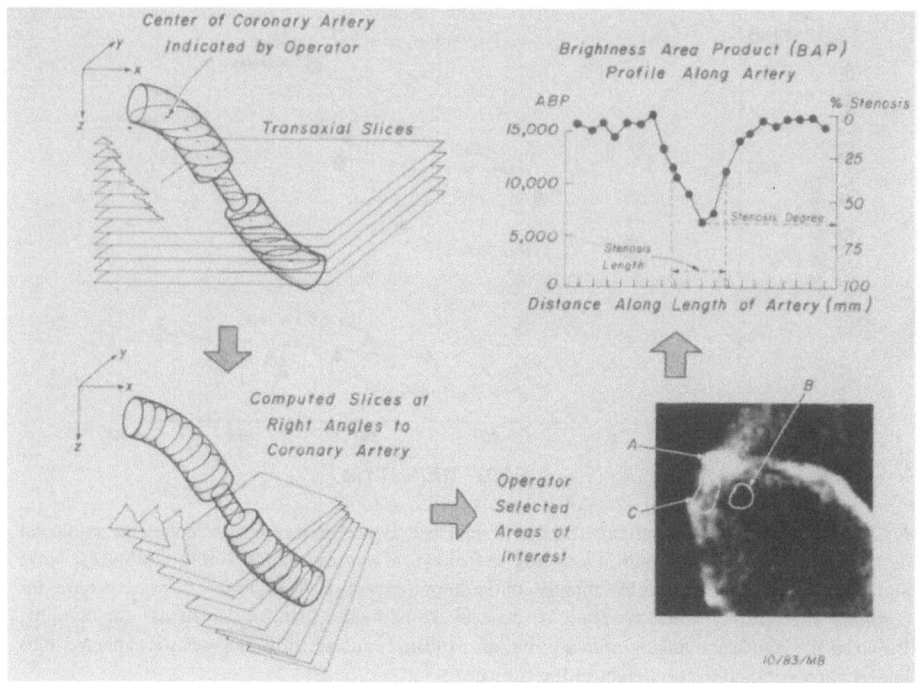

Figure 6. Measurement of percent area stenosis and stenosis length with the DSR. Using the spatial coordinates of vessel cross sections derived from transverse (or sagittal or coronal) sections (upper left panel) from which oblique sections perpendicular to the centerline of the vessel were computed (lower left panel). In each of those oblique sections, samplings of myocardial (C) and blood (B) density (image brightness) were obtained and the integrated brightness within the region of coronary artery cross sections (A) was measured (right lower panel). The calculated integrated brightness due to contrast medium in the stack of cross sections along the vessel lumen was plotted as a function of distance along the centerline of the vessel. Percent area stenosis was obtained from the ratio of prestenotic and minimal stenotic integrated brightness. The stenosis length was measured as the full width at half maximum deflection of the integrated brightness profile (right upper panel). (Reproduced with permission from Block, M. *et al.*: Circulation 70(2), 1984: 209–216.

The principle of removing superposition of an undesirable structure, such as the contrast filled left ventricular chamber, is illustrated in Figure 7. Three-dimensional image processing is necessary to achieve this selective erasure effect. It cannot be achieved by 2-D image processing. Even energy selective imaging would not eliminate the superposition of the chambers on the coronary arteries, or of the coronary arteries upon themselves. The ability to avoid superposition of the coronary arteries upon themselves is illustrated in Figure 8. Although only two angles of view are presented here, many others can be readily generated.

As illustrated in these figures, the general anatomy and presence and location of stenoses of the coronary arterial tree can be obtained for the entire tree with only a single injection and scan. Once the location of a stenosis has been

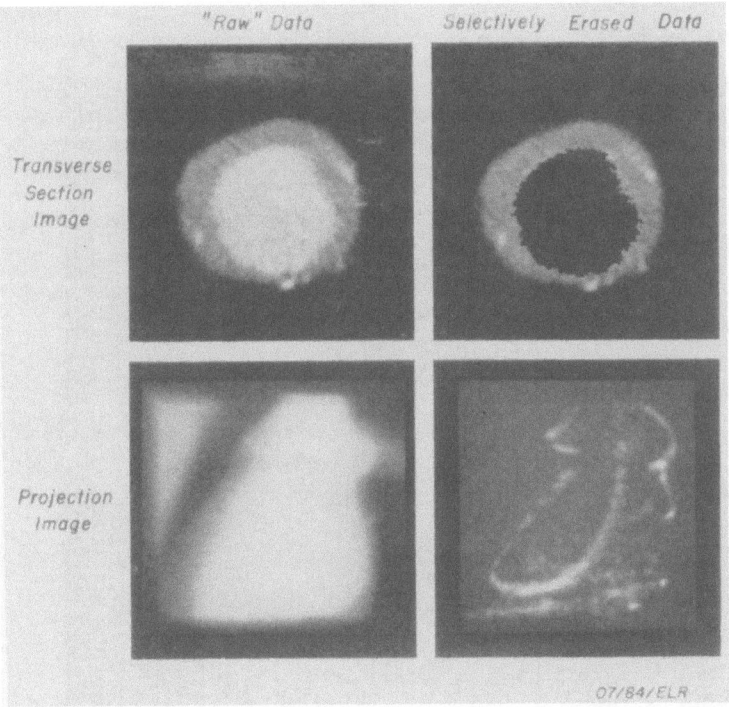

Figure 7. Illustration of selective erasure prior to projection imaging. *Upper Panels* – Images of selected thin cross sections of the left ventricular region of the radiological phantom. In the left panel the contrast agent in the LV chamber shows as a round bright area and the cross section of the contrast filled coronary arteries and catheter show as bright spots in the gray myocardium. Lung shows as dark area around the heart. In the right panel the contrast in the left ventricular chamber and anterior chest wall have been selectively erased – leaving all other structures in the image untouched. *Lower panels* – Projection images of the entire heart. In the left panel all cross section images were left untouched prior to projection. In the right panel all cross sections were processed as in the right upper panel prior to projection. Note that the coronary arteries and catheter are clearly discernable only in the projection of the selectively erased cross sections.

determined then quantitative measurements of the vessel's diameters and stenosis length can be made using the brightness area product method. Such an analysis for the catheter illustrated in Figure 3 is presented in Figure 9.

Conclusion

The desirable technical characteristics for a tomography based coronary artery imaging scanner can be defined once the size of the smallest coronary artery to be visualized and a stenosis in it is defined. For most clinically relevant situations it will probably be sufficient to quantitate a 25–50% stenosis in a 2 mm coronary

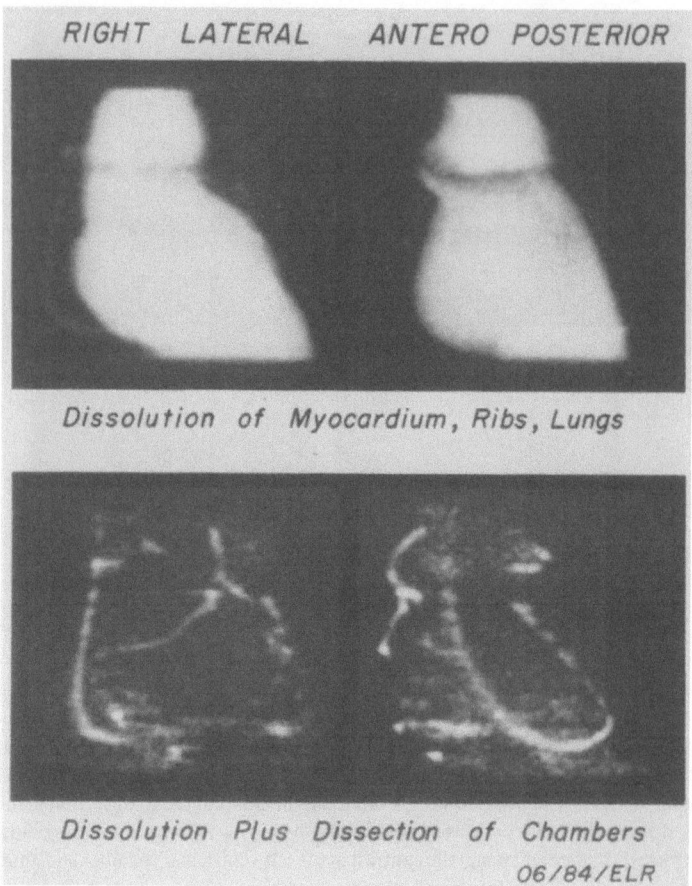

Figure 8. Upper Panels – Projection dissolution images generated from single volume image generated with DSR. Note that despite dissolution of the surrounding tissues (with 'CT' numbers different from iodine containing 'blood') visualization of contrast filled catheter lumen or coronary arteries remains poor when these are superimposed on the iodine containing chambers. *Lower Panels* – The projection dissolution images have been processed by operator 'erasure' of the cardiac chambers and aortic root which are clearly defined in the original images of the transverse slices making up the volume image. Reprojection after this erasure eliminates the superposition problem completely and allows ready visualization of the coronary arteries and the catheter lumen.

artery opacified following a bolus injection of up to 2 ml/kg roentgen contrast agent into the right ventricular outflow tract. In order to get sufficient photons in the transmitted X-ray beam, so that photon noise is less than half the deflection in the transmitted beam due to the contrast agent in the 2 mm coronary artery, we must use ECG-gated reconstruction. Our experience is that about four sequential diastoles should be scanned with an aperture time of approximately 0.12 seconds in each cycle. At normal heart rates spanning the four diastoles (i.e., three cardiac cycles), the DSR would rotate approximately 180° in the 2 seconds. Under these

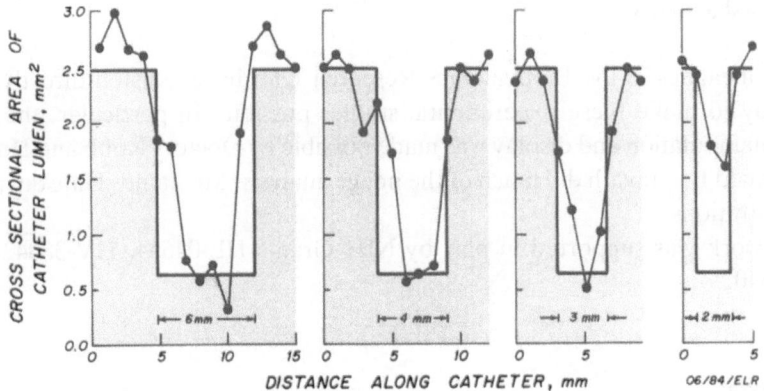

Figure 9. Comparison of the 1.8 mm lumen diameter catheter cross-sectional areas measured form DSR images and the known diameters. These data illustrate that the basic principle of contiguous thin slices, can be used to measure stenoses under conditions closely resembling a coronary arteriogram in an adult human. These scan data were obtained with the stenosed catheter lumen at right angles to the transaxial scan plane, the most challenging circumstance for tomographic imaging.

conditions the scan information from all cameras is spread fairly evenly around 360°, thereby minimizing reconstruction artifacts and providing sufficient numbers of angles of view for achieving the signal-to-noise ratio required for accurate visualization and measurement of the coronary arteries.

Gated adding will generally also be necessary so that most of the bolus of contrast agent passes each point along the epicardial coronary arteries during the composite scan. In this way, the average concentration of the contrast agent is approximately the same for all coronary arteries. This condition is necessary for absolute measurement of the coronary artery cross-sectional area.

In order to achieve the efficiency of conversion of X-ray photons to detected photo electrons and to achieve the dynamic range of the electronic representation of the X-ray image to a level needed for right sided injection coronary arteriography, we are currently upgrading the current DSR image chains. The important new features of this image chain will be the high efficiency of the objective lens (numerical aperture of 0.48) and a Charge Coupled Device (CCD) TV camera. The CCD TV camera should enable us to achieve our goal because it has a higher dynamic range and has essentially no lag as compared to the image isocon camera tube currently in use in the DSR (8). As the desired coronary artery may be oriented in a plane parallel to the scan plane of the DSR the scanned slice thickness should be no thicker than half the width of the 50% stenosed coronary artery – i.e., ~0.5 mm. This can be achieved with a 512 × 512 element CCD camera.

Acknowledgements

Many colleagues in the Biodynamics Research Unit have assisted directly and indirectly to make these experimental studies possible. In particular, the 3-D image manipulation and display was made possible by Doctors Robb and Harris. Mr. Donald L. Cravath did much of the image analysis. Mr. James Hanson made the illustrations.

This work was supported in part by NIH Grants HL-04664, HV-38042 and RR-02540.

References

1. Ritman EL, Robb RA, Harris LD: Imaging physiological functions. Experience with the Dynamic Spatial Reconstructor. Praeger, New York, 1985.
2. Ritman EL, Kinsey JH, Harris LD, Robb RA: Some imaging requirements for quantification of structure and function of the heart. In: MD Short, DA Pay, S Leeman and RM Harrison (Eds.) Physical Techniques in Cardiological Imaging, Adam Hilger Ltd. Bristol, 1983: 189–198.
3. Behrenbeck T, Kinsey JH, Harris LD, Robb RA, Ritman EL: Three-dimensional spatial, density and temporal resolution of the dynamic spatial reconstructor. J Comput Assist Tomogr 6, 1982: 1138–1147.
4. Harris LD, Robb RA, Yuen TS, Ritman EL: Noninvasive numerical dissection and display of anatomic structure using computerized x-ray tomography. SPIE 152, 1978: 10–18.
5. Block M, Bove AA, Ritman EL: Coronary angiography with the dynamic spatial reconstructor. Circulation 70(2), 1984: 209–216.
6. Bove AA, Block M, Smith HC, Ritman EL: Evaluation of coronary anatomy using high-speed volumetric computed tomographic scanning. Am J Cardiol 55, 1985: 582–584.
7. Block M, Liu Y-H, Harris LD, Robb RA, Ritman EL: Quantitative analysis of a vascular tree model with the dynamic spatial reconstructor. J Comput Assist Tomogr 8, 1984: 390–400.
8. Kinsey JH, Hansen CR, Roessler RW, Rhyner MH, Ritman EL: Technical characteristics of the X-ray video imaging chain of the DSR system. In: PH Heintzen, R Brennecke (Eds.): Digital Imaging in Cardiovascular Radiology. Georg Thieme Verlag Stuttgart, 1983: 41–56.

CT of the heart

Martin J. Lipton, M.D.

Summary

Advances based upon the detector elements instead of X-ray film have greatly increased the power of X-ray imaging. Computed tomography (CT) creates cross-sectional rather than projected images. Recently, high speed CT devices have been developed for cardiovascular studies. The Cine-CT scanner employs a scanning electron beam deflected on an extended tungsten target ring. Fast scans of 50 millisecond exposures at multiple levels can provide information concerning blood flow in vessels and tissues, myocardial wall motion, valve integrity, coronary bypass graft patency and proximal coronary artery anatomy. Cine-CT dynamic scanning can also provide volume imaging with small quantities (0.05–1.5 ml/kg) of contrast medium administered via peripheral vein injections.

Cine-CT provides simultaneous measurements of cardiac dimensions and function and is rapidly becoming a new tool for quantitating myocardial blood flow, cardiac chamber volumes and wall mechanics. The future outlook is very promising for this three-dimensional cine-CT technique with high spatial resolution. High speed CT should provide unique diagnostic information and as the technology continues to improve at a rapid speed, this new imaging modality could be a challenge for angiography.

Introduction

A significant shortcoming of all present imaging methods for diagnosing ischemic heart disease including invasive coronary arteriography, echocardiography and techniques requiring physiological gating similar to nuclear medicine and magnetic resonance is their inability to provide the combination of three-dimensional display and high spatial, density and temporal resolution.

Angiocardiography is the most trusted technique and it has not been replaced despite remarkable advances in the noninvasive imaging fields. Myocardial ischemia is characterized by data analysis of the opacified left ventricle (length, area and volume) and analysis of contours. The advantages of cineangiography include the ability to see the whole chamber (wide field of view) at sampling speeds in excess of 16 frames per second. The movie format is an excellent method of reviewing and quantitating cardiac function. Coronary arteriography depicts vessel contours and enables stenosis to be quantitated. However, coronary arteriography is by no means ideal, apart from its invasive nature. It estimates myocardial blood flow very indirectly and this often late relative to the patient's disease. Computed tomography is now emerging as a technique with the potential for providing improved sensitivity and specificity for diagnosing atherosclerotic coronary artery occlusive disease (11–12). This chapter reviews the arguments supporting this contention and describes the present and future prospects for this new modality.

Electron beam Cine-CT scanner

The problems preventing fast scanning in a conventional body scanner are heat load limitations and the angular momentum of the rotating X-ray tube. The new design replaces the X-ray tube with a magnetically deflected electron beam. The two important advantages are first, that the ultimate scan speed is limited only by the need to obtain a sufficient number of photons in a short time and not by mechanical constraints; and secondly, by scanning one or more of the four target rings it is possible to obtain multiple tomographic sections. Technical details of the Cine-CT scanner which produces a very intense beam of electrons in the range

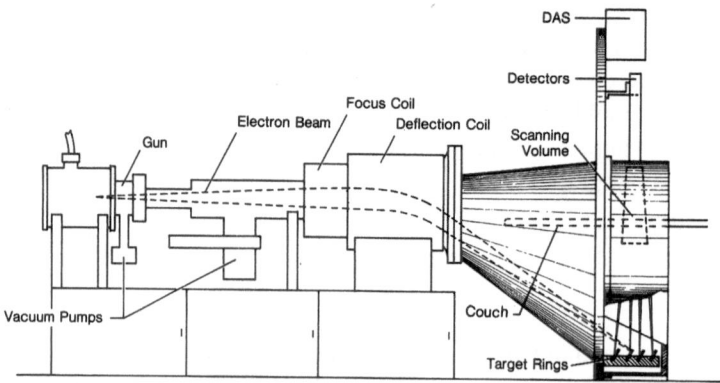

Figure 1. Cross-sectional diagram of the C-100 Cine-CT scanner at the University of California, San Francisco. Deflection of an intense beam of electrons totally replaces the mechanical gantry motion of conventional whole body CT scanners. X-rays are produced with a series of 4 tungsten target rings (180 cm diameter) that cover a semicircle below the patient. This design provides for high scanning speed, multi-plane images, and continuous multilevel scanning with reduced heat load limitations. There are, furthermore, no moving parts.

of 750 mA are available in the literature (12–15). Figure 1 shows the Cine-CT scanner design and illustrates the two rings of solid state detectors, which produce two simultaneous 8mm thick CT scans each time one tungsten target ring is swept by the focused electron beam. The exposure time is currently 50 milliseconds and scans can be obtained at any intervals up to 17/second. The scan reconstruction time is presently 10 seconds. Eight levels can be scanned within 240 milliseconds without the need for table incrementation, although this capability is also available. This scanner has a much wider aperture than any conventional CT or magnetic resonance imager, and in combination with a mobile table, allows patient angulation so that various cardiac tomographic imaging planes, including the short axis view, can be directly imaged.

Cine-CT scanning techniques

A Cine-CT study can be performed as a rapid patient procedure. The first requirement is correct patient positioning and accurate localization of the appropriate anatomical scan levels. The left ventricle is usually examined in the short-axis plane. This is accomplished by swivelling the table 20° so that the feet are moved to the right with the patient lying supine. Additionally, the table is tilted to elevate the head approximately 15 to 25 degrees.

Electrocardiographic monitoring is used so that the scan exposures can be triggered at selected phases of the cardiac cycle. A short intravenous catheter (Deseret Co., 5 cm long plastic needle) is placed in a peripheral vein in either the anticubital fossa or an external jugular vein. Eight localizing scans are then exposed to check the imaging plane and anatomical level and these are reviewed.

Contrast medium administration and scanning options

CT scanning of the heart should be considered as a greatly modified angiographic procedure and therefore, good results are consistently obtained only by standardizing the technique. A flow study is performed first by injecting 0.3 ml per kg body weight of contrast medium (usually 20–35 ml) at a flow rate of 5 ml/second. A flow controlled injector (Mark IV, Medrad Corp.) is used in our laboratory which allows highly reproducible and accurate injection procedures necessary for quantitative analysis of the image data. Fifty millisecond scans are obtained at eight contiguous levels; all are exposed during the same phase of the cardiac cycle, usually systole, on either every heart beat or every second or third beat. Ten scans are usually obtained at each of the 8 levels with one 20–25 ml bolus injection in adults, thus, the ten scans cover 10, 20 or 30 seconds as illustrated in Figure 2a. There is considerable display flexibility as the images are stored and displayed in the digitized format.

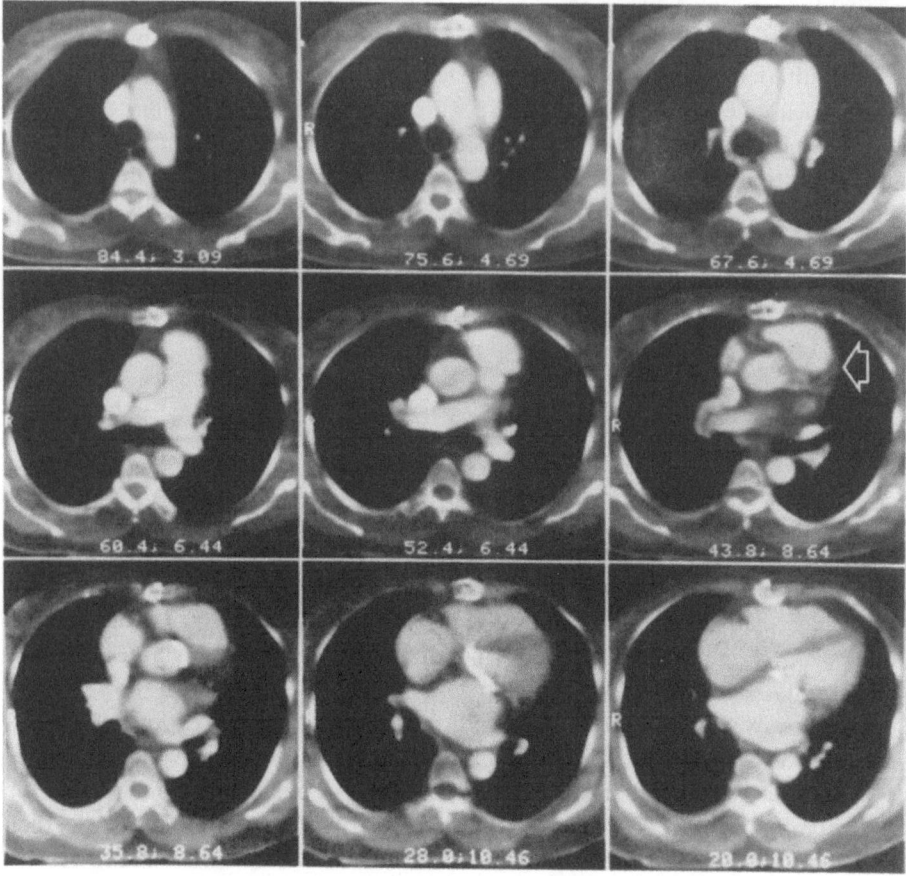

Figure 2a. Illustration of a collection of 9 contiguous 8 mm thick scans in a patient with valve prosthesis in the mitral and aortic areas. These scans were selected from a dynamic CT flow study at times when both right and left sided vascular structures were contrast enhanced. Note how relatively free from motion streak artifacts these images are despite the prosthesis. Also, the resolution is adequate for identifying the proximal right and left main coronary arteries and its proximal main branches on the image at 8.64 seconds (arrow). The left number in the images represents the spacing at 8 mm with a 1–2 mm gap between rings.

Figure 2b is a geometric on-line magnification of the 6th scan (8.64 sec) of the series in Figure 2a showing the proximal coronary arteries. Figure 3 illustrates a typical scan sequence at one of these eight levels from a dynamic flow-mode Cine-CT series. The circulation time is readily obtained from these scans as each scan is registered in time and anatomical site; the sequence is displayed on the monitor with each image. This circulation time is used to direct the next phase of a Cine-CT study, which is the scan acquisition in the movie mode. The flow mode of operation, as will be seen, is also the basis of quantitating vessel, cardiac chamber and tissue blood flow using gamma variate curve analysis.

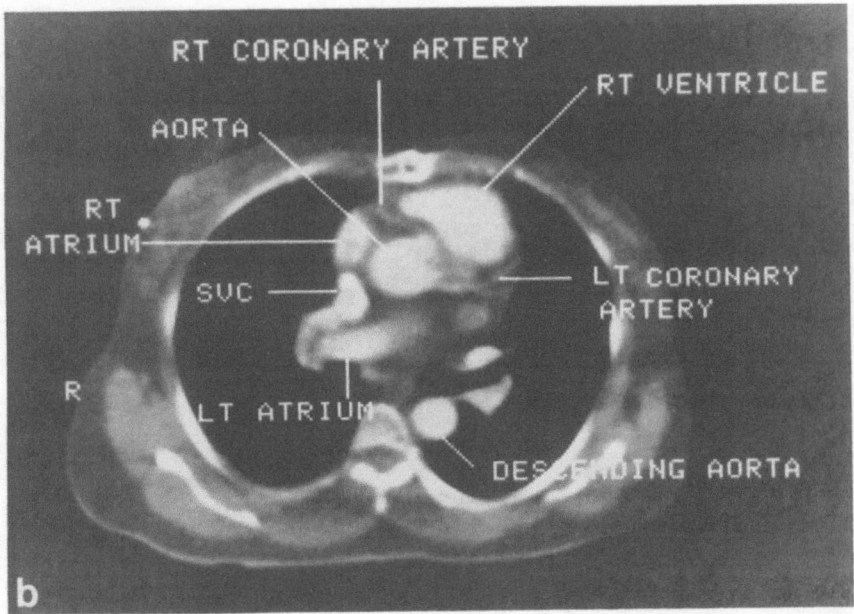

Figure 2b. This image showing the left main, left anterior descending, left circumflex and main right coronary artery is the same image as the one arrowed in Figure 2a. Magnification of this type is possible instantaneously with digitized Cine-CT images.

The movie mode involves a separate injection of contrast medium with high speed scanning at the rate of 17 images/sec at 4, 6 or 8 levels during biventricular contrast enhancement. The scan acquisition period is short, usually between 1 and 4 heart beats. The patient is instructed to hold his or her breath in inspiration during the short scanning period. Cine-CT is easily performed in the immediate post-operative period and also in relatively ill patients, because the procedure is rapid and not demanding on the patient.

The scans acquired at 17/second are ECG-monitored to ensure that end diastole and end systole are obtained for each level. The Cine-CT monitor can display the ECG and indicates the exposure times of each scan on its time base. Usually 8 or 12 levels are scanned to cover the whole ventricular muscle mass and cavities. The CT images are then displayed sequentially as a closed loop movie on the cathode ray oscilloscope for each level, and are also displayed as individual images at various phases of the cardiac cycle. This cinematographic mode demonstrates the changes in cardiac chamber dimensions throughout the cardiac cycle and also enables myocardial wall thickness and thickening to be studied, both qualitatively and quantitatively as shown in Figures 4a and 4b.

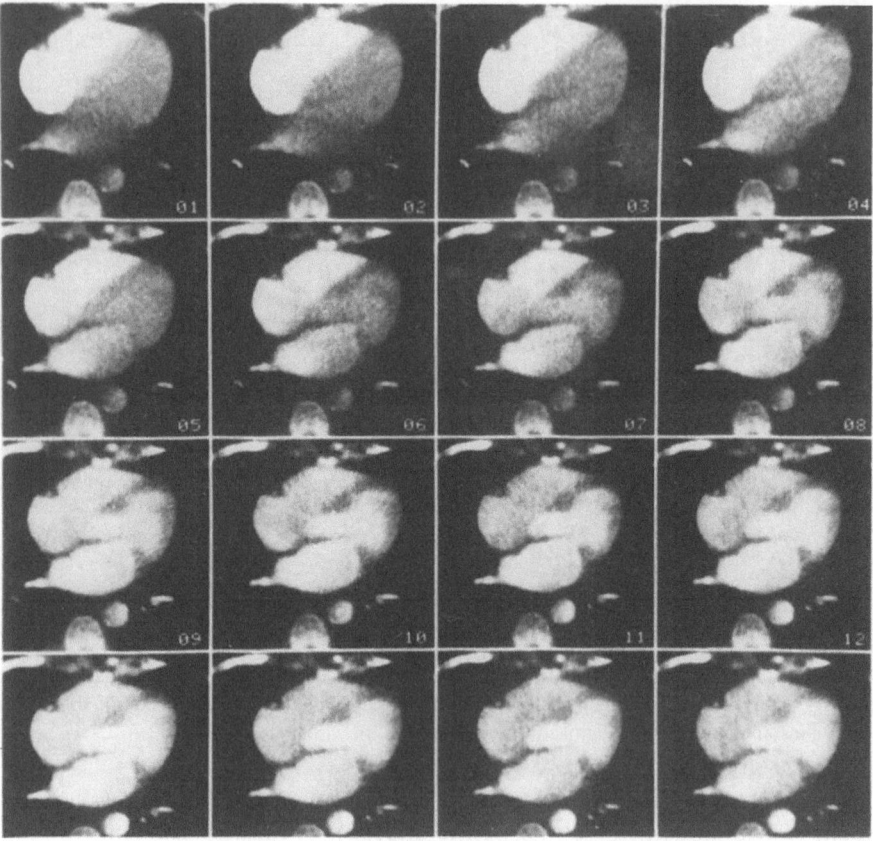

Figure 3. A sequence of 12, Cine-CT 50 millisecond exposures are shown illustrating the dynamic or flow-mode using a 20 ml bolus of Conray 400 injected into a peripheral vein. Contrast enhancement occurs progressively from right atrium to left atrium and finally, the left ventricle and descending thoracic aorta are maximally enhanced. This imaging plane demonstrates the mitral valve. All the CT scans in this sequence were exposed in diastole using ECG triggering. This ensures good slice registration on the matrix for data analysis.

Quantitative Cine-CT methods

Left ventricular volumes

The high spatial and density resolution of CT allows the endocardial as well as the epicardial boundaries to be planimetered using a track ball guided cursor and computer assisted software programs. This technique is illustrated in Figure 5. The areas of the outlined ventricular cavities are printed on the monitor as each level is planimetered, and are recorded on film using a multiformat camera. The end-diastolic and end-systolic volumes, and subsequent global and regional ejec-

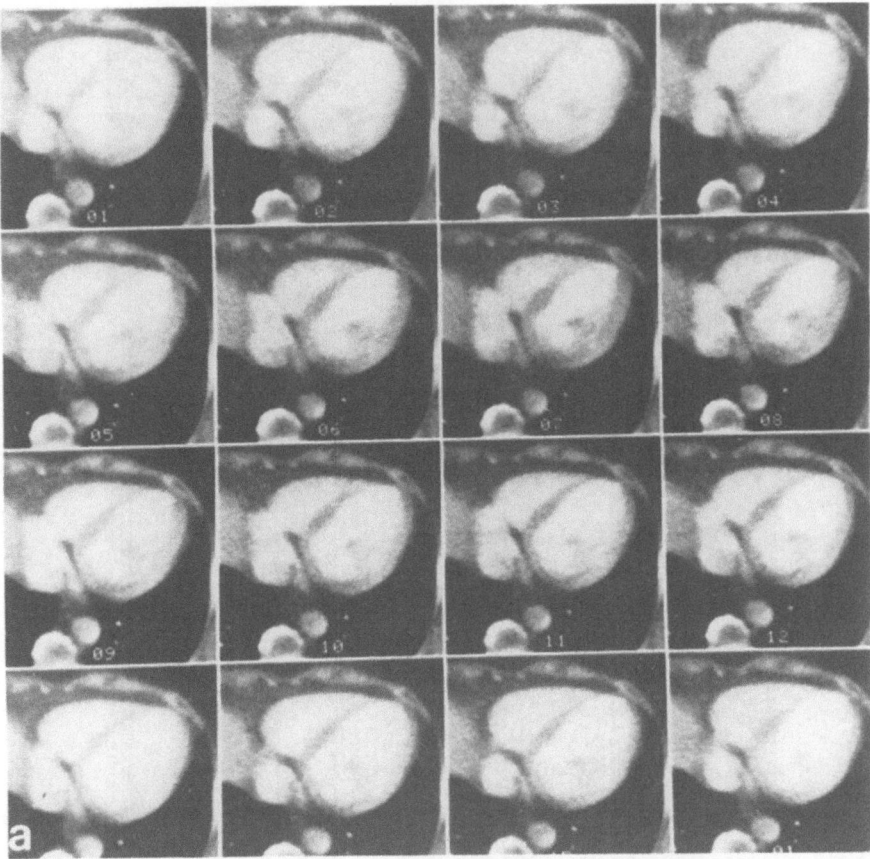

Figure 4a. This figure illustrates the movie mode of operation of the Cine-CT system. Sixteen CT images from a series during contrast enhancement in a patient with a previous antero-septal infarct. Various phases of the cardiac cycle are seen. Diastole is represented in the top left panel, numbered 1, while scan 8 is in systole.

tion fractions are obtained by Simpson's rule. Computed tomography measurement of left and right ventricular volumes have been shown to be independent of chamber orientation unlike angiocardiography and echocardiography which require geometric assumptions in their calculations (16–18). Global and regional ejection volume measurements are currently being validated for Cine-CT in man with biplane angiography.

Measurements of left ventricular mass by Cine-CT

The ability to define the endocardial and epicardial wall edges accurately and reproducibly by CT techniques has been validated previously for septal wall

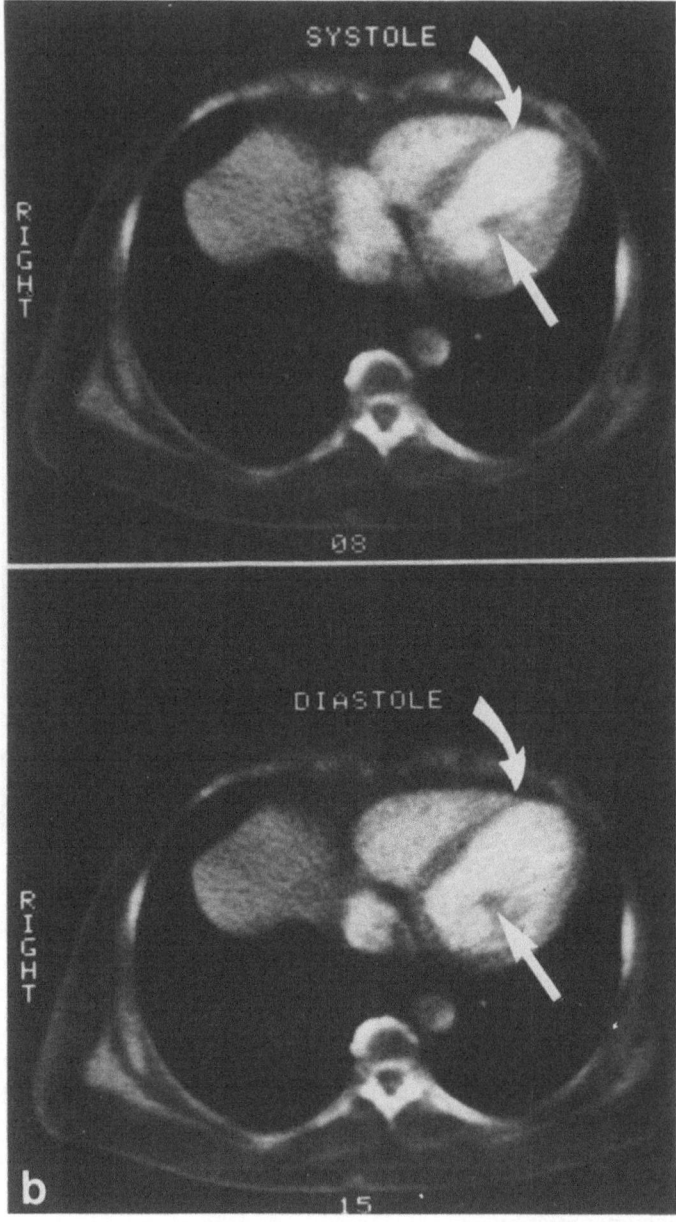

Figure 4b. Systolic and diastolic CT scans from Figure 4a and magnified. Note the absence of normal motion as well as myocardial wall thickening in the anterior wall and the anterior portion of the septum, which are markedly thinner than in other regions (curved arrow). The right atrium, and ventricle are also well defined, and their motion characterized. The right diaphragm and lobe of the liver can be seen adjacent to the heart at this scanning level. The posterior papillary muscle explains the increased density within the left ventricle in this plane (straight arrow).

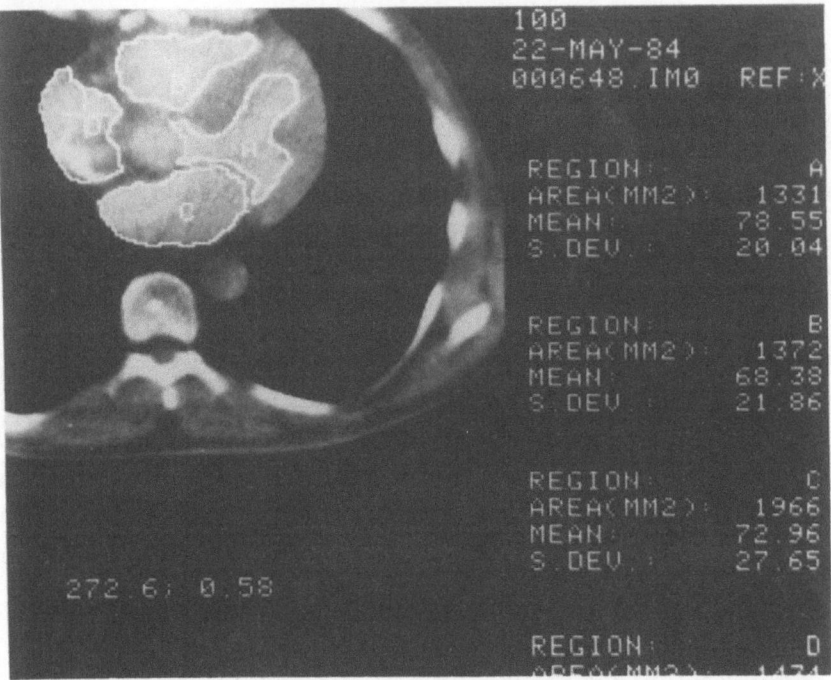

Figure 5. Endocardial boundary detection was enhanced using a half-contour method and enables the cardiac chambers to be outlined with a light pen. Dividing the difference between diastolic and systolic areas by the diastolic area provides the ejection fraction for this 8 mm thick slice. Chamber volumes are calculated by summation of areas at multiple levels and multiplication by level spacing according to Simpson's rule.

thickness and myocardial mass in animals (19–24). A recent study showed that left ventricular mass in dogs can be measured with Cine-CT more precisely than by any other invasive or noninvasive technique (25). Several centers which have recently acquired Cine-CT scanners are also performing various validation studies of chamber and wall dimensions in man, and validating their results against other established and proven modalities. The tomographic advantages of Cine-CT imaging are significant, particularly in conditions in which hypertrophy is asymmetrical as in some types of myopathies (Figure 6).

The role of Cine-CT in myocardial infarction

Acute myocardial infarction has been studied extensively since 1975 by earlier generation CT scanners (26–27). Laboratory studies have indicated that the infarct is seen within hours; first as a contrast enhancement perfusion defect, then within a few minutes as delayed enhancement in the surrounding infarct zone,

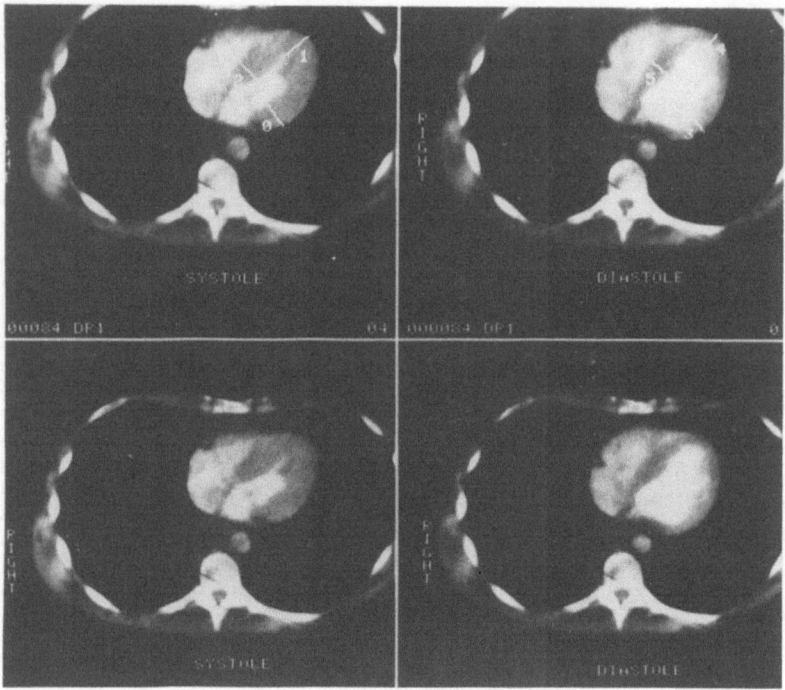

Figure 6. Systolic and diastolic images are seen in a patient with hypertrophic cardiomyopathy. The images in the upper panels are the same as below, but have been analyzed to determine regional wall thickness and thickening during the cardiac cycle. Wall thickening is readily appreciated from the movie display and is an excellent index of ischemia. Cine-CT is able to measure the percentage of change with precision. Once the operator defines the points, the computer displays these data numerically on the monitor alongside these images.

and with ECG gated-CT (and now Cine-CT) as regions with motion abnormalities of the adjacent myocardial wall (28). Similar studies confirm that these changes also occur in man (29). These reports have also indicated that CT can accurately size the infarct area (26). Until now, the use of slow CT has been limited by the single slice configuration and poor slice registration due to the need for sequential breath holding, as well as multiple injections of contrast medium. The C-100 overcomes these difficulties as so much data can be collected with each injection.

Chronic myocardial infarction

The effects of ischemia on wall thinning and contractility can be quantitated by Cine-CT. In a recent study at the University of California, San Francisco,

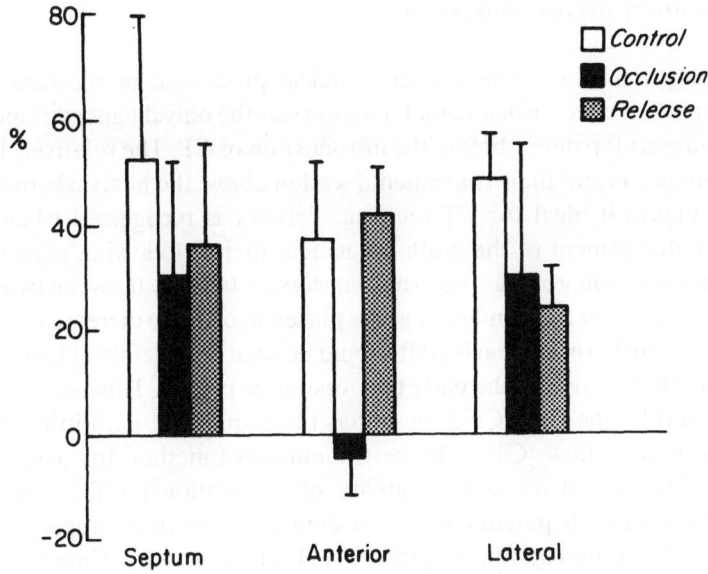

Figure 7. Graphic representation of end-diastolic and end-systolic wall measurements in five dogs for the control (C), occlusion (O) and release (R) states in the septal, anterior and lateral walls. There is a marked decrease in systolic thickness of the anterior wall during acute occlusion of the left anterior descending coronary artery.

comprising 24 patients, Cine-CT provided a reliable assessment of regional wall motion based on left ventricular cavity dynamics (Figures 4a and b). Abnormal contraction patterns by CT correlated in 90% (100/110) of the segments with the findings of biplane left ventriculography (30). It is likely that by adding wall thickening measurements the Cine-CT evaluation should be even more sensitive in characterizing ischemic dysfunction as illustrated in Figure 6. The sequelae of infarction, namely, thrombus and aneurysm formation can also be detected and quantitated by CT (9, 31).

Exercise and pharmacological Cine-CT stress testing

Wall mechanics have been quantitated and validation by Cine-CT which can measure wall thickening and thinning during acute ischemia (32). Figure 7 illustrates these results. Myocardial wall thickness is measured in this manner at all levels from cardiac apex to base. Supine exercise, using a bicycle ergometer attached to the Cine-CT table for exercise stress testing is presently being evaluated. Interventions with various pharmacological vasodilators are also being explored with Cine-CT to determine whether significant coronary artery disease can be quantitated by changes in wall mechanics (32–33).

Coronary artery bypass graft patency

This application of CT was the first clinical procedure in the heart to gain acceptance. Selective cardiac catheterization was the only diagnostic modality for determining graft patency before the introduction of CT. The relatively large size of the vein grafts and their convenient location above the heart where motion is minimal makes it ideal for CT imaging. Patency is recognized when there is contrast enhancement of the grafts coincident or just following peak enhancement of the ascending aorta. It is usually necessary to study between two and four levels depending on the number of grafts placed in order to increase the certainty of patency. Furthermore, each graft should be seen adequately at two levels. CT is particularly valuable in the early post-operative period. Time-density analysis as generated by the Cine-CT scanner has the promise of permitting the quantification of graft flow. CT is the best noninvasive method for detecting graft patency. The specificity and sensitivity of conventional CT in determining saphenous vein graft patency has been demonstrated to be approximately 95 percent (34). Internal mammary grafts can also be evaluated. Cine-CT by virtue of multilevel scanning allows all levels (4–8) to be scanned with only one bolus of contrast medium. This allows for a rapid study and also enables a Cine-CT left ventriculography study to be performed during the same procedure. The accuracy of Cine-CT should be high – it is presently being evaluated. Cine-CT offers a further exciting prospect – the measurement of graft flow.

Measurements of blood flow

No present imaging modality can measure regional myocardial blood flow in absolute terms with any degree of precision. Radioactive microsphere measurements in animals is the best available laboratory method known and requires sacrificing the animal. Thallium-201 imaging in man provides useful but nonetheless, only relative estimates of regional myocardial perfusion. Nearly all our techniques for evaluating ischemic heart disease are in fact, indirect, including coronary arteriography and left ventriculography.

Blood flow measurements which are to be clinically useful may be considered in two groups, blood flow through the cardiac chambers and vessels such as the carotid arteries and coronary bypass grafts and secondly, and much more difficult – blood flow measurements in tissue.

Cardiac output has been measured and validated by Cine-CT (35). This capability was assessed in a study of anesthetized dogs using the gamma-variate curve derived from a flow-mode sequence of scans. The area under this curve shown in Figures 8a and 8b reflects the cardiac output, which is given by the Stewart-Hamilton equation:

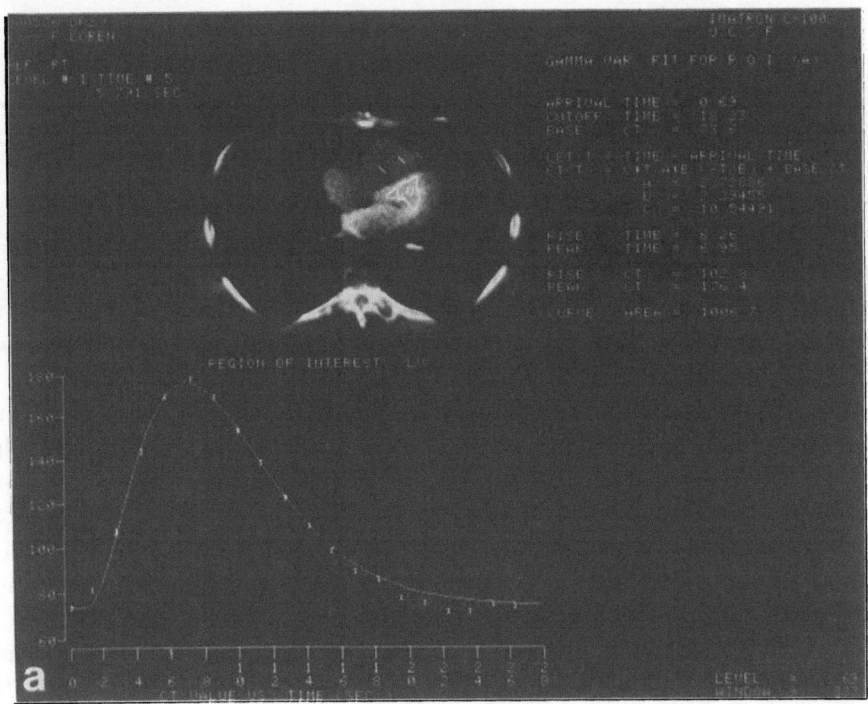

Figure 8a. Single axial 50 msec image from triggered or flow sequence when contrast bolus is present in left ventricle. Following the placement of a region of interest over left ventricular cavity, computer plots time/mean CT number (density) curve. These points are then fit to a standard theoretical curve (gamma variate), which corrects for secondary recirculation peak, if present. After performing the fit, the computer calculates various bolus parameters, including the rise time, peak time and area under curve.

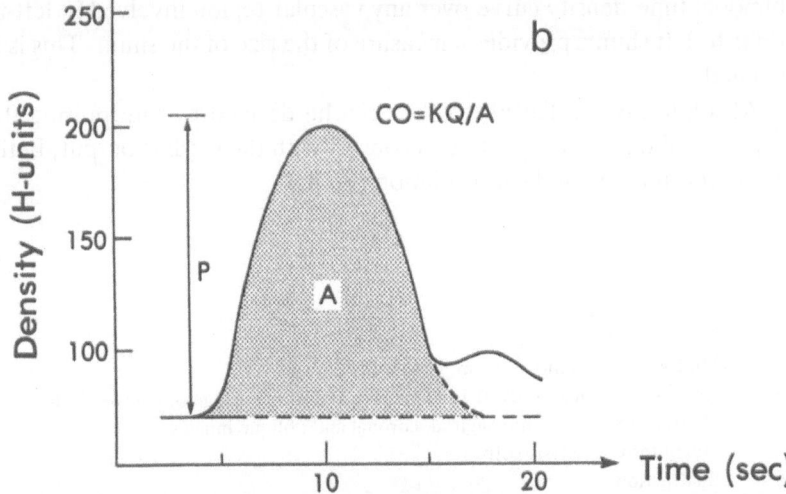

Figure 8b. Cardiac output can be determined from area under left ventricular curve (A) as in Figure 8a, if quantity of iodinated contrast medium injected (Q) is known.

$$CO = \frac{X}{\int c(t) \cdot \delta t}$$

where CO is the cardiac output, X is the quantity of indicator injected into the system and $c(t)$ is the concentration at the sampling site at time t. This concentration is given in terms of density, because a linear relationship exists between indicator (iodine) concentration and CT numbers over the physiological range. This densitometry was validated for the Cine-CT scanner in phantom experiments (36). The accuracy of Cine-CT was validated against simultaneous thermodilution measurements of cardiac output and the results showed an excellent correlation ($r = .92$); the mean percent difference between these techniques was 9.7% over a range of 1.5–6.3 l/min (35).

Vessel flow can also be characterized using high speed CT scanning using at least two methods. One approach is to obtain curves for example, from each carotid artery obtained simultaneously and using the first derivative of this to explore the relationship between slope and arterial occlusive disease. The results are being compared with pre- and post-operative angiographic findings. The carotid arteries are well seen by Cine-CT and digital subtraction capability is on-line and helpful in identifying, for example, the vertebral arteries, Table 1.

The ability to acquire flow curves at multiple levels from the same bolus injection allows the peak arrival time to be measured along a vessel. Figure 9 illustrates how the velocity can be calculated for each carotid artery. Other techniques can also measure velocity, but the cross-sectional images of CT permit the areas of the vessels to be measured accurately at each level, hence, the potential for measuring absolute carotid blood flow is apparent. Studies in our laboratory in a flow phantom indicate the reliability of this technique (36), and animal and patient evaluation data are being analyzed. The ability to obtain a bimodal time-density curve over any vascular region involved in left-to-right or right-to-left shunts provides a measure of the size of the shunt. This is also being studied.

Absolute myocardial blood flow can be derived by interpreting the relative myocardial time-density curve in concert with the cardiac output, both of which are determined by indicator dilution (37–41).

Table 1. Cine-CT capability.

1.	Rapid scan time, 50 msec.
2.	Multi-slice capability, 8 or more simultaneously.
3.	Repeat multi-slice study at 1 sec (or faster) during passage of contrast bolus.
4.	3D transformations into sagittal, coronal and oblique images.
5.	Quantitative analysis software.
6.	Subtraction.
7.	Functional image analysis and display.

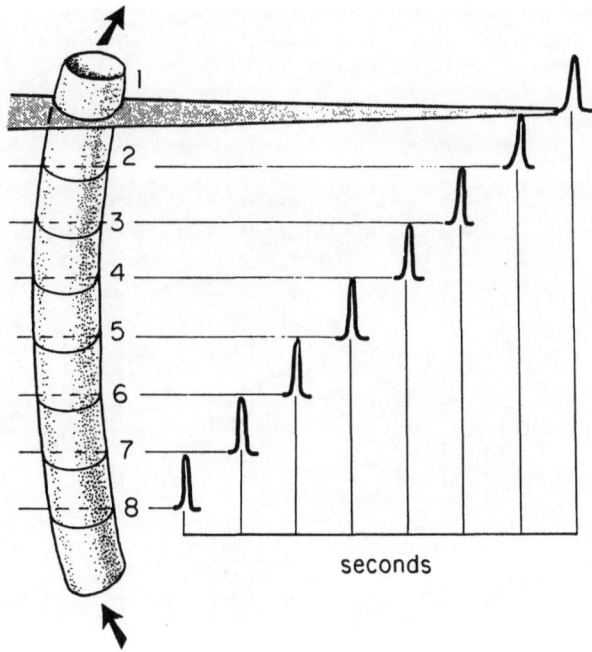

Figure 9. Illustrates the CT time-density curves generated at 8 contiguous levels from a multi-level Cine-CT flow sequence. The diagram represents a vessel-like carotid artery. The peak arrival time is given for each flow curve, hence, the velocity profile can be measured in cm/sec. Blood flow can be estimated from the velocity if the vessel area is known. This is readily calculated from the many cross-sectional CT images.

For any given contrast injection, as indicated above, measurement of the area under the time-density curves of the aorta and left ventricle is constant and representative of cardiac output (35). Absolute flow can then be calculated for any myocardial region as the ratio of peak enhancement of the time-density curve in that region to the area under the aortic or ventricular time-density curves (Figures 8a, 10a and 10b).

This formula assumes that the myocardial contrast washout time is longer than the width of the aortic or ventricular time-density curve. This is true in the myocardium because transit time through the capillary bed is longer than the duration of the systemic venous contrast bolus injection. The theoretical basis which underlies this concept has been discussed previously, but the only realistic approach is with 3D imaging techniques which allow accurate sampling. Mullani and Gould have demonstrated that regional blood flow can be measured by external detectors with a 3D isotope imaging technique (43). The equations derived for Cine-CT are similar to their theory. This formula has been validated in a tissue flow phantom in our laboratory and is currently being evaluated in dogs by radioactive microspheres. Studies performed at UCSF in collaboration with

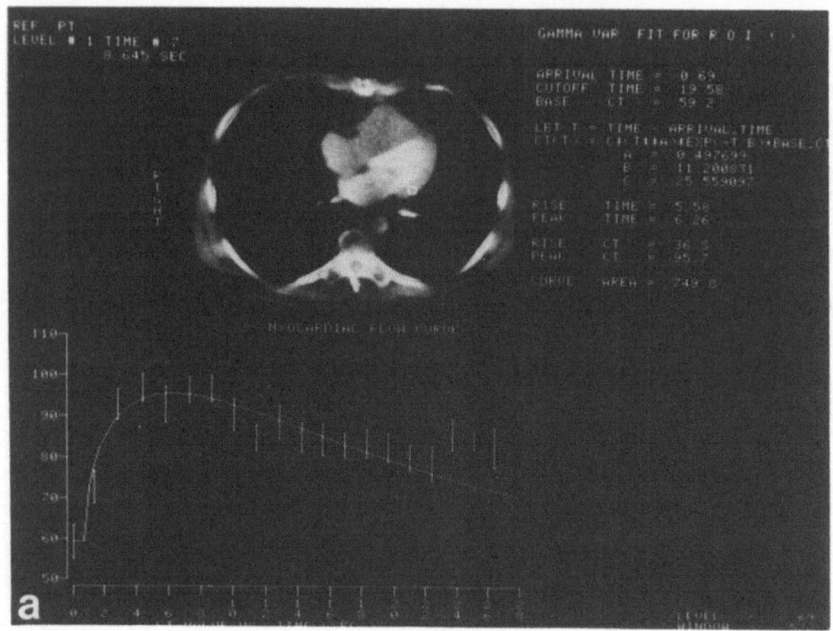

Figure 10a. Myocardial perfusion curve generated over lateral wall from patient with previous anterior myocardial infarction. Curve analysis provides peak height.

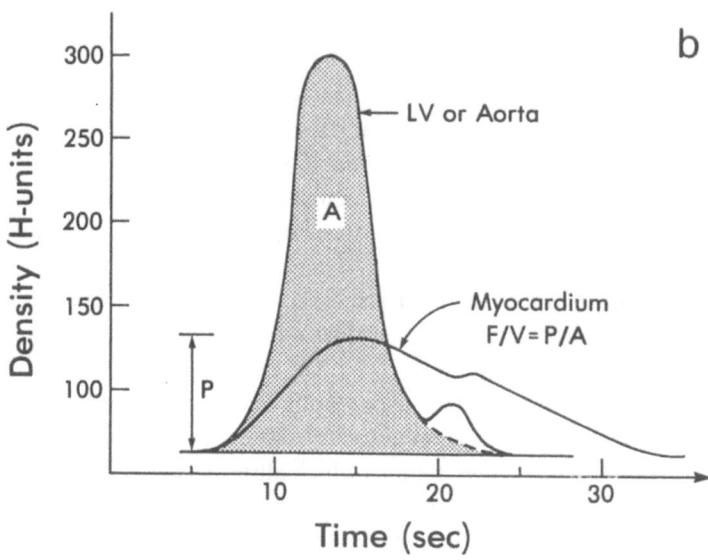

Figure 10b. Blood flow (F/V) in any myocardial region can be calculated as ratio of the peak of the time-density curve in that area (P) to the area under the aortic or left ventricular time-density curve (A), which is representative of cardiac output.

the Iowa University Medical Center look very promising (44). Another study reported the correlation of absolute myocardial flow measurements with changes in wall contractility during acute ischemia, produced by occluding a coronary artery in dogs (42). Useful CT measurements of regional myocardial perfusion with and without interventional pharmacological vasodilation have been demonstrated previously using labelled microspheres (45). There is therefore, the realistic prospect of measuring blood flow in man using high speed multilevel CT. The method has also been applied in the kidney where Cine-CT measurements of renal tissue flow correlated with radioactive microspheres (r=0.93) over a wide physiological range (46).

The future of direct measurements of flow by Cine-CT will depend upon the

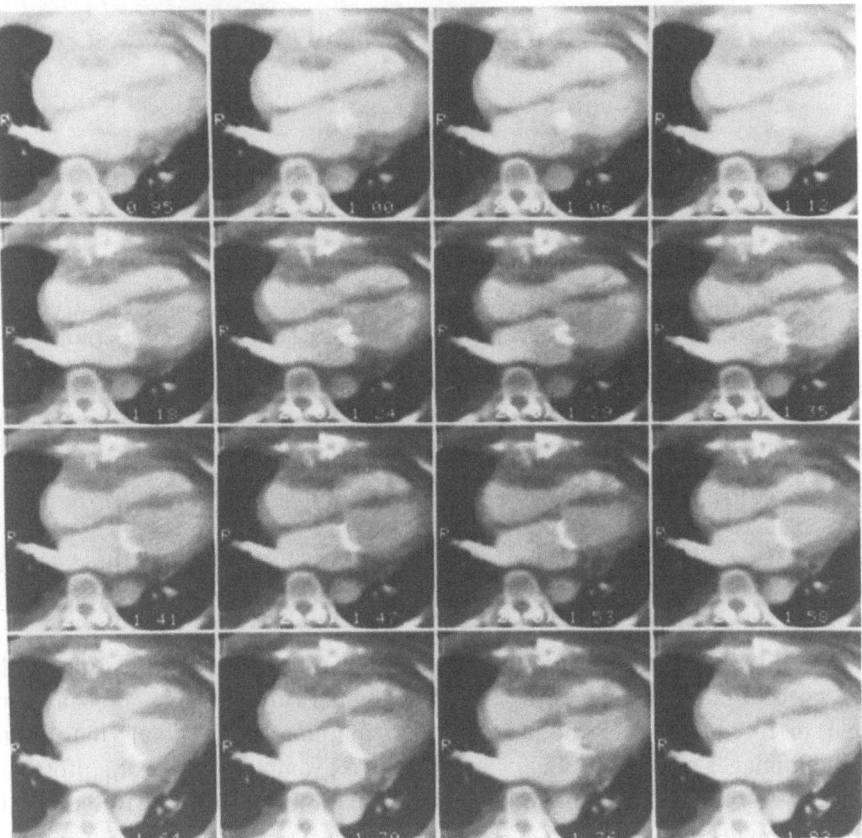

Figure 11. St. Jude mitral prostheses demonstrated by the movie mode (17 images/sec). This is one of 4 levels scanned simultaneously. The movement and position of the struts which are radiopaque is well seen. The velocity of their motion can also be estimated. Note that the prosthesis is not obscured by streak artifacts which are a major cause of extensive image degradation with slow conventional CT. The four cardiac chambers are all seen by contrast enhancement; 30 ml of Hypaque 60 was infused into a peripheral vein at 3 ml/sec.

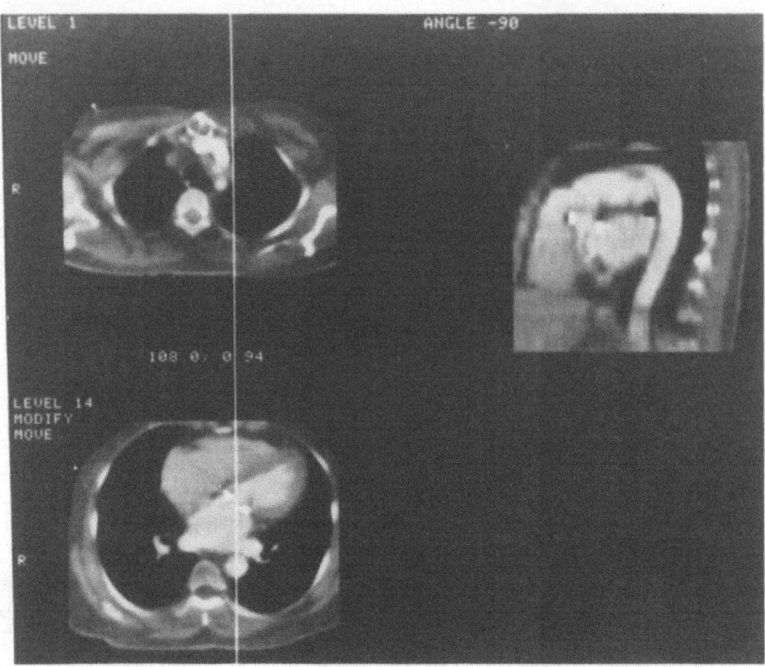

Figure 12. This figure demonstrates the ability of high speed CT to acquire contiguous levels through the whole chest if necessary during one injection, and with one bolus of contrast medium in the patient illustrated in Figure 2 with aortic and mitral prosthetic valves. Note that the aorta is seen over a wide region similar to a projected angiographic image. This ability of CT to reconstruct any imaging plane once a cubic matrix of CT data has been acquired with good registration is a unique and powerful capability. It allows many acquired as well as congenital lesions of the heart and great vessels to be analyzed and characterized.

results of studies now in progress, but the prospect of this new modality for improving the diagnosis and management of patients with coronary artery occlusive disease is exciting.

The Cine-CT scanner has demonstrated that it has a definite role in the diagnosis of many cardiac disorders, including pericardial, valve and congenital heart disease (47–54). The ability of the high sampling rates for analyzing motion, present images similar to cineangiography. An example is given of a prosthetic valve (Figure 11). An example of a transformation image is illustrated for the aorta in Figure 12.

Conclusions

Computed tomography represents the optimal theoretical approach to X-ray imaging. This conclusion arises from CT's capacity to solve the fundamental limitation of all forms of X-ray imaging, the superimposition of anatomical structures. Since CT is a fully three-dimensional method, this problem is addressed in a manner not subject to the risks, complications and technical limitations of selective angiography, subtraction angiography, tomography and many other techniques. The optimism therefore, for Cine-CT imaging of the heart is well founded. Apart from the demonstration of anatomical structures in any plane and in real time in movie format, this new generation of CT scanners offers a unique potential for measuring myocardial perfusion. This can be evaluated in two ways: by measuring myocardial wall thickening, which is a sensitive indicator of blood flow and, by assessing time-density changes due to the passage of contrast agent through thin slices of myocardium. Neither of these techniques can be performed adequately at present with noninvasive or even by invasive techniques. Feasibility studies, however, have demonstrated that this should indeed be possible using fast CT scanning (55–57). The radiation exposure of current whole body scanners is low (58). The Cine-CT scanner's radiation exposure to the patient is comparable or less; hence, this will not be a practical limitation.

Obviously, further controlled clinical studies are needed to validate Cine-CT's capability for general clinical purposes and comparisons will be necessary with established angiographic, echocardiographic and nuclear medicine techniques. Further studies are also needed in animals as well as patients to determine the sensitivity and specificity of Cine-CT. Should Cine-CT reach its anticipated potential, electron beam systems of the type described may not only replace present 3rd and 4th generation CT scanners for general purposes, but also may become a complementary or even the primary screening and diagnostic cardiac imaging technique of the future.

References

1. Lipton MJ, Higgins CB: Evaluation of ischemic heart disease by computerized transmission tomography. Radiology Clinics of North America 18, 1980: 557–576.
2. Moncada R, Baker M, Salinas M, Demos TC, Churchill R, Love L, Reynes C, Hale D, Cardosso M, Pifarre R, Gunnar RM: Diagnostic role of computed tomography in pericardial heart disease: Congenital defects, thickening, neoplasms, and effusions. Am Heart J 103, 1982: 263–282.
3. Higgins CB, Carlsson E, Lipton MJ: CT of the heart and the great vessels: Experimental evaluation and clinical application. Futura Publishing Co., Mount Kisco, New York, 1983.
4. Lackner K, Thurn P: Computed tomography of the heart. ECG-gated and continuous scans. Radiology 140, 1981: 413–420.
5. Doppman JL, Rienmuller R, Lissner J, Cyran J, Bolte H-D, Strauer BE, Hellwig H: Computed tomography in constrictive pericardial disease. J Computed Assisted Tomography 5, 1981: 5–11.
6. Bohn J, Reinmüller R, Seiderer M, Strauer BE: The non-invasive determination of the end-diastolic volume of the left ventricle: a comparison of cineangiographic, two-dimensional echocardiographic, multiple gated angiographic and computertomographic techniques. Z Kardiol 72, 1983: 438–447.
7. Masuda Y, Yoshida H, Morooka N, Takahashi O, Watanobe S, Inagaki Y, Uchiyama G, Tateno

Y: ECG synchronized computed tomography in clinical evaluation of total and regional cardiac motion: Comparison of postmyocardial infarction to normal hearts by rapid sequential imaging. Am Heart J 103, 1982: 230–238.

8. Godwin JD, Hefkins RL, Skiöldebrand CG, Federle MP, Lipton MJ: Evaluation of dissections and aneurysms of the thoracic aorta by conventional and dynamic CT scanning. Radiology 136, 1980: 125–133.

9. Tomoda H, Hoshiai M, Furuya H, Shotsu A, Ootaki M, Matsuyama S: Evaluation of left ventricular thrombus with computed tomography. Am J Cardiol 48, 1981: 573–577.

10. Reinmüller R, Ontyd J, Krappel W, Strauer B-E: Infarktbedingte Veränderungen des links-ventrikulären Myokards in der kardialen Computertomographie. Fortsch Röntgenstr 138, 1983: 403–411.

11. Ritman EL, Robb RA, Johnson SA, Chevalier PA, Gilbert BK, Greenleaf JF, Sturm RE, Wood EH: Quantitative imaging of the structure and function of the heart, lungs and circulation. Mayo Clinic Proc 53, 1978: 3–11.

12. Boyd DP, Gould RG, Quinn JR, Sparks R: A proposed dynamic cardiac 3-D densitometer for early detection and evaluation of heart disease. IEEE Trans Nucl Sci 26, 1979: 2724–2727.

13. Boyd DP: Future technologies, transmission CT in radiology of the skull and brain: technical aspects of computed tomography. TH Newton and DG Polk (Eds.), St. Louis, MO. CV Mosby, 1981: chapter 13.

14. Boyd DP, Lipton MJ: Cardiac computed tomography. Proc IEEE 71, 1983: 298–307.

15. Peschmann KR, Couch JL, Parker DL: New developments in digital X-ray detection. In: Digital Radiography, SPIE Proceedings 314, 1981: 5054.

16. Lipton MJ, Hayashi TT, Boyd D, Carlsson E: Measurement of left ventricular cast volume by computed tomography. Radiology 127, 1978: 419–423.

17. Lipton MJ, Hayashi TT, Davis PL, Carlsson E: The effects of orientation on volume measurements of human left ventricular casts. Invest Radiol 15, 1980: 469–474.

18. Ringerts HG, Rodgers B, Lipton MJ, Cann C, Carlsson E: Assessment of human right ventricular cast volume by CT and angiocardiography. Invest Radiol 20, 1985: 29–32.

19. Skiöldebrand CG, Ovenfors C-O, Mavroudis C, Lipton MJ: Assessment of ventricular wall thickness in vivo by computed transmission tomography. Circulation 61, 1980: 960–965.

20. Skiöldebrand CG, Lipton MJ, Mavroudis C, Hayashi TT: Determination of left ventricular mass by computed tomography. Am J Cardiol 49, 1982: 63–70.

21. Teicholz LE, Kreule T, Herman MV, Gorlin R: Problems in echocardiographic volume determinations: Echocardiographic – angiographic correlations in the presence or absence of asynergy. Am J Cardiol 37, 1976: 7–11.

22. Schiller NB, Skiöldebrand CG, Schiller EJ, Mavroudis CC, Silverman NH, Rahimtoola SM, Lipton MJ: Canine left ventricular mass estimation by two-dimensional echocardiography. Circulation 68, 1983: 210–216.

23. Peck WW, Maruini GBJ, Slutsky RA, Mattrey RF, Higgins CB: In vivo assessment by computed tomography of the natural progression of infarct size, left ventricular muscle mass and function after acute myocardial infarction in the dog. Am J Cardiol 53, 1984: 929–935.

24. Iwasaki T, Sinak LJ, Hoffman EA, Robb RA, Harris LD, Bahn RC, Ritman EL: Mass of left ventricular myocardium estimated with dynamic spatial reconstructor. Am J Physiol 246, 1984: H138–H142.

25. Feiring AJ, Rumberger JA, Reiter SJ, Skorton DJ, Collins SM, Lipton MJ, Higgins CB, Ell S, Marcus ML: Determination of left ventricular mass in dogs with rapid-acquisition cardiac Computed tomographic scanning. Circulation 72, 1985: 1355–1364.

26. Adams DF, Hessel SJ, Judy PF, Stein JA, Abrams HL: Computed tomography of the normal and infarcted myocardium. Am J Roentgenol 126, 1976: 786–791.

27. Doherty PW, Lipton MJ, Berninger WH, Skioldebrand CG, Carlsson E, Redington RW: Detection and quantitation of myocardial infarction in vivo using transmission computed tomography. Circulation 63, 1981: 597–606.

28. Slutsky RA, Mattrey RF, Long SA, Higgins CB: In vivo estimation of myocardial infarct size and left ventricular function by prospectively gated computerized transmission tomography. Circulation 67, 1983: 759–765.

29. Kramer PH, Goldstein JA, Herfkens RJ, Lipton MJ, Brundage BH: Imaging of acute myocardial infarction in man with contrast-enhanced transmission tomography. Am Heart J 108, 1984: 1514–1523.

30. Lipton MJ, Farmer DW, Killebrew E, et al: Evaluation of regional myocardial function with fast CT in patients with prior myocardial infarction. Radiology, 1985: in press.

31. Goldstein JA, Schiller NB, Lipton MJ, Ports TA, Brundage BH: Evaluation of left ventricular thrombi by contrast-enhanced computed tomography and two-dimensional echocardiography. Am J Cardiol 57, 1986: 757–760.

32. Farmer D, Lipton MJ, Higgins CB, Ringertz H, Dean PB, Sievers R, Boyd DP: In vivo assessment of left ventricular wall and chamber dynamics during transient myocardial ischemia using cine computed tomography. Am J Cardiol 55, 1985: 560–565.

33. Rumberger JA, Feiring AJ, Skorton DJ, et al: Patterns of regional left ventricular endocardial motion in normal dogs as demonstrated by rapid acquisition computed tomography: Circulation, 1985: in press.

34. Brundage BH, Lipton MJ, Hefkens RJ, Berninger WH, Redington RW, Chatterjee K, Carlsson E: Detection of patent coronary bypass grafts by computed tomography: A preliminary report. Circulation 61, 1980: 826–831.

35. Garrett JS, Lanzer P, Jaschke W, et al: Noninvasive measurement of cardiac output by Cine-CT. Am J Cardiol, 1985: in press.

36. Jaschke W, Gould R, Assimakopoulos PA, et al: Flow measurements with a high speed CT scanner. Invest Radiol, 1985: submitted.

37. Sapirstein LA: Regional blood flow by fractional distribution of indicators. Am J Physiol 193, 1958: 161–168.

38. Zierler KL: Equations for measuring blood flow by external monitoring of radioisotopes. Circ Res 16, 1965: 309–321.

39. Thompson HK, Starmer CF, Whalen RE, McIntosh HD: Indicator transit time considered as a gamma variate. Circ Res 14, 1964: 502–515.

40. Nassi M, Brody WR: Regional myocardial flow estimation using computed tomography. Med Phys 8, 1981: 302–307.

41. Klingensmith III WC: Regional blood flow with first circulation time-indicator curves: A simplified, physiologic method of interpretation. Radiology 149, 1983: 281–286.

42. Lipton MJ, Dean PB, Farmer D, Ringertz HG, Higgins CB: Measurement of regional myocardial blood by cine computed tomography. Circulation 70, 1984: II-169. (Abstract)

43. Mullani NA, Gould KL: First-pass measurements of regional blood flow with external detectors. J Nucl Med 24, 1983: 577–581.

44. Rumberger JA, Fiering AJ, Lipton MJ, Higgins CB, Marcus ML: Measurement of myocardial perfusion by ultrafast CT. JACC 5, 1985: 500. (Abstract)

45. Doherty PW, Skiöldebrand CG, Redington RW, Berninger WH, Lipton MJ: Measurement of regional changes in myocardial perfusion using dynamic computed tomography and contrast medium. Acta Radiol Diagn 24, 1984: 297–303.

46. Jaschke W, Cogan MG, Sievers R, Gould R, Lipton MJ: Measurement of renal blood flow by cine computed tomography. Submitted, Kidney International, 1985.

47. Doppman JL, Reinmuller R, Lissner J, Cyran J, Bolte HD, Straver BE, Hellwig H: Computed tomography in constrictive pericardial disease. Journal of Computed Assisted Tomography 5, 1981: 1–11.

48. Moncada R, Salinas M, Churchill R, Love L, Reynes C, Demos TC, Hale D, Schreiber R: Patency of saphenous aortocoronary-bypass grafts demonstrated by computed tomography. New Engl J Med 303, 1980: 503–505.

100

49. Lipton MJ, Higgins CB: Computed tomography: The technique and its use for the evaluation of cardiocirculatory anatomy and function. In: Pediatric Cardiac Imaging. WF Friedman, CB Higgins (Eds), Saunders Publishers, Philadelphia, 1984: 120–134.

50. Fisher M, Lipton MJ, Higgins CB: Magnetic resonance imaging and computed tomography in congenital heart disease. Sem. Roentgen. 20, 1985: 272–282.

51. Lipton MJ, Higgins CB, Farmer D, Boyd DP: Cardiac imaging with a high speed Cine-CT scanner. Preliminary results. Radiology 152, 1984: 579–582.

52. Lipton MJ, Herfkens RJ: Computed tomography of the heart and pericardium. In: CT of the Body. A Moss, G Gamsu, H Genant (Eds.), WB Saunders, Co., Philadelphia, PA, 1983: 401–425.

53. Inagaki Y, Masuda Y: Diagnosis of cardiovascular disease by CT. Igaku-Shion Ltd, Tokyo, Japan, 1983.

54. Farmer DW, Lipton MJ, Webb WR, Ringertz H, Higgins CB: Computed tomography in congenital heart disease. J Comp Assist Tomogr 8, 1984: 677–687.

55. Lanzer P, Dean PB, Lipton MJ, Sievers R, Botvinick E, Higgins CB: Effects of intravenous administration of iotrol, iosimide and diatrizoate on systemic and coronary circulation in dogs. Invest Radiology, 1984: in press.

56. Lanzer P, Garrett J, Sievers R, Gould R, Botvinick E, Lipton M, Higgins C: Wall thickening dynamics; assessment by Cine computed tomography. Circulation 72 (Supp III), 1985: III–180 (Abstract).

57. Garrett JS, Jaschke W, Aherne T, Higgins CB, Lipton MJ: Quantitation of intracardiac shunts by Cine-CT. Circulation 72 (Supp III), 1985: III–27 (Abstract).

58. Brasch RC, Boyd DP, Gooding CA: Computed tomography scanning in children: comparison of radiation dose and resolving power of commercial CT scanners. Am J Roentgenol 131, 1978: 95–101.

Part II: Quantitative coronary cineangiography

Part II: Quantitative contact linguistics

Quantitation of coronary artery stenosis severity: Limitations of angiography and computerized information extraction

J. Richard Spears and T. Sandor

Summary

Accurate, reproducible assessment of angiographic coronary luminal dimensions would facilitate management of patients with obstructive atherosclerosis and would expedite studies of interventions in atherosclerosis. In this chapter, we discuss our experience with many of the limitations of angiography which had to be addressed during the development of a computerized image analysis system for extraction of quantitative morphometric information from digitized cine-angiograms. A mathematical definition of the position within the angiographic image edge gradient which corresponds to the anatomic vessel boundary was found to be independent of many radiographic variables. Contrast medium concentration, however, had a small but predictable effect on this definition and, hence, on diameter measurement. Diameter measurements may be made with this system with an error of less than 100 microns, once temporal fluctuations in the imaging system, such as quantum mottle and film grain, are taken into account by multi-frame averaging. Likewise, studies of the reproducibility of diameter measurements, including between clinical angiographic procedures, suggest that a 3% variation or less of a 3 mm vessel is achievable in prospective studies if multi-frame analysis is performed. Potential problems with extrapolation of cross-sectional area from diameter information are discussed as is the use of densitometry for direct rotationally invariant measurement of relative cross-sectional area. Important future goals of image processing of coronary angiograms are improved automation and greater information extraction. Accordingly, recently developed techniques for automatic vessel centerline recognition and for potential tomographic reconstruction of complex luminal shapes from a small number of radiographic views are presented.

Introduction

Ischemic cardiac events occur in patients with coronary atherosclerosis primarily when the coronary lumen is compromised. Coronary angiography, by providing anatomic information regarding luminal dimensions of the coronary arterial tree (1), has therefore revolutionized our understanding of ischemic heart disease. The technique has been invaluable in the diagnosis and prognosis of the disease in individual patients, and it has been indispensable in the treatment of patients with coronary bypass surgery and balloon angioplasty. From the viewpoint of researchers interested in the evaluation of the efficacy of any intervention on the course of plaque encroachment on the coronary lumen, the use of sequential angiograms should greatly reduce the population size, duration, and cost/effectiveness of studies of a large number of potentially useful interventions, compared to conventional studies wherein data is generated solely by clinical endpoints.

In general, information provided by the angiogram is highly reliable, and it is unusual when the clinical picture, including noninvasive testing, is discordant with the findings at angiography. One might speculate that the reliability of the angiogram is, in part, responsible for the fact that its limitations have been recognized gradually only after many years of clinical application. Some important limitations are listed in Table 1. In this chapter, we discuss our experience, both published and previously unpublished, with many of these limitations during the development of an automated system for computerized analysis of digitized cineangiograms.

Radiographic view

Even when a vessel segment of interest is well-filled with contrast medium, free of overlapping branches, and intersected by the X-ray beam perpendicular to its centerline, underestimation of lesion severity can occur because of an inadequate radiographic view. A thin, shelf-like lesion for instance, may not be appreciated until it is viewed within a few degrees of its profile view (Figure 1). Virmani *et al.* in a postmortem study (2) recently described a group of patients succumbing from sudden death who were found to have ostial ridges or shelves which partially obstructed either the right or left coronary arteries; the authors speculated that, during exercise, aortic root dilatation could have increased the degree of obstruction from these ridges, which were contiguous with the wall of the aorta. Since these ridges were more likely to be present when a coronary artery arose at an acute angle from the aortic root, it is apparent that these thin shelves cannot be visualized when the proximal segment of the coronary artery is viewed perpendicular to the direction of the X-ray beam. Failure to opacify the aortic side of the shelf, of course, further compounds the difficulty in angiographic visualization of this pathology.

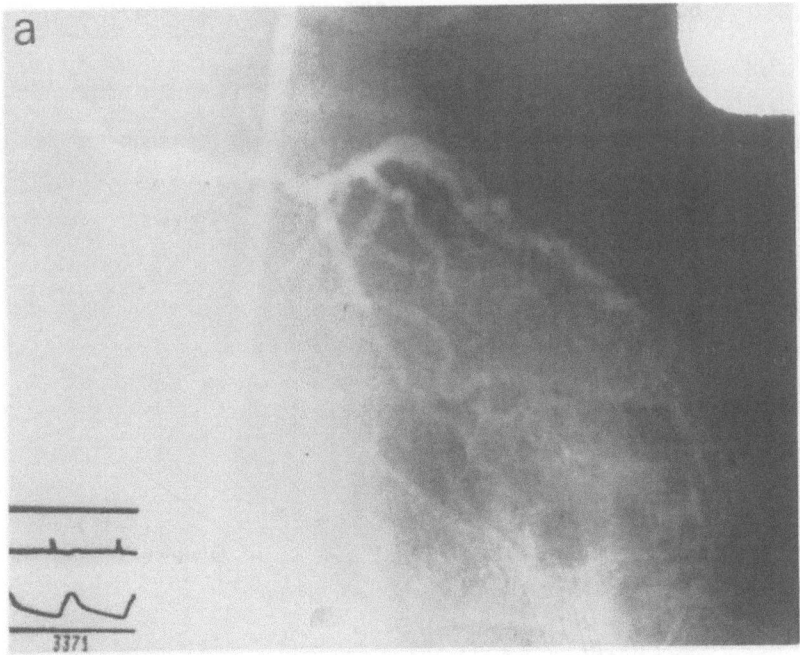

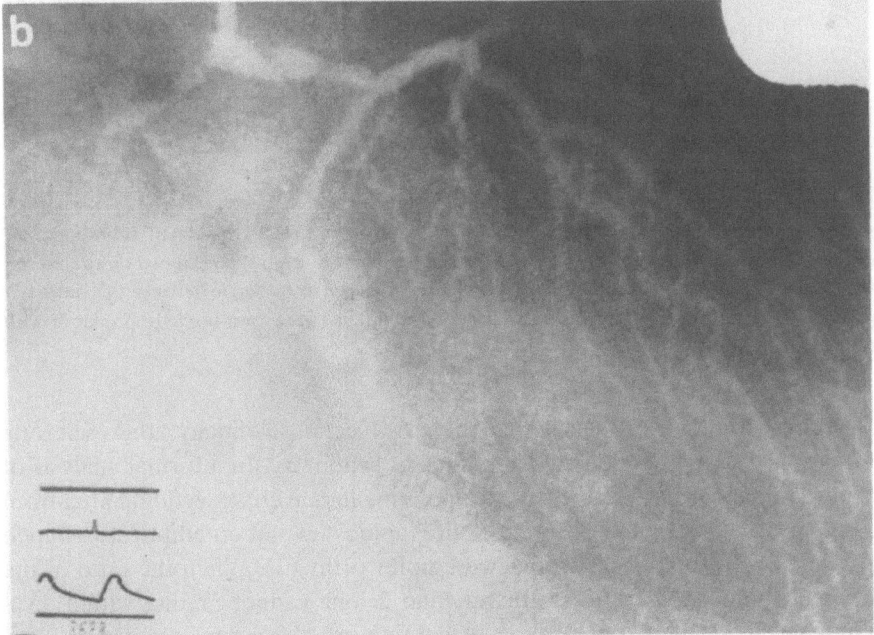

Figure 1a)b). Left coronary angiogram, AP (a) and shallow RAO-caudal (b) views. Although the views differ by only 20°, the true severity of the shelf-like lesion in the left mainstem artery is apparent only in (b).

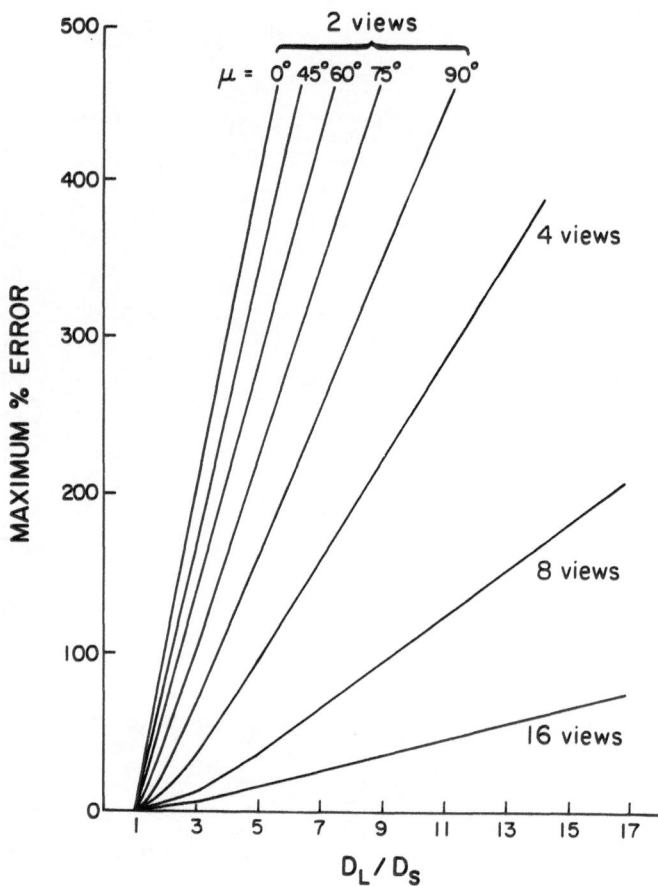

Figure 2. Potential maximum percent error of cross-sectional area extrapolated from apparent diameters versus degree of ellipticity, D_L/D_S (true major/minor axis ratio). When two views are used in the estimate of area, the maximum potential error is reduced as the angle between the views (μ) approaches 90°. This error is further reduced when additional views are used. Reproduced with permission from Spears *et al.* (3).

A more common problem is that the cross-sections of many atherosclerotic coronary artery lumina deviate from circular symmetry. In a formal analysis of the potential error incurred when extrapolating lumen cross-sectional area from the apparent diameters in different radiographic views of an elliptically-shaped cross-section, several observations were noteworthy (3). When the ratio of the true major/minor axis ratio is greater than 2, one cannot predict within 95% confidence limits that the error in estimating cross-sectional area from 2 arbitrarily oriented perpendicular views will be less than 20%. As the degree of ellipticity increases, the maximum potential error likewise increases (Figure 2). For example, when the actual major/minor axis ratio is 5, the maximum potential error is approximately 160% when 2 orthogonal radiographic views are used. For radiographic views <90° apart, the maximum potential error increases. Of interest is the fact that, when 2 orthogonal views of an elliptical lumen are available, extrapolated cross-sectional area cannot be underestimated, unlike the situation wherein the 2 views are separated by less than 90°. Thus, when only 2 views are available, an attempt should be made to make them 90° apart. Ideally, additional radiographic views will reduce the maximum potential error further, but from a practical viewpoint, there are few coronary segments for which more than 2 adequate views separated by more than 30° can be obtained. Since the probability of overestimating cross-sectional area of a highly elliptical lumen is much greater than that of underestimating the area, it is prudent clinically to use the smallest of the diameters noted in estimating percent area stenosis, rather than averaging diameters from multiple views. When one considers that any deviation of lumen shape from an ideal ellipse will only serve to increase the probability of overestimating cross-sectional area from apparent radiographic diameters, this assertion is strengthened further.

Computerized image analysis of coronary angiograms

Accuracy of diameter measurements

The necessity for reliable, reproducible quantitative information regarding luminal pathology from atherosclerosis has spurred the development of computerized analysis of digitized radiographic images (4–16), first developed at the Biomedical Image Analysis Laboratory of the Jet Propulsion Laboratory in conjunction with USC Medical Center for an objective measure of radiographic luminal irregularity (4, 5, 7). The efforts of our group have been directed primarily at extraction of quantitative indices of luminal dimensions from digitized coronary cineangiographic frames. Objective measurement of lumen diameter, the most fundamental index, requires that the location of the anatomic vessel edge be defined within the edge gradient of the angiographic vessel image. Theoretically, one might achieve this goal from knowledge of the point spread function of each component of the imaging chain. When one considers that temporal variation in the size of the focal spot may occur and that unpredictable biologic variables (Table 1), such as contrast medium concentration, may influence the size and shape of the edge gradient, a strictly mathematical approach to this problem appeared unrealistic. We therefore took the following empiric approach. Three spatially disparate positions within the edge gradient were defined mathematically, and computer-derived measurements of diameter were compared with the known anatomic diameter of each of a series of cylindrical model lumina. Analysis of covariance was used to determine whether the slope or intercept of the regression equations relating the measured and known diameters were affected by a wide variety of radiographic variables (14). Only one variable of practical importance, contrast medium concentration, was found to have a statistically significant effect on the regression equations. As contrast medium concentration decreased from 100% to 25% Renografin-76, computer-derived diameter measurements also decreased on the order of 100–300 microns for vessels 2–6 mm in diameter. When 5 experienced angiographers at our institution measured the diameters of the same phantom vessels at 10× magnification with a calibrated optical reticle, the diameter measurements of each angiographer were likewise affected (p<.05) to a similar degree by contrast medium concentration. Of interest was the observation that such manual measurements (n = 560) showed considerable intra- and interobserver variability. It appeared that angiographers differed in their guess at the location of the anatomic edge within the edge

Table 1. Limitations of Angiography

I.	Inadequate Angiographic View
	• Poor contrast medium filling
	• Vessel segment severely foreshortened
	• Overlapping branches
	• Minimum diameter not seen
	• Poor radiographic contrast
	• Mach Bands
II.	Diameter Information Inadequate
	• Irregular lumen geometry
	• Reference segment narrowed or ectatic
	• Vessel wall not visualized
III.	Biologic Variation
	• Blood-contrast medium mixing
	• Vasomotor tone
	• Intra-arterial pressure
	Pulsatile variation
	Contrast medium injection
	• Myocardial blush and filling of small adjacent vessels, including vasa vasorum
	• Vessel motion
IV.	Failure to Extract Precise Information
	• Visual methods unreliable, particularly for estimation of diameter percent stenosis in 30–70% range.
	• Visual estimates of enface plaque stenosis severity by gray scale evaluation unreliable
	• Manual-visual methods of diameter measurement tedious for multi-segment, multi-frame analysis.
V.	Complex Relation Between Lumen Geometry and Flow
	• Angiography provides potentially highly accurate, reproducible anatomic information but frequently unreliable physiologic information (Reference 31).

gradient, although the position selected was relatively reproducible for each observer over a large range of vessel sizes and over time. By contrast, computer-derived diameter measurements were not only highly reproducible (mean absolute variability <2% for a 3 mm vessel), but were also accurate to within 60 microns for each vessel for the fastest edge detection algorithm, first described by Selzer et al. (5), which consisted of finding the maximum first-derivative of a second degree polynomial fitted to gray scale values of consecutive pixels within a window which 'moved' across the densitometric vessel profile.

Reproducibility of diameter measurements

In the foregoing studies, each computer-derived diameter measurement represented the mean value from 8 consecutive cineframes of a contrast medium-filled phantom vessel. Multiple diameter measurements of the identical vessel segment were obtained to reduce variability due mainly to quantum mottle and film grain. A good example of the effects of these variables on the edge gradient can be seen in a single cineframe of a cylindrically-shaped model lumen filled with contrast medium; the edge gradient contour and, hence, the location of the anatomic edge within the gradient appear to vary axially along the lumen. At each axial location the error in the measured diameter resulting from such statistical fluctuations should be reduced by a factor roughly equal to $(n)^{1/2}$, where n = the number of diameter measurements over multiple cine exposures. In addition, averaging adjacent scan lines, oriented perpendicular to the vessel centerline, should likewise reduce variability in diameter measurements due to quantum mottle and film grain. We currently digitize cineframes with a Spatial Data Systems (Goleta, CA) EyeCom digitizer interfaced to a Vax 11/780 computer (Figure 3). Each image is digitized 4 times to reduce the effects of noise in the process of digitization. A scanning resolution of approximately 10 microns/pixel is achieved by optical magnification with a vidicon camera, and a window of interest within a potential 640×480 scanning array is digitized 8 bits deep. Because of the approximate 8 fold minification of vessel dimensions on cine, each pixel represents approximately 80 microns of antomic vessel dimension.

Variability in diameter measurement, as a result of digitizing system noise, is approximately 1% (±1 s.d.) for a 3 mm phantom vessel, as assessed by digitizing the identical vessel segment from a single cineframe multiple times (Figure 4). When the diameter of this vessel segment was determined over many consecutive cineframes (Figure 5), a variability of approximately 4% (±1 s.d.) was noted. Frame-to-frame changes in the image of the same vessel segment, principally as a result of quantum mottle and film grain, thus produced considerably more variability than than inherent in the process of digitization alone. It should be emphasized that the 4% variability was noted despite ideal exposure conditions, i.e., a homogeneous background, a fixed 100% concentration of Renografin 76,

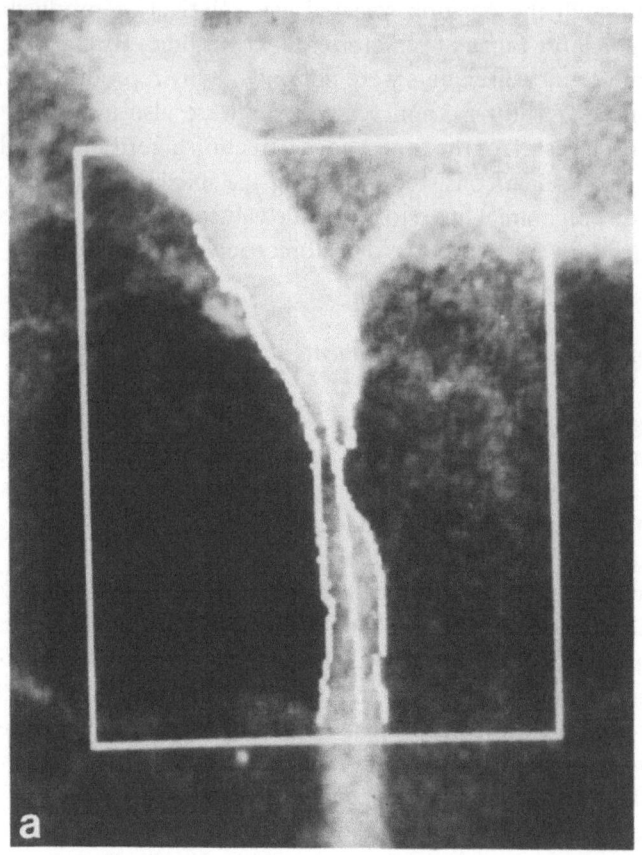

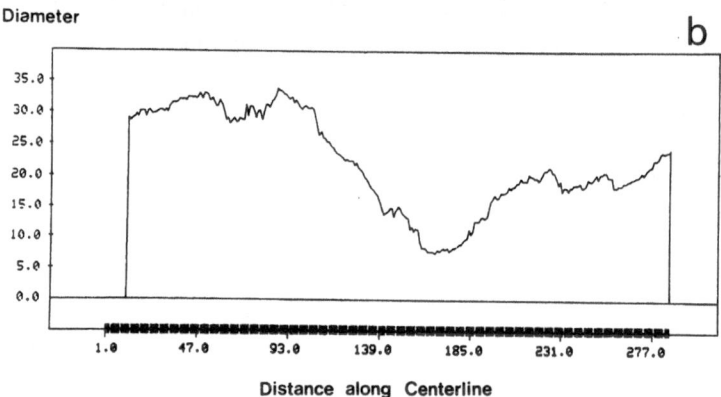

Figure 3a)b). Portion of cineframe of right coronary artery, RAO view. Following digitization of operator-defined region of interest (window), automatic edge tracking with a maximum slope algorithm is performed (a), and vessel diameter, perpendicular to the centerline, is displayed as a function of distance along the centerline (b). Reproduced with permission from Spears *et al.* (14).

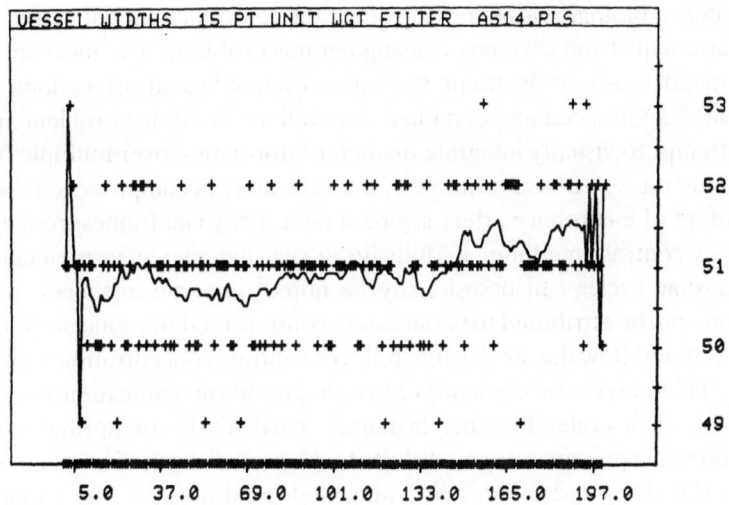

Figure 4. Repeated diameter measurement (200×) of the same segment of a contrast medium-filled 3 mm cylindrical phantom from a cineframe. Digitizing system variability was approximately 1% (±1 s.d.).

and no motion of the phantom vessel. In view of this intrinsic frame-to-frame variability, it is not surprising that, when 8 consecutive frames were used to measure the mean diameter of a vessel phantom at one axial location, an inter-study variability of only approximately 2% was found as previously noted.

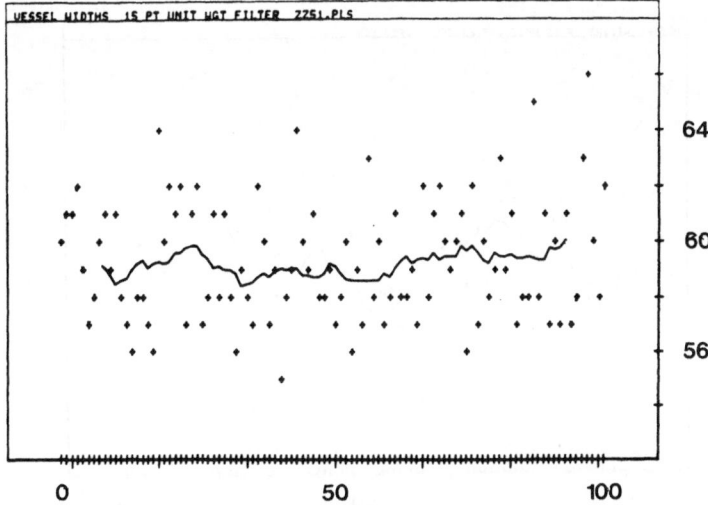

Figure 5. Repeated diameter measurement of the same segment as in Figure 4, but over 100 consecutive cineframes. The increased variability, approximately 4% (±1 s.d.), compared to that inherent in the process of digitization, resulted principally from quantum mottle and film grain.

A number of biologic variables may affect the reproducibility of vessel diameter measurements from coronary cineangiograms (Table 1). The most important of these, in most cases, is the frame-to-frame variation in contrast medium mixing with blood. Experienced angiographers are well aware of this problem and will usually attempt to visually integrate diameter information over multiple frames. Figure 6 illustrates a clinical example of the variability in computerized diameter measurement of a coronary artery segment over many cineframes from a single injection of contrast medium. Periodicity in the diameter measurements over several cardiac cycles can occasionally be noted; in some instances, periodic fluctuations can be attributed to variations in contrast medium concentration (the increase in blood flow during diastole reduces contrast concentration and, therefore, vessel diameter measurement) or in radiographic magnification as the heart rotates with each cycle. In other instances, particularly for normal coronary arteries, pulsatile pressure may contribute to the periodicity in diameter measurement. In the dog, under carefully controlled conditions, a 5% variation in coronary arterial diameter of a 3–4 mm epicardial segment can be noted angiographically (17). That this variation was secondary to the pulsatile nature of arterial pressure was confirmed by measuring intraluminal diameter continuously, on-line with a semiconductor based caliper, the Feldstein arterial contour transducer (Figure 7). Angiographic variation in diameter measurements from digitized cineframes were often apparent, in this ideal laboratory setting, only after application of autocorrelation techniques to data sets available for 5–14 cardiac cycles per injection. The shorter period of injection as used clinically precludes meaningful application of such statistical techniques, so that periodicity

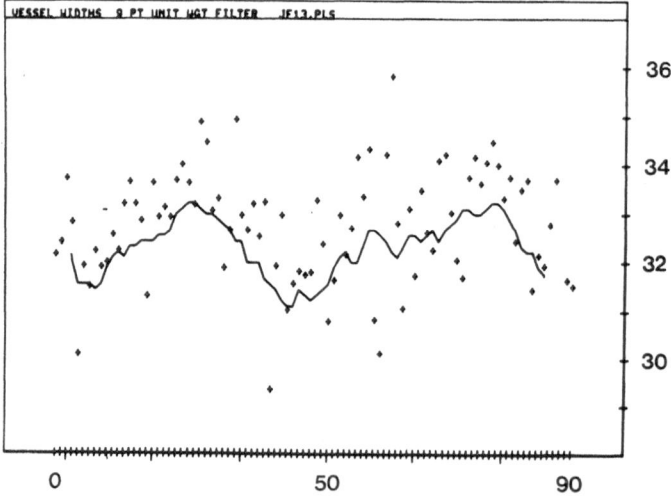

Figure 6. Diameter measurement of an identical vessel segment on each of 90 consecutive frames during contrast medium filling of a patient's right coronary artery. The apparent periodicity (approximately 45 frames in cycle length) corresponded to the heart rate.

in diameter measurements with a frequency similar to the cardiac cycle is difficult to detect or quantify in the clinical setting. Such information might be of value, however, because of the potential for assessing coronary compliance from the angiogram.

The injection of contrast medium per se may affect diameter measurements. Measurement of downstream intra-arterial pressure during contrast medium injection in coronary arteries of anesthetized dogs in our laboratory demonstrates a 10–20 mmHg rise in pressure which may increase lumen diameter. In addition, we have found that a second injection of contrast medium, 5 minutes after an initial injection, is associated with an increase in angiographic lumen diameter of 5% (17). During the latter part of all coronary angiographic injections, contrast medium filling of myocardial capillaries and small adjacent side-branches may cause spurious changes in angiographic luminal diameter measurements. Additionally, atherosclerotic coronary arteries have a rich network of vasa vasorum (18) which, when filled during a late phase of a contrast medium injection, can slightly alter the shape of the edge gradient.

When only one cineframe of a series obtained during a coronary injection of contrast medium is used for angiographic analysis, an end-diastolic frame is usually selected (6). We feel that this approach is less than ideal for several reasons. Coronary flow is greatest during diastole, so that contrast medium concentration is often less than during systole. Unless cine exposure is performed with electrocardiographic gating, the 'end-diastole' frame is at best a temporal approximation. Although one might assume that cardiac motion is minimal near end diastole, the converse is true for coronary segments which lie in the A–V grooves. In fact, rapid swinging of these segments frequently occurs between atrial and ventricular systole, particularly noticeable in RAO views.

A more rational approach to selection of cineframes for angiographic diameter analysis appears to us as follows: Selection of frames should be made on the basis of maximal contrast medium filling with no overlapping branches in a view which does not severely foreshorten the vessel segment of interest. In order to reduce variability from quantum mottle, film grain, inhomogeneities of contrast medium concentration, etc., at least 5–10 frames from a single injection should be analyzed and the measurements averaged. An additional advantage to multi-frame analysis is the fact that vessel motion from one frame to the next results in variable background tissue density, so that the effect of spurious densities on the edge gradient and on the entire transverse densitometric profile as a result of background tissue inhomogeneity will be reduced.

In order to assess the efficacy of any intervention in atherosclerosis on luminal dimensions, an objective measure of the latter must be highly reproducible over time. From the foregoing discussion, it is apparent that potentially many radiographic and biologic variables may alter measured luminal dimensions, either artifactually or anatomically. We therefore examined the reproducibility of diameter measurements by computerized image analysis of coronary stenoses between

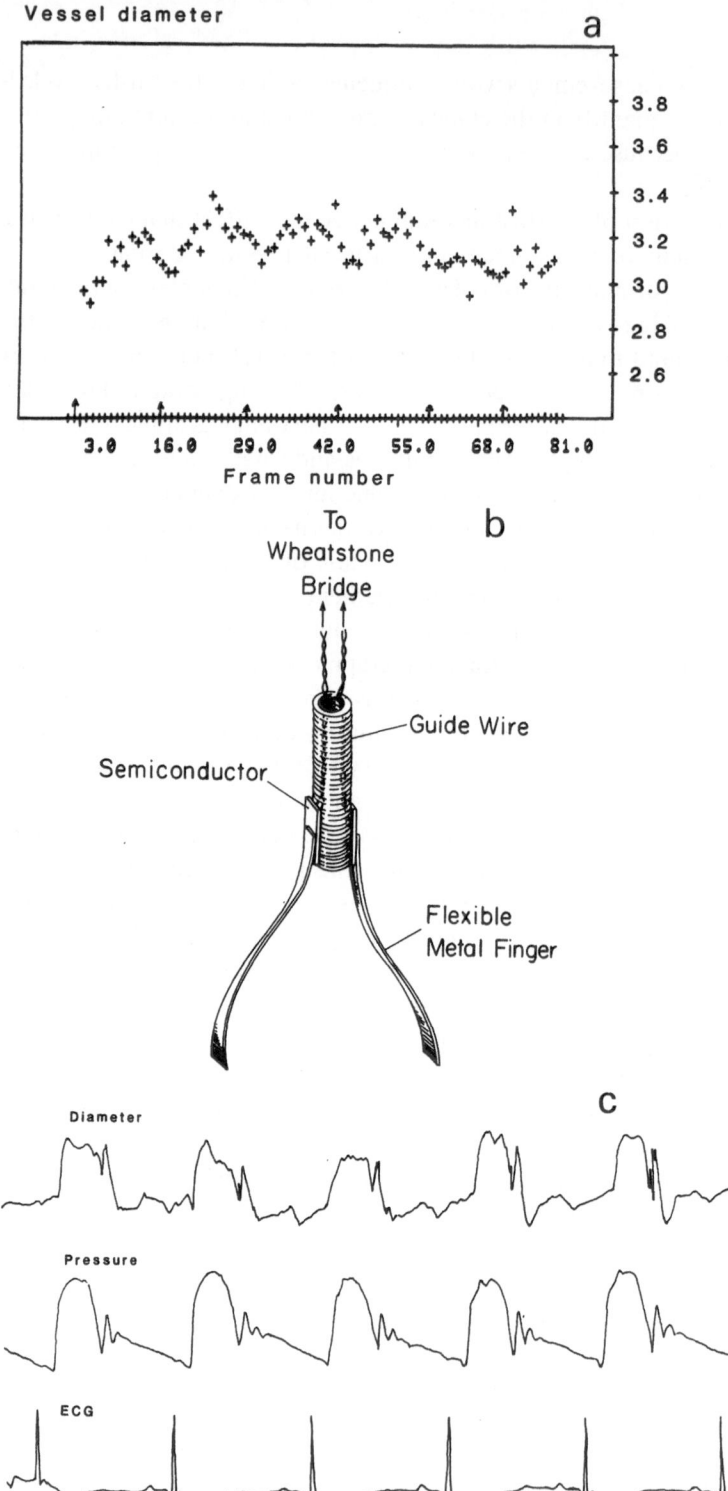

Vessel diameter

a

3.8
3.6
3.4
3.2
3.0
2.8
2.6

3.0   16.0   29.0   42.0   55.0   68.0   81.0
Frame number

b

To
Wheatstone
Bridge

Guide Wire

Semiconductor

Flexible
Metal Finger

c

Diameter

Pressure

ECG

Figure 7a)b)c). a) Pulsatile variation in angiographic diameter of an anesthetized dog's circumflex coronary artery over 6 cardiac cycles. Troughs in diameter measurement corresponded to the R-wave (arrows) of the ECG. b) Feldstein intra-arterial diameter displacement caliper. As fingers are displaced, pressure is exerted on semiconductors with a resultant change in electrical resistance. c) Caliper recording of intra-arterial diameter along with intra-arterial pressure recording in coronary artery of same dog as in 'a'. A parallel relationship between pressure and diameter is noted.

clinical angiographic studies (19). The study was retrospective and, therefore, represented a worst case situation wherein sources of variability in the measurements were potentially exaggerated. No attempt was made to control vasomotor tone, reproduce the identical radiographic view, or employ the same catheterization approach. The assumption was made that no change in atherosclerotic progression/regression occurred during the 1–4 week interval (mean = 2 weeks) between the 2 angiographic studies per patient; patients were selected from a pool of patients treated with either PTCA or thrombolytic therapy with intra-coronary streptokinase (SK) infusion. Selection of patients was made on the basis of having a routine follow-up angiogram available within 1 month of the initial procedure and the presence of a coronary stenosis in an artery not directly treated with either PTCA or SK as indicated in a written catheterization report. Of 10 patients selected in this manner (SK = 5 patients, PTCA = 5 patients), only one pair of films provided an inadequate view of the lesion of interest and could not be

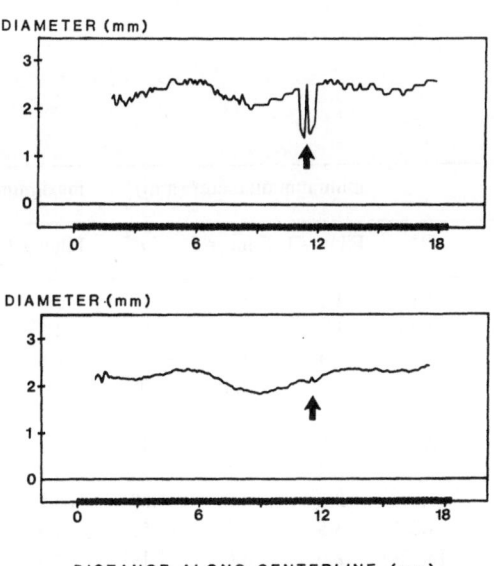

Figure 8. Diameter profile of a vessel segment from a single cineframe of a clinical coronary angiogram (top panel) versus the diameter profile averaged over 10 consecutive cineframes (bottom panel). The effect of artifacts in diameter measurement as a result of blood-contrast mixing, quantum mottle, etc. are reduced by multi-frame averaging (arrow).

analyzed by automated edge tracking of the vessel image. Similar radiographic views from each study were always selected for each stenosis analyzed.

For each stenosis measurement, 10 sequential cineframes during peak contrast medium filling in an optimal view were analyzed. Following automated edge tracking within a digitized window of interest by the moving window maximum slope algorithm (14), the centerline was identified as the midpoint between vessel edges. A fourth degree polynomial was fit to these points and scans perpendicular to the centerline were used to measure diameter as a function of distance along the vessel centerline. The same digitizing window was used for each subsequent frame of a series, and the diameter profile of each frame was moved along the abscissa (distance along centerline) until a least squares best fit match of values along the ordinate (diameter values) was found with ordinate values of the previous diameter profile (Figure 8). Thus, a running average of the diameter profile was constructed automatically over 10 consecutive frames, despite frame-to-frame variation in vessel position within the digitizing window secondary to cardiac motion. The maximum and minimum vessel diameters were extracted from each analysis, and absolute dimensions were obtained by using the known dimensions of the catheter shaft in conjunction with image analysis of a 1 cm segment of the latter over 5 consecutive frames. In order to reduce errors associated with analysis of the catheter shaft, the assumption was made that radiographic magnification was unchanged in each pair of angiograms.

Reproducibility of percent stenosis and vessel dimensions between studies was

Table 2.

Pt	% stenosis			minimum diameter (mm)			maximum diameter (mm)		
	Film #1	Film #2	D*	Film #1	Film #2	D*	Film #1	Film #2	D*
JC	32%	35%	− 3.1%	1.9	1.8	.15	2.8	2.7	.10
VS	62%	64%	− 2.3%	1.7	1.7	.06	4.5	4.7	− .13
RS	23%	29%	− 6.7%	2.1	2.4	− .29	2.8	3.4	− .66
PK	33%	32%	1.5%	2.3	2.4	− .05	3.5	3.5	.00
BB	41%	49%	− 7.9%	2.1	1.8	.26	3.5	3.6	− .05
HC	29%	30%	− 0.6%	4.0	3.9	.13	5.7	5.5	.13
TP	53%	51%	2.2%	2.4	2.6	− .22	5.1	5.3	− .21
HG	48%	47%	1.0%	3.2	3.2	.00	6.1	6.2	− .12
PG	25%	21%	4.2%	3.5	4.0	− .52	4.6	5.0	− .42
Mean	39%	40%	[3.3%]	2.6	2.6	[.19]	4.3	4.4	[.20]
s.d.	±14%	±14%	±4.1%	±0.8	±0.9	±.25	±1.2	±1.2	±.25
r+	.96			.96			.98		

* D = Film 1 – Film 2.
+ Pearson correlation coefficient between films 1 and 2.

surprisingly good (Table 2). The mean absolute difference in absolute, anatomic dimensions between studies was approximately ± 200 microns for both maximum and minimum diameters, and a close correlation for each measurement was found between studies (r > 0.95). These results are encouraging, particularly in view of the retrospective nature of the study and the possibility that anatomic changes in lumen caliber might have occurred between studies.

It is reasonable to expect that variability in computerized diameter measurements, not intrinsic to atherosclerotic progression/regression, can be reduced further by angiographic studies performed in a prospective manner. Thus, if vasomotor drug history preceding and during the initial angiographic study is reproduced in the second study, and identical radiographic views, angiographic technique, and magnification are used for each pair of angiograms, it should be possible to reduce inherent variability in the diameter measurements to 100 microns or less, e.g. 3% of a 3 mm vessel. We would like to emphasize that such optimism is probably warranted, however, only if multi-frame analysis is used.

Significant further reduction in diameter measurement variability would require subpixel precision in identification of the vessel edges. We have recently demonstrated, with the application of Monte Carlo methods for generation of the probability distribution of the noise of each measured pixel within the densitometric vessel profile, that a potential spatial resolution of 1/6 of a pixel for a 3 mm vessel is achievable (20).

Densitometric analysis of luminal cross-sectional area

A transverse densitometric scan is required to locate the vessel edge within the edge gradient of the digitized vessel image by most currently available image processing systems. As mentioned previously, contrast medium concentration affects both visual and automated methods of edge recognition. This observation is a clear example of the principle that densitometric information between vessel edges may affect the apparent location of the latter and, thereby, the measured diameter. Thus, highly accurate diameter measurement requires analysis of the entire densitometric scan across vessel image edges. More importantly, however, densitometric analysis can potentially provide a rotationally invariant measure of relative cross-sectional area (21). In addition, densitometric measurement of relative cross-sectional area can be accurate despite an irregular luminal geometry, such as a crescent-shaped lumen, unlike estimates of cross-sectional area from diameter measurements alone.

Several important assumptions are made when a densitometric analysis is performed. The actual parameter which cannot be angiographically measured directly is the thickness of contrast medium within a vessel lumen, and the assumption is made that contrast medium concentration is constant throughout the lumen cross-sections of the stenotic and adjacent reference segments. Most investigators have also assumed that a linear relationship exists between film optical density and contrast medium thickness (8,16). Nonlinearities in this relationship occur, however, because of spectral hardening of the polyenergetic X-ray beam, image intensifier gamma, vignetting, and veiling glare, and, for film-based recordings, the characteristic (Hurter-Driffield) curve of film. While a strictly mathematical approach can be used to correct for nonlinearities in the film response under carefully controlled conditions (22), the response of the image intensifier varies temporally with automatic brightness control and spatially during panning over a field heterogenous in tissue thickness, thus rendering a priori correction difficult for cineangiographic systems. The relationship between film gray scale and contrast medium thickness can be calibrated precisely during radiographic exposure, however, by use of a rotating wedge technique (23, 24), wherein sequential steps of a wedge are superimposed during contrast medium injection over a field position of constant tissue thickness, such as lung tissue during held inspiration, and a parametric analysis of wedge step thickness vs. gray scale changes provides a continuous series of calibrations over time. Fortunately, such studies have demonstrated a near-linear relationship between contrast medium thickness and cinefilm gray scale over the central portion of the sigmoidal curve. Thus, errors in use of the assumption of linearity occur primarily at the ends of the gray scale. Linearity should not be assumed, therefore, when performing a densitometric analysis of a large vessel, well filled with contrast medium, particularly when the vessel is foreshortened or overlaps the diaphragm or spine; likewise, a similar analysis of a coronary segment immediately adjacent to over-exposed lung field may be associated with significant error.

Under ideal conditions, densitometric measurement of relative cross-sectional area can provide a measure of percent stenosis which is more accurate than area percent stenosis estimated from diameter measurements (23), even when the lumen is circular. Densitometric measurements in the usual clinical setting, however, are less immune than diameter measurements to the effects of vessel foreshortening, background tissue inhomogeneity, and superimposition of small branches. For highly curved coronary artery segments, an orthogonal view may be required to correct for errors in densitometric measurement of percent area stenosis, when the stenotic and reference segments do not lie within the same plane. Inhomogeneities in background tissue thickness may result in an error in the use of the commonly used assumption (22, 23) that a linear trend in tissue thickness is present between vessel edges. As mentioned previously, multi-frame averaging of densitometric measurements will reduce the magnitude of this error by providing a variable background as a result of vessel motion. At present, the only solution to the problem of superimposition of small branches is careful selection of frames to be analyzed.

Despite such difficulties in obtaining accurate densitometric measurements of luminal cross-sectional area, the effort expended is valuable because many important coronary segments, such as the left main coronary artery, cannot be visualized well in more than one view, and failure to appreciate the severity of an enface plaque may otherwise occur (25). Even when a segment can be well visualized in multiple views, underestimation of lesion severity may occur in the use of diameter measurements alone when lumen geometry is highly irregular. A common example of this problem is the coronary lumen following balloon angioplasty. A shaggy or hazy appearance of the lumen and/or overt evidence of a dissection are found commonly after PTCA, and diameter measurements may greatly underestimate the severity of the residual stenosis (26).

Future directions

Vessel curvature and the presence of overlapping branches are the dominant variables which interfere with both visual and objective analysis of lesion severity from high quality coronary angiograms. A fully three-dimensional description of the coronary vasculature, including lumen cross-sectional area and shape at each position along the vessel centerline, would be quite valuable clinically. The densitometric information present in each view of an angiographic study could theoretically be used to provide projection data for tomographic reconstruction of a lumen crosssection, but conventional CT reconstruction techniques require a large number of views, far greater than that available from a conventional angiographic study. We therefore investigated the potential utility of the MENT (maximum entropy) algorithm developed by Minerbo (27, 28); this algorithm requires only a few views and is less subject to streaking artifacts present in other algebraic reconstruction techniques. Figure 9 illustrates the fidelity of the 3 and 5 view reconstructions of a double lumen phantom when transverse densitometric scans from digitized cine images provided the projection data for the MENT algorithm. These results are encouraging, and the fact that this algorithm has been successfully used to reconstruct defects of individual pins within a to-mographic reconstruction of a crosssection of a 36 pin nuclear reactor core from a small number of views (29) suggests that a similar reconstruction of planes across the myocardium, within which multiple vessels are present, may be possible. Many problems would have to be solved before such clinical application of the MENT algorithm could be realized, including vessel motion, inhomogeneities of blood-contrast medium mixing, and registration of identical points along the centerline in multiple angiographic views to provide reliable sets of projections. Solution to the latter problem will be simultaneously useful for reducing the magnitude of the other two problems by facilitating multi-frame averaging of each densitometric projection.

Automatic recognition of the vessel centerline is an important first step in the registration of equivalent points along the centerline from multiple views and would also have immediate utility in reducing the amount of operator interaction in conventional analysis of vessel morphometric indices. A technique which

120

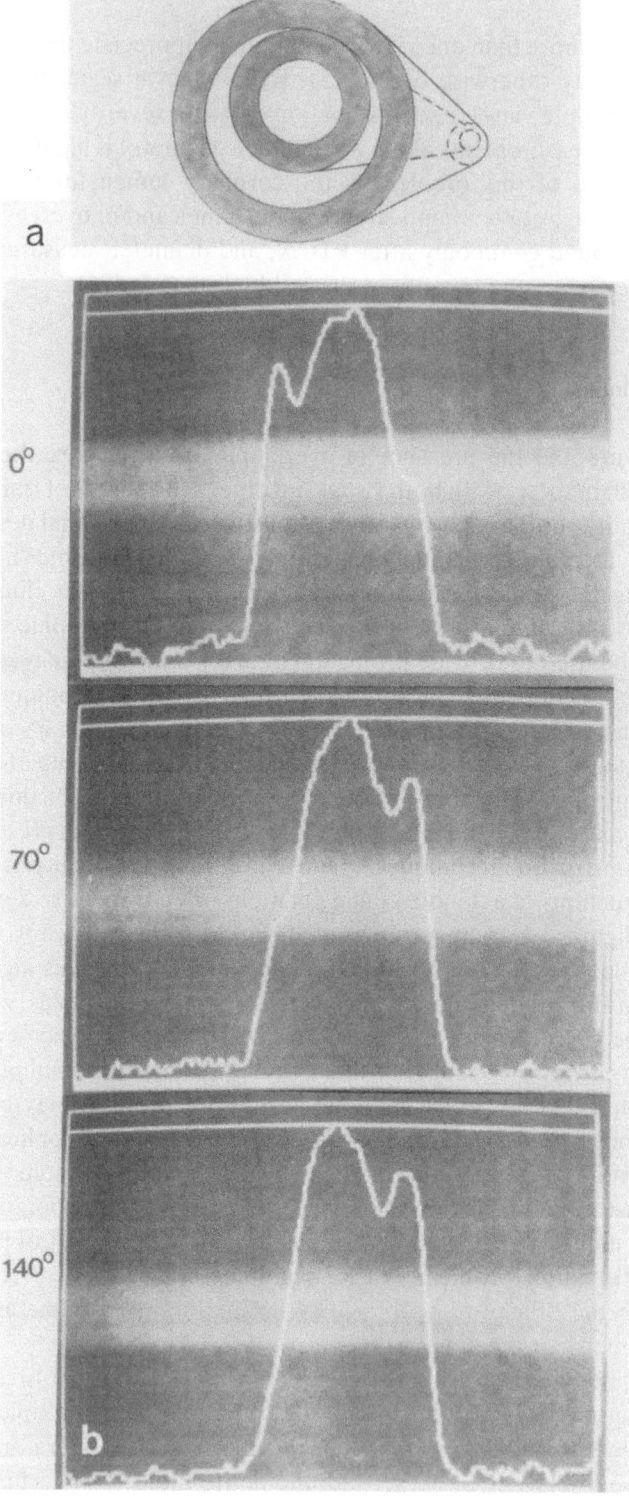

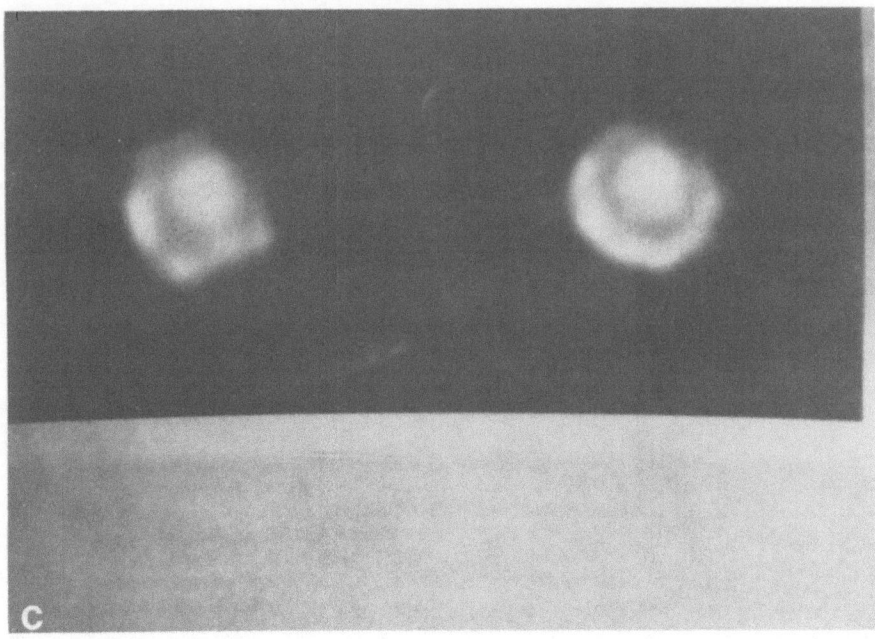

Figure 9a)b)c). MENT reconstruction of double lumen. a) A 3 mm phantom was filled with Re-nografin-76 to provide a circular lumen eccentrically located within a crescent-shaped lumen to simulate the complex lumen geometry frequently seen after PTCA. b) Transverse densitometric scans (perpendicular to the vessel long axis) are shown superimposed over each cineframe from each radiographic view used to provide projection data. c) Three (left) and five (right) view MENT reconstructions of the lumen crosssection are shown. Reproduced with permission from Spears *et al.* (28).

shows promise in this regard was developed by M.A. Fischler *et al.* (30), who described an algorithm for extraction of linear features from a wide variety of scenes. We have successfully applied this algorithm to coronary angiograms as illustrated in Figure 10. The algorithm has been incorporated in our vessel edge tracking programs, and vessel diameter and area analysis may be initiated solely by the operator indicating the proximal and distal ends of a vessel segment of interest without the need for further operator interaction. The centerline was previously found as the midpoint between detected edges, and since the latter have a much lower signal-to-noise ratio than the vessel long axis, fewer errors in centerline recognition now occur in the presence of increased noise such as from adjacent branches, high grade stenoses, and vessel tortuosity. In the future, pattern recognition techniques could be applied to the delineated centerlines throughout an angiographic field for completely automatic recognition and analysis of coronary luminal images.

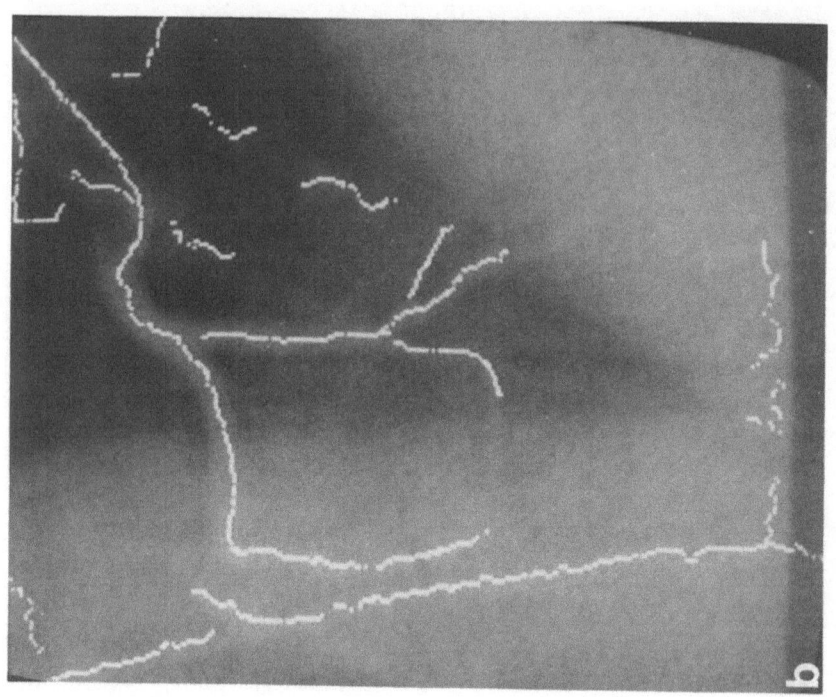

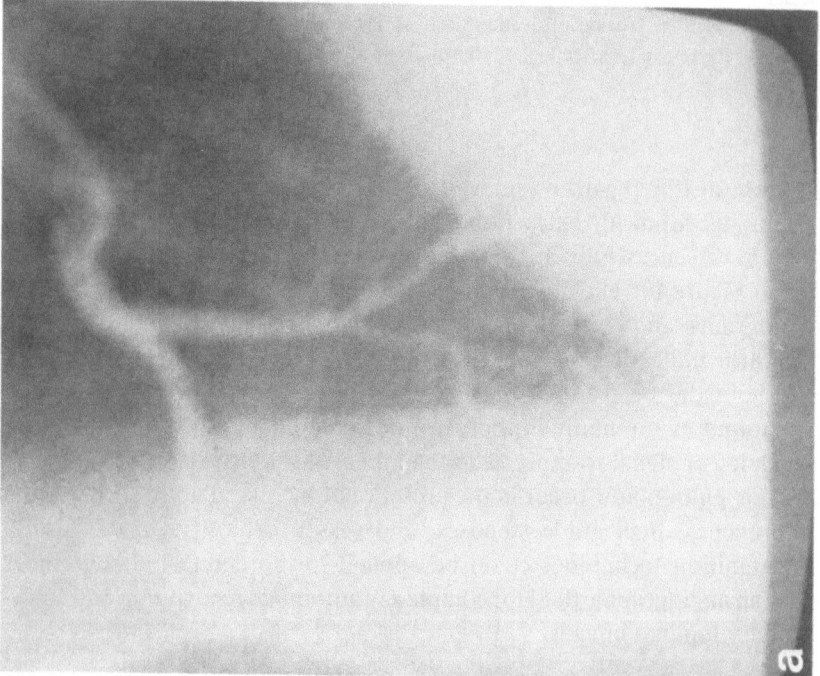

Figure 10. Automatic recognition of vessel centerline. Application of a linear feature extraction algorithm developed by Fischler *et al.* (29) to digitized coronary cineframes (a) allows delineation of the centerline of all major coronary branches, (b) as illustrated in digitized cineframe of LAO view of left coronary artery.

Acknowledgement

The authors are indebted to Carol Anne Centauro for expert preparation of the manuscript.

References

1. Sones FM, Shirey EK: Cine coronary arteriography. Modern Concepts of Cardiovasc Disease 31, 1962: 735–738.
2. Virmani R, Chan PKC, Goldstein RE, Robinowitz M, McAllister HA: Acute takeoffs of the coronary arteries along the aortic wall and congenital coronary ostial valve-like ridges: association with sudden death. JACC 3, 1984: 766–771.
3. Spears JR, Sandor T, Baim DS, Paulin S: The minimum error in estimating coronary luminal cross-sectional area from cineangiographic diameter measurements. Cathet Cardiovasc Diagn 9, 1983: 119–128.
4. Crawford DW, Beckenbach ES, Blankenhorn DH, Selzer RH, Brooks SH: Grading of coronary atherosclerosis. Atherosclerosis 19, 1974: 231–241.
5. Selzer RH, Blankenhorn DH, Crawford DW, Brooks SH, Barndt R Jr: Computer analysis of cardiovascular imagery. Proceedings of the Caltech/JPL Conference on Image Processing Technology, Data Sources and Software for Commercial and Scientific Applications. Pasadena, Nov. 3–5, 1976: 1–20.
6. Brown BG, Bolson E, Frimer M, Dodge HT: Quantitative coronary arteriography. Estimation of dimensions, hemodynamic resistance, and atheroma mass of coronary artery lesions using the arteriogram and digital computation. Circulation 55, 1977: 329–337.
7. Crawford DW, Brooks SH, Selzer RH, Barndt R, Beckenbach ES, Blankenhorn DH: Computer densitometry for angiographic assessment of arterial cholesterol content and gross pathology in human atherosclerosis. J Lab Clin Med 89, 1977: 378–392.
8. Sandor T, Als AV, Paulin S: Cine-densitometric measurement of coronary arterial stenoses. Cathet Cardiovasc Diagn 5, 1979: 229–245.
9. Booman F, Reiber JHC, Gerbrands JJ, Slager CJ, Schuurbiers JCH, Meester GT: Quantitative analysis of coronary occlusions from cine-angiograms. Comput Cardiol 1979: 177–179.
10. Reiber JHC, Gerbrands JJ, Booman F, Troost GJ, Boer A den, Slager CJ, Schuurbiers JCH: Objective characterization of coronary obstructions from monoplane cineangiograms and three-dimensional reconstruction of an arterial segment from orthogonal views. In: Applications of Computers in Medicine, MD Schwartz (Ed). IEEE Cat No TH0095-0, 1982: 93–100.
11. Sanders WJ, Alderman EL, Harrison DC: Coronary artery quantification using digital imaging processing techniques. Comput Cardiol, 1979: 15–19.
12. Kirkeeide RL, Fung P, Smalling RW, Gould KL: Automated evaluation of vessel diameter from arteriograms. Comput Cardiol 1982, 215–218.
13. Spears JR, Sandor T, Als A, Malagold M, Markis J, Paulin S: Accuracy of computer vs. visual measurement of vessel diameter from cineangiograms. Circulation 64, 1981: 130 (Abstract).
14. Spears JR, Sandor T, Als AV, Malagold M, Markis JE, Grossman W, Serur JR, Paulin S: Computerized image analysis for quantitative measurement of vessel diameter from cineangiograms. Circulation 68, 1983: 453–461.
15. Siebes M, Gottwik M, Schlepper M: Qualitative and quantitative experimental studies on the evaluation of model coronary arteries from angiograms. Comput Cardiol 1982: 211–214.
16. Nichols AB, Gabrieli CFO, Fenoglio JJ, Esser PD: Quantification of relative coronary arterial stenosis by cinevideodensitometric analysis of coronary arteriograms. Circulation 69, 1984: 512–522.

17. Sandor T, Spears JR, Paulin S: Densitometric determination of changes in the dimensions of coronary arteries. Proc Conf Digital Radiography, SPIE 314, 1981: 263–272.

18. Barger AC, Beewkes R III, Lainey LL, Silverman KJ: Hypothesis: vasa vasorum and neo-vascularization of human coronary arteries. A possible role in the pathophysiology of atherosclerosis. N Engl J Med 310, 1984: 175–177.

19. Spears JR, Sacks FM, Arvidson E, Sandor T, Paulin S: Reproducibility of computer assessment of coronary lesion severity between angiographic studies. Circulation 68 (Suppl III), 1983: III–43.

20. Sandor T, Spears JR: Statistical considerations on the precision of assessing blood vessel diameter in cine coronary angiography. Comp Biomed Res (in press 1985).

21. Spears JR, Crawford DW, Serur J, Grossman W, Paulin S: A catheterization technique for reproduction of human atherosclerotic lumen within the dog coronary artery in-vivo. Cath Cardiovasc Diagn 9, 1983: 219–229.

22. Crawford DW, Brooks SH, Barndt R Jr, Blankenhorn DH: Measurement of atherosclerotic luminal irregularity and obstruction by radiographic densitometry. Invest Radiol 12, 1977: 307–313.

23. Sprears JR: Rotating step wedge technique for extraction of luminal cross-sectional area information from single plane coronary cineangiograms. Acta Radiologica Diag 22, 1981: 217–225.

24. Spears JR, Sandor T, Serur J, Paulin S: Computer aided densitometric evaluation of coronary cineangiograms. In: Radiological Functional Analysis of the Vascular System. Heuck HW (Ed). Springer-Verlag, New York 1983: 195–206.

25. Isner JM, Kishel J, Kent KM, Ronan JA, Jr, Ross AM, Roberts WC: Accuracy of angiographic determination of left main coronary arterial narrowing. Circulation 63, 1981: 1056–1064.

26. Serruys PW, Reiber JHC, Wijus W, Brand M, Koojman CG, Katen H, Hugenholtz PG: Assessment of percutaneous transluminal coronary angioplasty by quantitative coronary angiography: Diameter versus densitometric area measurements. Am J Cardiol 54, 1984: 482–488.

27. Minerbo G. MENT: A maximum entrophy algorithm for reconstructing a source from projection data. Comput Graph Image Proc, vol. 10, 1979: 48–68.

28. Spears JR, Sandor T, Kruger R, Hanlon W, Paulin S, Minerbo G: Computer reconstruction of luminal cross-sectional shape from multiple cineangiographic views. IEEE Trans Med Imag MI-2, 1983: 49–54.

29. Sanderson JG: Reconstruction of fuel pin bundles by a maximum entropy method. IEEE Trans Nucl Sci, NS–26, 1979: 2685–2686.

30. Fischler MA, Tenenbaum JM, Wolf HC: Detection of roads and linear structures in low-resolution aerial imagery using a multisource knowledge integration technique. Comput Graph Image Proc 15, 1981: 201–223.

31. Gould KL: Quantification of coronary artery stenosis in vivo. Circ. Res 57, 1985: 342–353.

A second look at quantitative coronary angiography: some unexpected problems

Robert H. Selzer, A. Shircore, P.L. Lee, L. Hemphill and D.H. Blankenhorn

Summary

There are currently more than ten research groups, including ours at JPL and USC, that are developing computer methods to quantify atherosclerosis from cineangiograms. There are variations in equipment and algorithms employed by the various groups but results in terms of accuracy and precision have been roughly similar. In the past six months, we have been investigating several sources of measurement variability that have received relatively little attention, but which we believe could cause significant errors if ignored. For example, we have observed substantial variability in the measurement of arterial dimensions due to vessel pulsation and to mixing artifacts of the radio-opaque contrast. The problems appear solvable but the solutions may create new problems by making the measurements more difficult and time consuming.

Introduction

A number of investigators have been working since 1977, on the development of automated techniques to quantify atherosclerosis (1–11). These include a method jointly developed by the Jet Propulsion Laboratory and the University of Southern California. The method is intended to assess changes in arterial disease of individuals in a clinical intervention trial designed to lower blood cholesterol. Each subject in the trial receives a coronary angiogram at the beginning of the study and one after 24 months. The angiographic conditions are kept as constant as possible to maintain exposure angles and other factors the same in the two films. Computer analysis involves digitization of the angiographic film frames, computer detection of the arterial boundaries and measurement of relative stenosis from the detected edges. Both native coronary arteries and bypass grafts are analyzed.

As originally planned, the first step in the processing sequence to assess change for a particular coronary segment was to locate end-diastolic frames on each angiogram showing the target segment in a matched view. In a test of the method, the process of matching end-diastolic frames was found to be more difficult than anticipated and as discussed below, the procedure was modified to allow segment matching with frames corresponding to other parts of the heart cycle. This solved the original problem (of finding matched frames), but raised the question of the effects of cyclic changes in the film image on measurement accuracy and precision.

To determine these effects, a study was carried out involving measurement of stenosis throughout the heart cycle for selected arterial segments. As a result of this study, a question arose concerning the effect of contrast wash-in and wash-out on the lumen measurements. This topic is also addressed in this chapter. Finally, a related problem of the effect of mixing artifacts on stenosis measurement is discussed and a possible solution to the problem described.

The problem

As previously mentioned, the computer measurement of coronary stenosis described in this paper is designed to detect possible effects of a cholesterol-lowering therapy on coronary atherosclerosis. Since atherosclerosis typically changes only one or two percent a year, it is important that the variability of the change detection method be low. Otherwise, the number of subjects that must be studied to reliably detect a treatment effect becomes large. As an example, in an earlier study (12), it was shown that for a one-year clinical trial with expected treatment effect of 2% per year, test significance level of 5% and power of 90%, a change in measurement precision from 2% to 4% (or from 4% to 6%) would require a 50% increase in subjects to be tested.

In a study of computerized stenosis variability (11), it became clear that a significant increase in precision could be obtained by measuring stenosis on several sequential frames and averaging the results. In that study, 3 to 5 frames were selected as the number to be processed and frames were chosen from the portion of the cinefilm corresponding to end-diastole, since the arteries have minimal curvature at this point and relative frame-to-frame movement of the arterial image is minimal.

End-diastolic frames suitable for processing are frequently not available. The most common problem is obscuration of the edges of the target artery segment by overlapping branches or other arteries and occasionally the end-diastolic frames are not uniformly opacified. Parenthetically, for large diameter bypass grafts, perfusion artifacts occur on film throughout the heart cycle. A possible solution to this problem is discussed later in the chapter.

Relaxation of the requirement to process only end-diastolic frames solves the problem of finding the target artery image clear of interferring shadows in most cases (some artery segments cannot be computer-processed under any conditions and must be analyzed by other means). However, consideration must now be given to the effects, if any, of cyclic phenomena such as arterial pulsation, on stenosis measurements.

If arterial dimensions undergo significant cyclic variations, the measurement of absolute stenosis is clearly dependent on the relative location within the cardiac cycle of the frame analyzed. The picture is not clear for relative stenosis measurement. In addition, the magnitude of effect of atherosclerosis on wall pulsation is not known. Furthermore, differences in pulsation response among different arteries may exist because of architectural differences such as the depth of the artery in the myocardium.

An argument can be made that to measure relative stenosis change over time, pulsation effects can be ignored as long as frames to be analyzed are selected from the *same* point in the cardiac cycles in each film. To some extent this is true, but if the cyclic changes in vessel measured diameter are large, the measured percent *change* in stenosis will still be phase dependent.

For some films studied, a low frequency trend in measured vessel diameter over a period of several cardiac cycles was detected that was not visually apparent to the eye. The vessel appeared uniformly opacified for two or three cardiac cycles after the wash-in period seemed complete and before contrast wash-out could be visually detected, but a gradual change in diameter was measured.

It is not clear if these trends represent real changes in arterial diameter (a reactive hyperemic response) or the response of the edge tracking process to changes in optical film density associated with variation in iodine concentration. To some extent, the reason for the changes are not important. Rather, it must be determined if the magnitude of the diameter change is significant and if so, can a correction be applied to minimize the variable effects of cycle selection.

The questions addressed by the study are the following:

For relative or absolute stenosis,

(1) What is the magnitude of measurement error due to random frame selection relative to the cardiac phase and,

(2) What is the magnitude of measurement variability due to low frequency diameter trend?

In this chapter, a description is given of the image processing hardware and software used for the coronary analysis and the method and results of the multi-frame processing study are discussed. In addition, a method to compensate for mixing artifacts in bypass grafts is described.

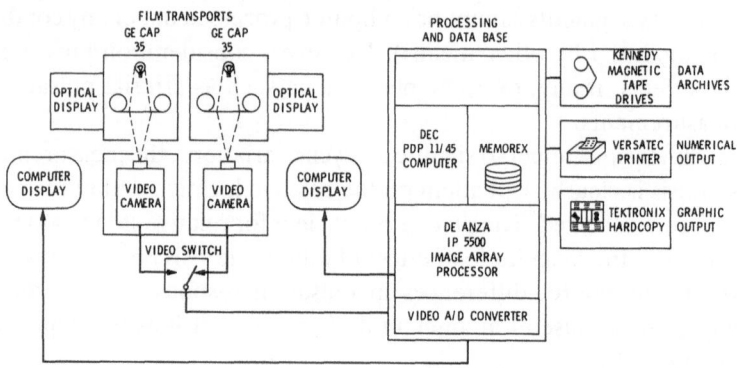

Figure 1. Image processing system used to quantify coronary stenosis.

Image processing system

A dedicated computer system at the Jet Propulsion Laboratory was utilized for the sequential frame analysis described in this chapter. This system includes a DEC PDP 11/45 computer, a De Anza IP5500 Image Array Processor, an interactive picture display system and a computer controlled Vanguard film transport in which the optical projection system has been removed and replaced with a vidicon TV camera/digitizer. A three-position turret lens provides magnifications of 1.0, 2.5, and 3.7 between the film and vidicon. At 1× magnification, the image of a 20 mm by 20 mm area of film is digitized into a 512 × 480 array of intensity values between 0 and 255. The effective 'horizontal' sample spacing at the film plane with 1× magnification is thus 20/512 = .0391 mm/pixel or 39.1 microns. The equivalent sample spacing at 2.5× and 3.7× is 15.6 microns and 10.6 microns, respectively. Magnification is selected to assure that a vessel to be analyzed is sampled from 30 to 50 times at each cross-section.

This system has been recently modified to utilize a pair of GE CAP 35 projectors instead of the single Vanguard M35C projector. We have found that the process of finding matching views of a vessel segment in two cineangiograms virtually *requires* simultaneous viewing of both films. A block diagram of the image processing system is shown in Figure 1.

Frame selection and digitizing

In the initial processing step, an operator views the cine film and searches for film frames in which each arterial segment is uniformly perfused, free of overlapping vessel images and roughly parallel to the imaging plane. Magnification is selected, the segment centered in the viewing area of the TV camera and the image digitized. To minimize video noise effects, each frame is digitized 16 times and the average is taken. Total time for digitizing is approximately one second.

Vessel tracking

The initial steps of the processing sequence after frame selection and digitizing are illustrated in Figure 2.
a.   illustrates the unmagnified image viewed during frame selection.
b.   shows the 2.5× optically magnified image used for analysis.
c.   illustrates operator selection of a segment with a cursor at a series of points along the vessel's centerline.

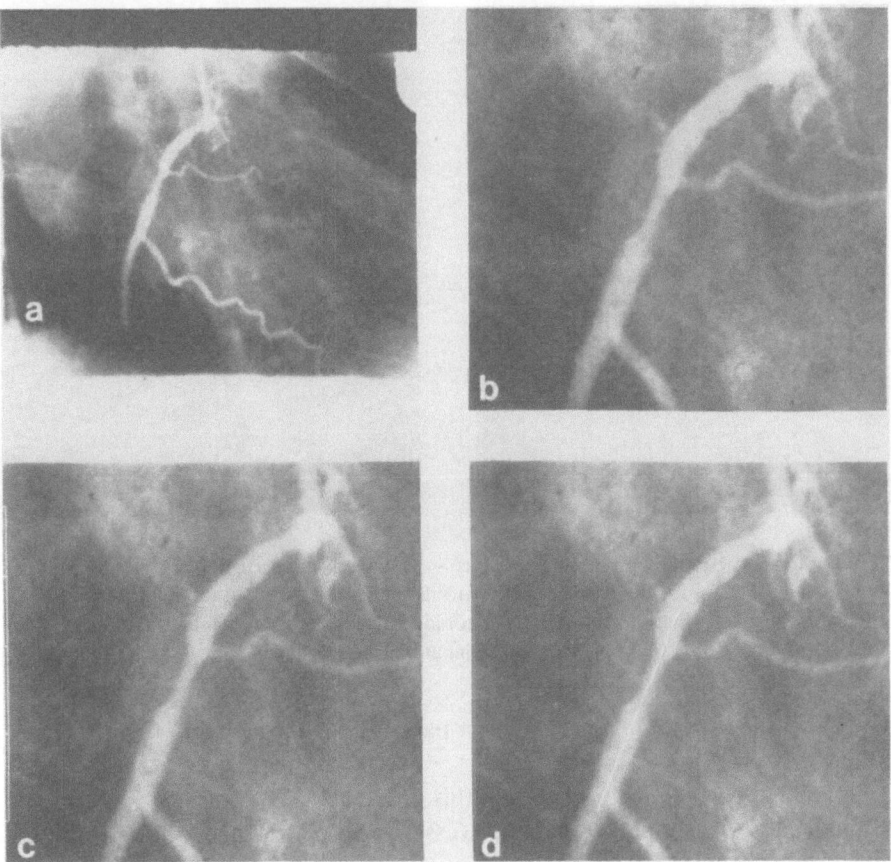

Figure 2. Current coronary processing sequence. (*Upper left*) Monitor image of entire frame. Magnification from film to TV input is 1.0×. (*Upper right*) After 2.5× magnification. (*Lower left*) Illustration of operator identification of vessel midpoints. Computer drawn midline curve, first pass (*Lower right*).

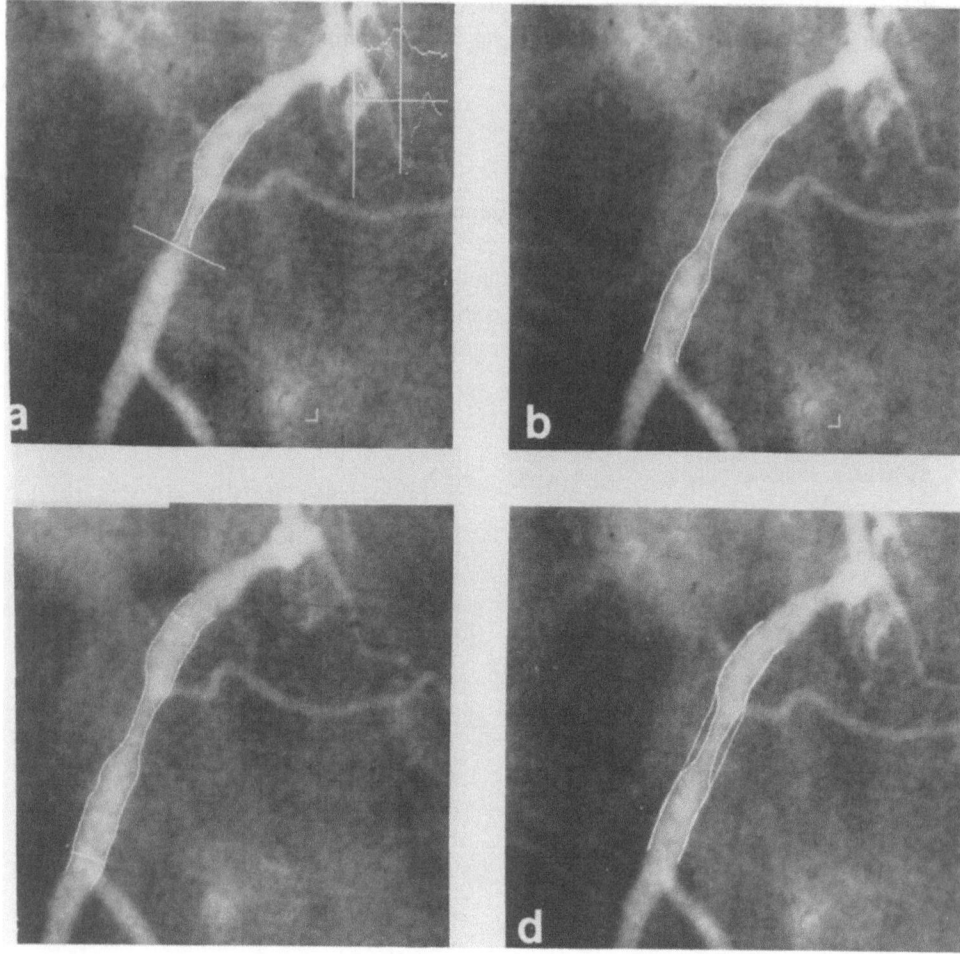

Figure 3. Current coronary processing sequence – continued. (*Upper left*) Partial edge tracking. Intensity and gradient for the most recently detected edges are shown to the right. (*Upper right*) Complete segment tracking. (*Lower left*) Operator identification of segment limits for measurements of lesions.(*Lower right*) After application of computer reference lumen.

d. shows the computer generated first-pass midline through the cursor-selected points.

Figure 3 shows the further steps in this process:

a. indicates the computer search for vessel edges perpendicular to the midline. Edges are selected as the points of maximum positive and negative gradient which is computed from the vessel intensity values by a second degree polynomial curve fitting algorithm. The profile and gradient curves for one processed line are shown in this figure.

The number of points used to compute the gradient varies from 7 to 13, depending on the measured average of the three previous diameters, and decreases as the vessel narrows. If this is not done, the diameter of narrow vessel sections is consistently overestimated because of the poor fit of the second degree polynomial to the vessel profile. The computed gradient values are smoothed over three to seven points and an exponential weighting function, centered at the prior edge location is applied to the smoothed gradient values before selection of the maximum and minimum values. The number of points smoothed varies in a manner similar to the variation of the gradient polynomial. The purpose of the weighting function is to discriminate against false gradient values from other vessel images close to the vessel being tracked.

b. shows the completed edge tracking. A second-pass midline is generated from the detected edges and the edge search repeated with the new midline. The purpose of the second pass is to minimize edge detection variability associated with operator selection of vessel midpoints.

c. indicates selection by the operator of proximal and distal limits of the segment.

d. shows the computer reference lumen which parallels the second-pass midline and has width equal to the 90th percentile of the segment diameters. This 90th percentile value, described below, represents the computer estimate of the pre-disease lumen width.

Figure 4 illustrates $D(3)$ and $D(90)$, the quantities used to represent the minimum and 'normal' vessel diameters, respectively, in the stenosis computation. $D(3)$ is the value of the 3rd percentile of the diameter plot and $D(90)$ is the value of the 90th percentile point.

The catheter image is also tracked to determine the scale factor to convert vessel diameter in picture elements to millimeters.

A rectangular grid with curves spaced one centimeter apart is radiographed and recorded with each cine film. The current version of the coronary measurement software locates the vertices of this grid image, computes the geometric distortion in the image and applies a correction to the frame being processed. This will also compensate for the difference in pixel to mm conversion in the horizontal and vertical directions. However, at the time of the sequential frame processing described in this paper, this correction was not in use but as previously described, an attempt was made to select segments for processing that were recorded in the low-distortion central part of the frame.

Tracking errors due to incompete contrast mixing

As previously indicated, edge tracking errors due to incomplete contrast mixture have been encountered, particularly with large diameter bypass grafts. This is illustrated in Figure 5. The upper images are unprocessed sequential frames of an

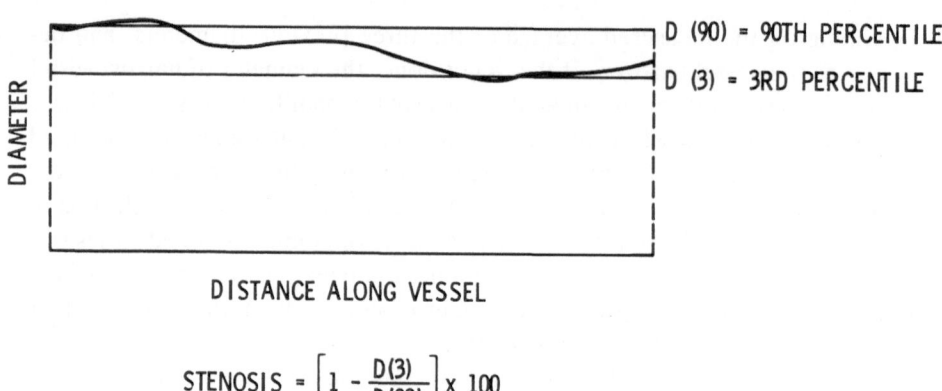

$$\text{STENOSIS} = \left[1 - \frac{D(3)}{D(90)}\right] \times 100$$

Figure 4. Definition of computed stenosis.

opacified bypass graft, while the lower images show the detected edges. Note the incomplete filling area indicated by the arrow in the upper left image which creates a false 'lesion' as shown in the detected edges.

If such an artifact is isolated and transient, bad frames can be skipped in favor of others where opacification is uniform. In some cases, however, all frames have artifacts. Figure 6 shows the diameter profiles of five sequential frames of this graft, which indicates nonuniform opacification in all frames.

An improved diameter profile of this vessel is obtained if the individual profiles are averaged but this still produces an erroneous result because the effects of a large defect will be reflected in the average profile. A better approach is to derive a composite profile whose value at each point is the maximum of the input values.

This algorithm has been implemented and the composite 'maximum' profile for the case shown in Figure 7. Before the composite was generated, profiles 2–5 were registered with profile 1 by translating each profile to the point which minimized the sum of the absolute differences.

This approach assumes that tracking errors only result in false vessel narrowing. A better approach that avoids this assumption and also improves the signal-to-noise ratio of the composite vessels is to examine the input diameters at each point, throw out the one or two lowest values and average the rest.

Sequential frame tracking

To minimize operator intervention, the vessel tracking programs have been modified to analyze a sequence of cineframes automatically. The first frame of a sequence is processed as described above with the operator minimally indicating the vessel midline points and the proximal and distal limits of the segment to be

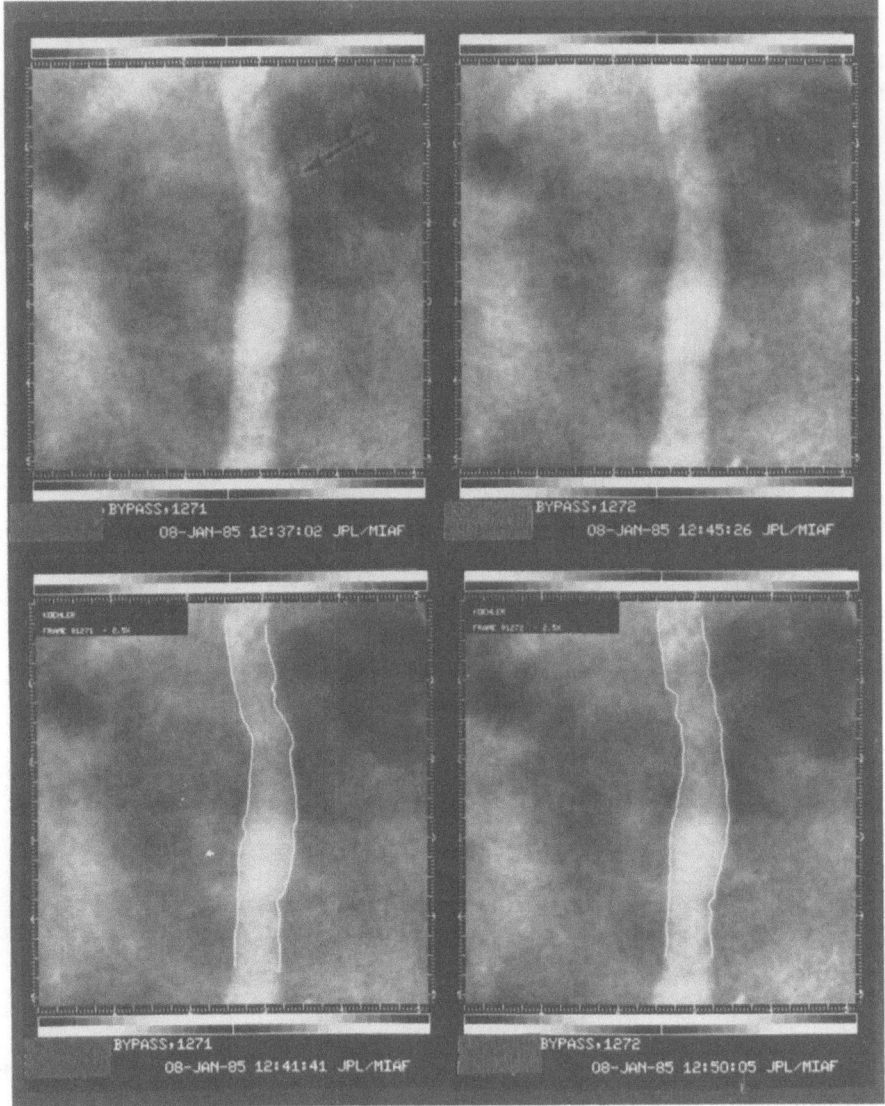

Figure 5. Sequential frames of bypass graft (upper), showing contrast filling artifact (arrow) and effect on edges (lower).

processed. After processing of the first frame is complete, the program retrieves the next sequential frame from disk memory and begins tracking by searching for edges along lines perpendicular to the computed midline of the first frame.

The relative position of the first detected edges along the vessel segment is kept constant by aligning each frame to a common landmark such as a nearby vessel

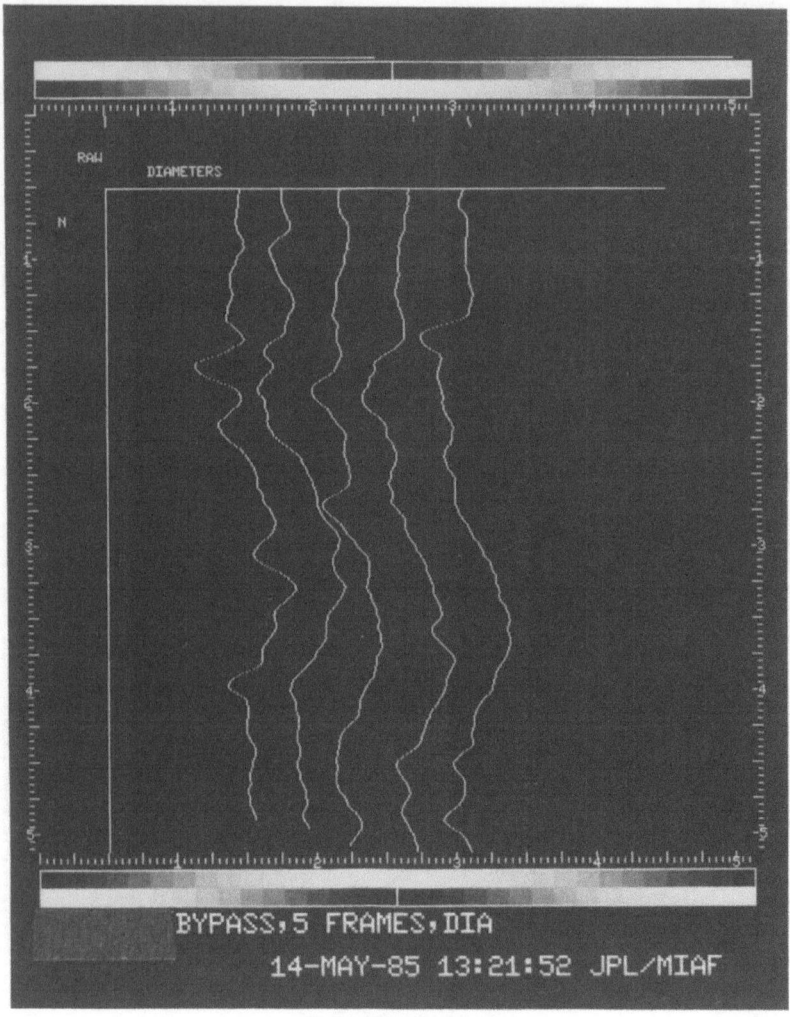

Figure 6. Diameter profiles for five sequential frames of bypass graft. Profiles are offset from each other.

bifurcation before digitization. When this is done, the segment to be analyzed appears in a nearly fixed position in the digitized frame sequence. An example of tracked edges for a right coronary artery of subject R is shown in Figure 8. In this case, the small branch above the tracked segment was used to register the images.

For each of the 100 to 140 frames in each sequence, the quantities D(3), D(90), average diameter and percent stenosis were calculated and plotted. In addition, the mean, standard deviation, linear regression line and standard-error-of-the-estimate (SEE) were computed.

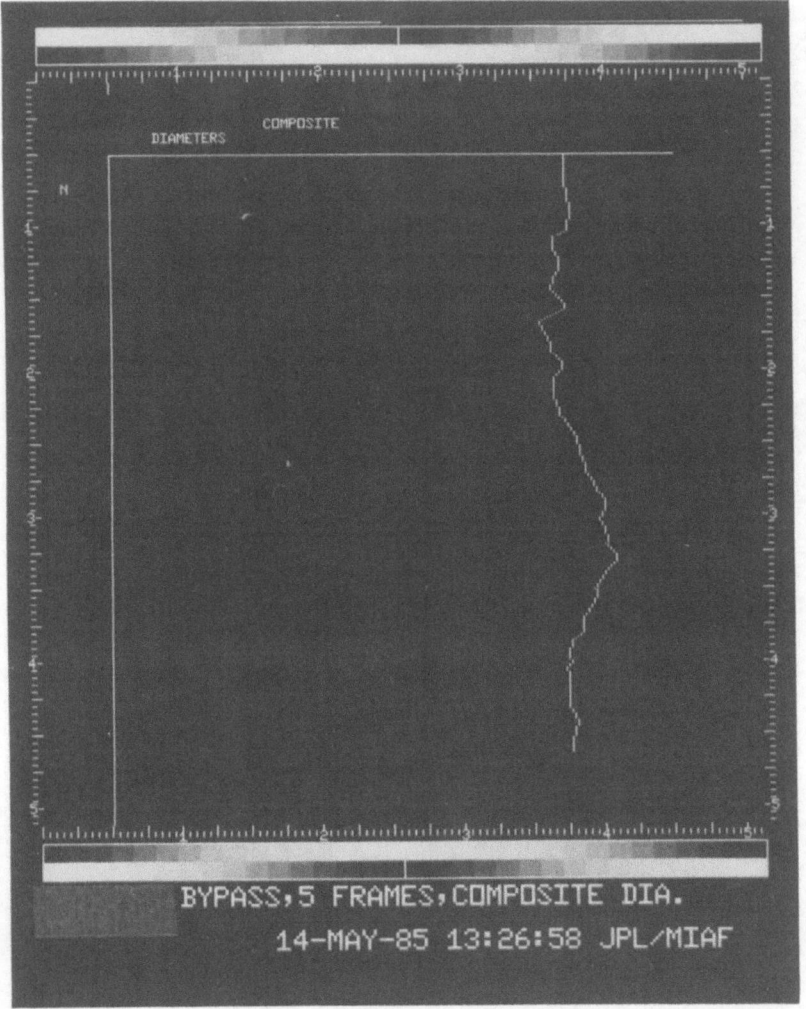

Figure 7. Composite diameter profile derived from data shown in Figure 6. Each point in the composite curve is the maximum of five corresponding input points. Profiles in Figure 6 were registered to each other before composite was derived.

Segment selection

Segments were selected for processing only if the following criteria were met:

1. The vessel segment visually appeared to be uniformly opacified for at least two complete heart cycles.
2. Segments were recorded within an area that approximately corresponds to

136

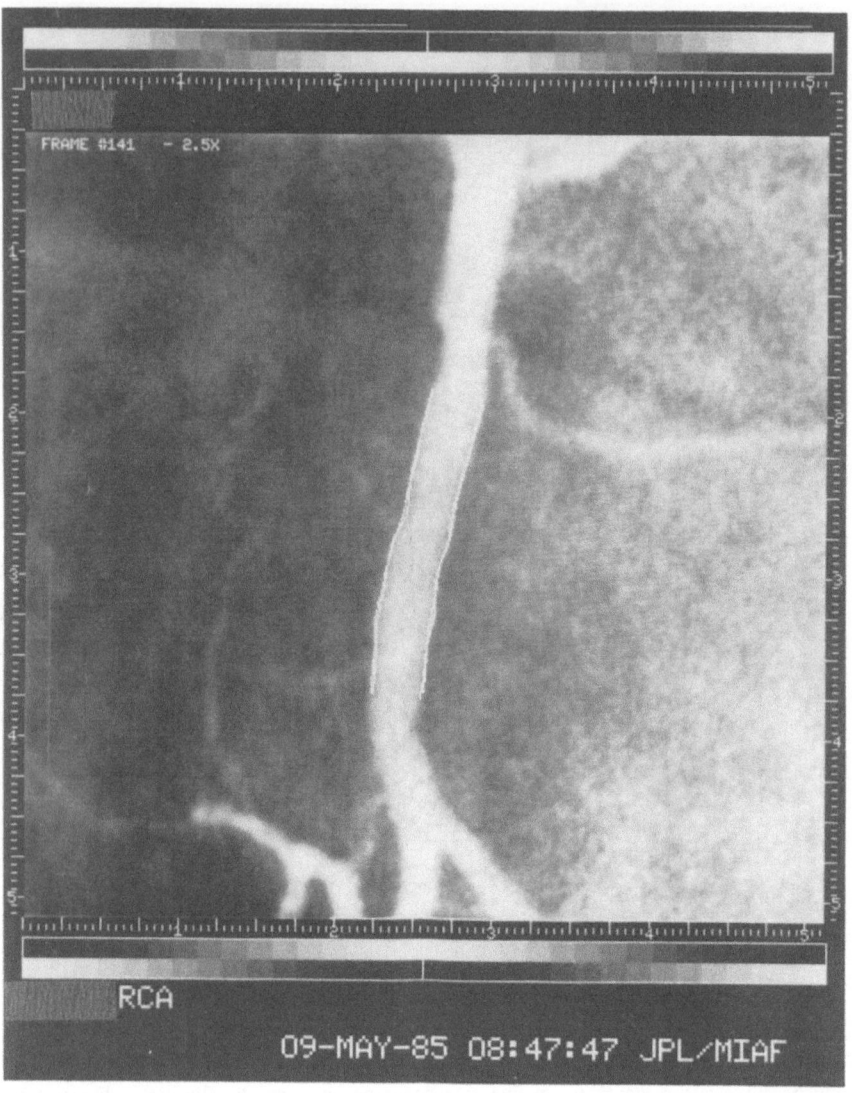

FRAME #141   - 2.5X

RCA

09-MAY-85 08:47:47 JPL/MIAF

Figure 8. Example of a tracked right coronary artery from the sequential frame analysis for subject R.

the central 50% of the image intensifier.

3.   Segments were free of branches or overlapping vessel shadows that might interfere with the edge tracking process.

Processing was applied to nine frame sequences which as shown in Table 1, includes examples of the left, right and circumflex arteries and right and left bypass grafts. Each segment was tracked through at least two complete cardiac cycles and in some cases for three.

The plots of D(3), D(90), average diameter and percent stenosis for the circumflex artery segment of subject T are shown in Figure 9. As can be seen from the marked end-diastolic (ED) and end-systolic (ES) frames, the 140 frames processed covered more than three complete cardiac cycles. Figure 10 shows the result of smoothing the data in Figure 9 with a five point averaging filter. Note that on the smoothed plots, a possible periodic effect and a slight negative linear trend has become apparent in the D(90) and stenosis plots. This was not a consistent pattern. In the case of subject M, the trend in D(90) was positive as shown in Figure 11.

To quantify trend, the slope of the linear regression line was computed for each plot as shown in Table 2. For diameters, these values are expressed in units of millimeters per cardiac cycle and for stenoses the slope values are in units of percent per cardiac cycle.

A degree of periodicity was usually detected in the average diameter and in D(90), but not consistently in D(3) or stenosis. An example is shown for subject GO in Figure 12.

The effect of periodic changes in the vessel image size on diameter and stenosis measurements is summarized in Tables 3 & 4. In Table 3, the standard deviation of the diameter values and stenosis are shown. Diameters are expressed in units of microns and stenosis in percent. Table 4 shows the standard error of the estimate which is defined as the square root of the residual variance of each quantity after the effects of linear trend have been subtracted.

Table 1. Vessel sequences processed.

Subject Vessel	GO LAD	T CXA	R RCA	B CXA	GU RT graft	D Left graft	M Left graft	S LAD	N RCA
Frames processed	92	140	140	120	143	139	135	120	110
Frames/cardiac cycle	39	40	43	37	43	54	66	60	53
Complete cycles	2.4	3.5	3.3	3.2	3.3	2.6	2.1	2.0	2.1
Approximate stenosis %	25	23	20	32	10	10	12	48	53

138

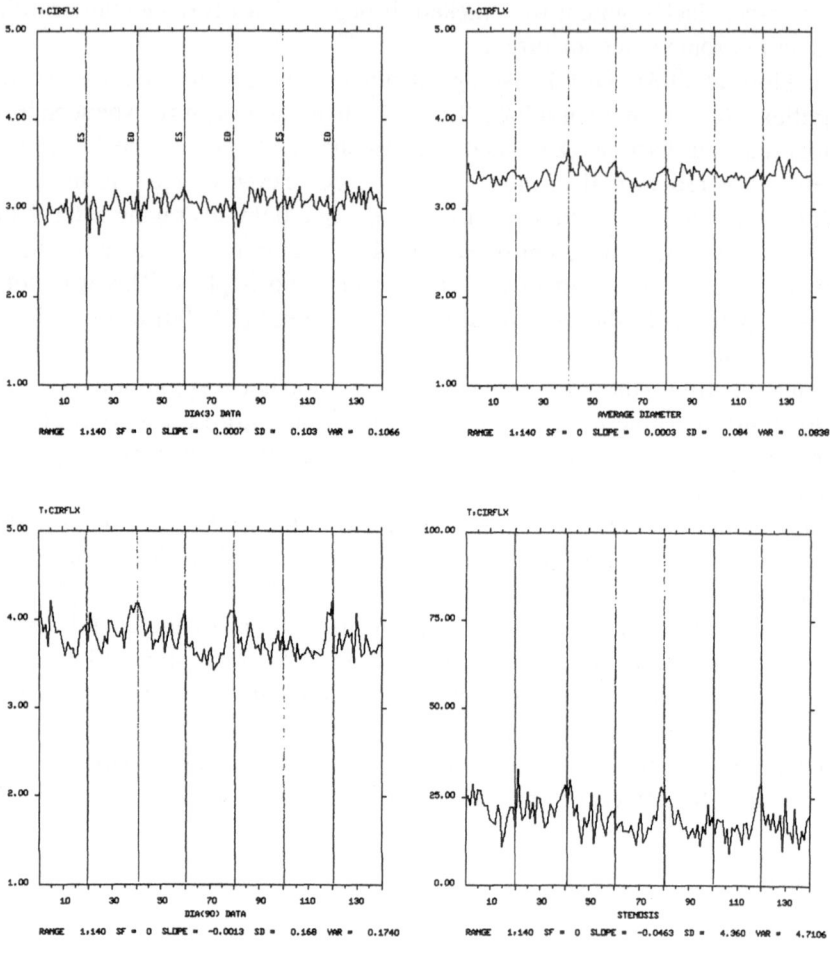

Figure 9. Subject T, circumflex artery. D3, average diameter, D90, stenosis, 5 points smoothing.

Discussion

The original intent of this study was to estimate the measurement variability for stenosis and diameter which will result from quasi-random frame selection. This is, if frames cannot be selected from a fixed point of the cardiac cycle such as end-diastole, how important are cyclic changes in the arterial images on the measurements. Cyclic effects on the image can be caused by pulsation, changes in the position of the arterial image relative to the field of the image intensifier and changes in three-dimensional orientation of the artery. In addition, there are slower cycle-to-cycle changes in the images associated with contrast material

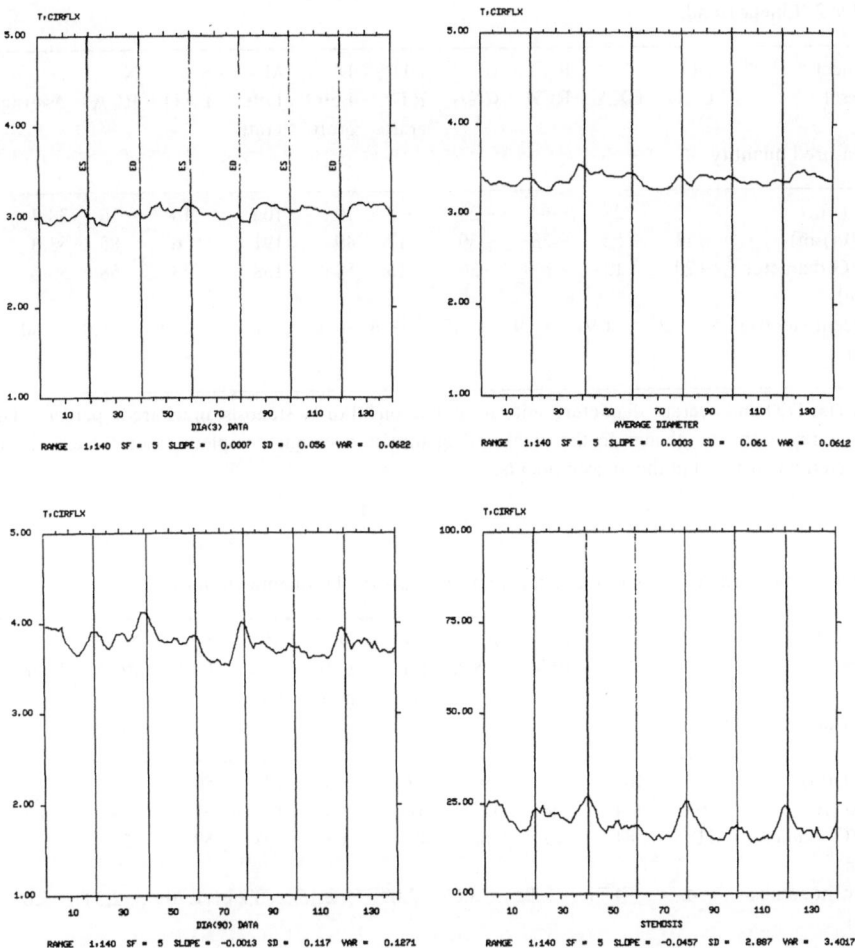

Figure 10. Subject T, Circumflex artery. D3, average diameter, D90, and stenosis, 5 points smoothing.

infusion and wash-out, possible changes in diameter due to reactive hyperemia and perhaps even subtle changes in image intensity due to the response of the automatic gain control to the cumulative amount of infused contrast material.

Studies of nine vessels obviously cannot provide a definitive answer to these questions of measurement variability. However, some general observations can be made. The average measured diameter change due to cycle-to-cycle trend is approximately 50 microns, while average percent stenosis change is 0.8. These are relatively small changes that will be difficult to detect and correct. Procedures may have to be employed in serial film comparison to match films relative to the time since contrast injection.

Table 2. Linear trend.

Subject Vessel Measured quantity	GO LAD	T CXA	R RCA	B CXA	GU RT graft	D Left graft	M Left graft	S LAD	N RCA	Average
D3 (μm)	− 16	28	− 64	− 26	− 4	70	106	− 18	− 16	38.7
D90 (μm)	− 12	− 52	− 38	− 30	− 17	49	191	6	85	53.3
AVG diameter (μm)	− 20	12	− 52	− 30	− 13	54	138	− 78	58	50.6
Percent stenosis (%)	.2	− 1.9	.9	.2	− .4	− .7	1.4	.5	1.0	.80

For D3, D90 and average diameter, units are in microns. For % stenosis, units are in percent. The values represent the change in the measured quantities over one complete cardiac cycle due to detected linear trend in the measurements.

Table 3. Standard deviation of diameters and stenosis for all sequential frames.

Subject Vessel Measured quantity	GO LAD	T CXA	R RCA	B CXA	GU RT graft	D Left graft	M Left graft	S LAD	N RCA	Average
D3 (μm)	138	107	115	97	59	106	133	50	97	100.2
D90 (μm)	106	174	88	125	67	60	141	67	123	105.7
AVG diameter (μm)	112	84	67	68	49	68	97	59	59	73.7
Percent stenosis (%)	4.1	4.71	2.91	3.66	2.09	2.15	3.28	1.70	2.54	3.02

Table 4. Standard error-of-the-estimate of diameters and stenoses for all sequential frames.

Subject Vessel Measured quantity	GO LAD	T CXA	R RCA	B CXA	GU RT graft	D Left graft	M Left graft	S LAD	N RCA	Average
D3 (μm)	138	103	145	95	59	92	118	49	97	95.1
D90 (μm)	106	168	84	123	66	59	87	68	113	97.2
AVG diameter (μm)	112	84	53	62	49	56	53	38	48	61.8
Percent stenosis (%)	4.1	4.36	2.86	3.69	2.09	2.09	3.22	1.68		2.49	2.96

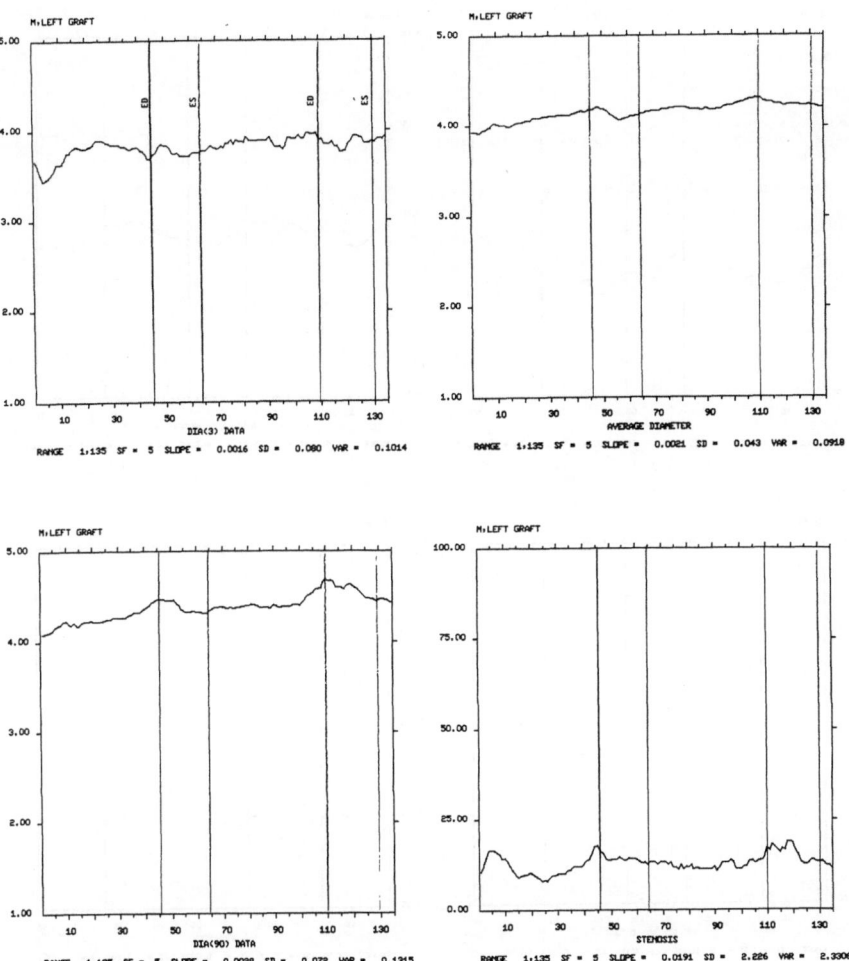

Figure 11. Subject M, left graft. D3, average diameter, D90, percent stenosis, 5 points smoothing.

The cyclic measurement effects within a cardiac cycle are somewhat greater than the cycle-to-cycle trend effects. As seen in Table 3, if a frame is selected at random from two or three apparently equivalently opacified cardiac cycles, the variability of the diameter measurement is approximately 100 microns and the stenosis measurement three percent. Note that removal of the trend has little effect, as shown in Table 4.

Comparison of the approximate stenosis size from Table 1 and the standard deviation of the stenosis measurement in Table 3 does not show any obvious relationship. Since a stenosis variation of 3% as defined above, in a 10% stenotic lesion is actually a 30% relative change in the measurement, the error due to

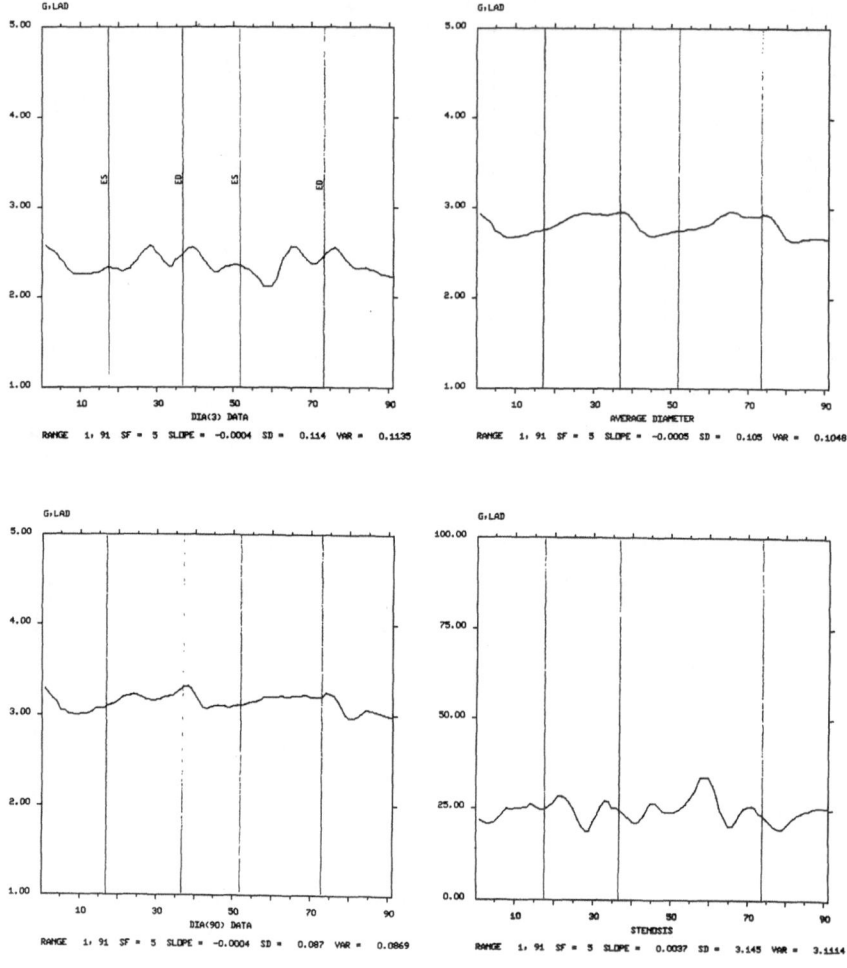

Figure 12. Subject GO, LAD D3, average diameter, D90, percent stenosis, 5 points smoothing.

cyclic image variation will likely be more important in the detection of change in early lesions than in detection of advanced lesions change.

From the frame-to-frame dispersion of diameter and stenosis values illustrated in Figure 9, it is clear that a major improvement in measurement variability can be achieved simply by measuring these quantities on two or more sequential frames and then averaging the results. The relative gain in precision as a function of cost from this approach may be considerably greater than that obtained by detection and correction of cyclic and trend effects.

Acknowledgement

This work was supported by the NASA Office of Life Sciences and by NIH/ NIHLBI. Grants HL-30390 and HL-23691.

References

1. Selzer RH, Blankenhorn DH, Crawford DW, Brooks SH, Barndt Jr R: Computer analysis of cardiovascular imagery. Proceedings of the Caltech/JPL Conference on Image Processing, Technology, Data Sources and Software for Commercial and Scientific Applications, Pasadena, California 1976: 6-1 - 6-20.
2. Selzer RH, Blankenhorn DH, Crawford DW, Brooks SH, Barndt Jr R: Computer measurement of arterial disease from angiograms. Proc Intern Conf on Signals and Images in Medicine and Biology. Biosigma 1978: 267-275.
3. Selzer RH, Blankenhorn DH: On the identification of the variation of atherosclerosis plaques, invasive and non-invasive methods. Proceedings at the 4th International Meeting on Atherosclerosis – Clinical Evaluation and Therapy. Bologna, Italy, November, 1981. Ed Lenzi & Descovich, MTP Press Limited, England.
4. Selzer RH, Blankenhorn DH, Brooks SH, Crawford DW, Cashin WL: Computer assessment of atherosclerosis from angiographic images. IEEE Trans Nucl Sc NS–29, 1982: 1198–1207.
5. Reiber JHC, Booman F, Tan HS, Slager CJ, Schuurbiers JCH, Gerbrands JJ, Meester GT: A cardiac image analysis system. Objective quantitative processing of angiocardiograms. Comp Cardiol 1978: 239–242.
6. Kishon Y, Yerushalmi S, Deutsch V, Neufeld HN: Measurement of coronary arterial lumen by densitometric analysis of angiograms. Angiology 39, 1979: 304–312.
7. Alderman EL, Berte LE, Harrison DC, Sanders W: Quantitation of coronary artery dimensions using digital image processing. In: Digital Radiography. WR Brody (Ed.) SPIE 314, 1981: 273–278.
8. Sandor T, Spears JR, Paulin S: Densitometric determination of changes in the dimensions of coronary arteries. In: Digital Radiography. WR Brody (Ed.) SPIE 314, 1981: 263–272.
9. Barth K, Decker D, Faust V, Irion KM: Die automatische erkennung und messung von stenosen der herzkranzgefässe im digitalen Röntgenbild. Digital Signal Processing Conference, Göttingen.
10. Reiber JHC, Kooijman CJ, Slager CJ, Gerbrands JJ, Schuurbiers JCH, Boer A den, Wijns W, Serruys PW: Computer assisted analysis of the severity of obstructions from coronary cineangiograms: A methodological review. Automedica 5, 1984: 219–238.
11. Cashin WL, Brooks SH, Blankenhorn DH, Selzer RH, Sanmarco ME, Benjauthrit B: Computerized edge tracking and lesion measurement in coronary angiograms; A pilot study comparing smokers with non-smokers. Atherosclerosis 52, 1984: 295–300.
12. Selzer RH: Atherosclerosis quantitation by computer image analysis. Conference on Clinical Diagnosis of Atherosclerosis. Quantitative Methods of Evaluation. MG Bond (Ed). Springer-Verlag, Stuttgart/New York 1983: 43–65.

Approaches towards standardization in acquisition and quantitation of arterial dimensions from cineangiograms

Johan H.C. Reiber, P.W. Serruys, C.J. Kooijman,
C.J. Slager, J.H.C. Schuurbiers and A. den Boer

Summary

Computer-based techniques have been and are being developed to obtain objective and reproducible parameters about the extent and severity of coronary artery disease from coronary cineangiograms. To evaluate changes in arterial dimensions over time repeated cineangiographies need to be performed and analyzed. However, the qualities of both the angiographic investigation and the computer analysis are hampered by various sources of variation.

In the angiographic data acquisition, the following sources of variation can be distinguished: (1) differences in the angles and height levels of the X-ray gantry with respect to the patient at the time of repeated angiography; (2) differences in vasomotor tone of the coronary arteries; (3) variations in the quality of mixing of the contrast agent with the blood; (4) differences in the angiographic image quality of the catheters; and (5) deviations in the size of the catheter as listed by the manufacturer from the true size.

Variations in the data analysis procedure are caused by: (1) quantum noise in the images; (2) electronic noise contributions in the video or otherwise converted images; (3) quantitation errors in the analog-to-digital conversion; (4) the effects of resampling the data along scanlines through the square grid of the digital data; (5) user variations in the definitions of the approximate centerline of the catheter and of the selected arterial segment; (6) possibly manual corrections to the otherwise automatically detected contours; (7) selection of reference positions; and (8) manual definition of starting and end points in selected arterial segments. To obtain reliable quantitative results from coronary cineangiograms, these variations should be minimized as much as possible.

In this chapter approaches towards standardized cineangiographic acquisition and analysis procedures are presented. It is shown that without these precautions taken, the variabilities in absolute coronary dimensions may increase dramatically. On the other hand, when the necessary precautions are taken, the variabilities in absolute dimensions from repeated cineangiographies and analyses

146

increase only by a factor of 1.5 to 2.2 as compared to those from repeated cinefilm analysis alone.

Introduction

Our laboratory has been involved over a long period of time in the development of techniques for quantitative analysis of coronary cineangiograms (1–5). These efforts have resulted in the design and implementation of the Cardiovascular Angiography Analysis System (CAAS), which is now commercially available (6). Applications of such an objective and reproducible technique for the assessment of coronary arterial dimensions include the evaluation of: 1) the efficacy of modern therapeutic procedures in the catheterization laboratory (7–10); 2) the effects of vasocactive drugs (11, 12); and 3) the effects of short- and long-term interventions on the regression of progression of coronary artery disease (13).

Since there are potentially many sources of error in the entire chain of angiographic investigation and quantitative analysis of the cinefilm product, precautions must be taken to reduce these errors as much as possible. It is the purpose of this paper: (1) to briefly describe the basic principles of the CAAS; (2) to present the results from a validation study of this technique; (3) to list the sources of variation in both the coronary angiographic and computer analysis procedures; and (4) to discuss our approaches towards standardized procedures of acquisition and analysis with the ultimate goal to minimize the effects of the error sources on the quantitative results.

CAAS methodology

The procedures for quantitative analysis of coronary arterial segments have been implemented on the CAAS, which runs under the multi-user RSX-11M Operating System. To analyze a coronary arterial segment in a selected cineframe, the cinefilm is mounted on the specially constructed cine-video converter (CIVICO) of our prototype CAAS or on the cine digitizer of the Pie Medical CAAS. Both cine-systems will be described briefly, since: (1) the validation data presented in this paper were obtained with our prototype system; and (2) the new cine digitizer represents new developments towards more reproducible and standardized digitization, in particular for densitometric applications.

With the CIVICO the selected cineframe is projected onto the target of a high-resolution video camera via a drum with six different lens systems, which allow for six different optical magnifications. The video camera is attached to a movable x-y stage, so that any area of interest in the cineframe can be selected with the appropriate magnification factor. The center square of the resulting video image is digitized in matrix size of 512 × 512 picture elements (pixels) with eight bits (256 levels) of brightness resolution.

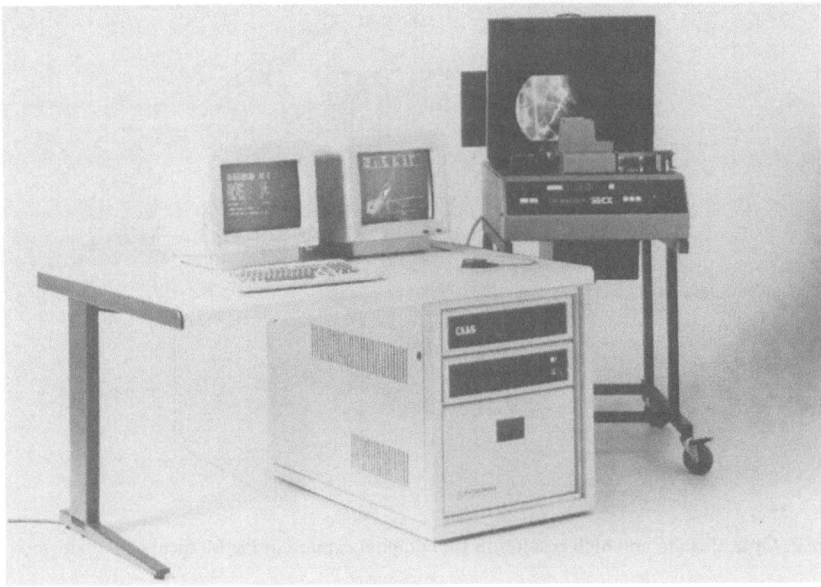

Figure 1. Pie Medical CAAS with cine digitizer.

The Pie Medical cine digitizer consists of a standard cineprojector (Tagarno 35CX) with a field-installable modification package for high resolution digitization of a selected cineframe (Figure 1). The modification package consists of a film guiding system, a specially developed optical chain and a high resolution CCD digital camera. The film guiding system ensures optimal flatness of the selected cineframe to be digitized. The optical chain has been designed for homogeneous light distribution over the cineframe to be digitized and a high resolution response of the projected cinefilm (Figure 2).

The monochromatic light source consists of an array of light emitting diodes (LED's) optimally suitable for high resolution imaging and densitometric analysis of the cinefilm. Any area of 6.9×6.9 mm in a selected cineframe (size 18×24 mm) can be digitized by the CCD-camera with a resolution of 512×512 pixels (13μm/pixel at the face of the CCD-linear array) with 8 bits of grey levels. Effectively, this means that the entire cineframe of size 18×24 mm can be digitized with a resolution of 1330×1770 pixels. The concept of this cine digitizer differs basically from that of the CIVICO. However, the resolution and quality of the digitized subimages used for contour detection and analysis are nearly identical, so that both systems perform equally well. Both systems have an automated brightness control of the light source, such that the full 8 bits range is utilized.

To analyze the dimensions of a coronary arterial segment quantitatively, the following steps need to be performed: (1) computation of the calibraton factor on the basis of the contrast catheter displayed in the images; (2) boundary detection

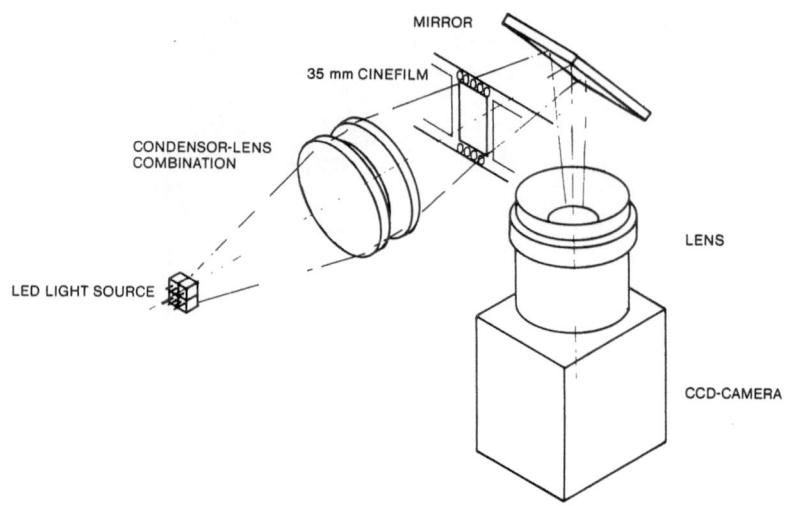

Figure 2. Optical chain and high resolution CCD digital camera in Pie Medical cine digitizer.

of the arterial segment; (3) computation of the diameter function from the detected and pincushion-corrected contour positions; (4) determination of the severity of a coronary obstruction in terms of absolute and relative parameters; and (5) determination of the mean diameter over one or more user-defined nonobstructed portions of this segment. These different steps will be described briefly in the following sections; further details have been described elsewhere (1–6).

Contour detection procedure

Calibration of the diameter data of the vessels in absolute values (mm) is achieved by computer detection of the outer boundaries of a user-selected portion of the optically magnified contrast catheter (optical magnification factor $2\sqrt{2}$ on CIVICO). The contour positions are corrected for pincushion distortion in the image. From these corrected positions a mean diameter value is determined in pixels; from the known size of the catheter the calibration factor can be calculated in millimeters per pixel. Figure 3 shows the contours detected along a portion of the optically magnified catheter.

Pincushion distortion from the image intensifier results in a position-dependent magnification of an object. Since the distortion cannot be described by a simple analytic function, a cineframe of a centimeter grid placed against the input screen of the image intensifier is used to assess the distortion. A correction vector for each pixel in the image can be obtained from the automatically computer-processed cineframe of the grid.

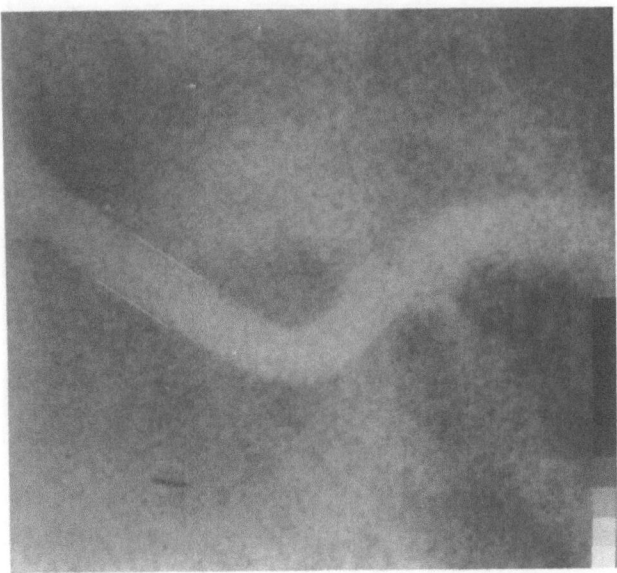

Figure 3. Optically magnified (2 √2×) catheter with detected boundaries superimposed.

The procedure for arterial contour detection requires the user to indicate a number of center positions in the optically magnified arterial segment (optical magnification factor 2). A smoothed version of this centerline determines the regions of interest of size 96 × 96 pixels encompassing the arterial segment to be transferred to the host processor (PDP 11/44 on prototype CAAS, LSI 11/73 on Pie Medical CAAS)) for edge definition. To decrease spatial fluctuations due to quantum noise, the digital data are smoothed spatially with a 5 × 5 median filter. Subsequently, the digital data are resampled along straight lines, denoted scanlines, perpendicular to the local centerline directions. Contours of the arterial segment along the scanlines are determined on the basis of the weighted sum of first and second difference functions applied to the resampled brightness information by so-called minimal cost criteria. If the user does not agree with part of the detected contours, these erroneous positions may be corrected interactively with the writing tablet.

Since the tentative centerline was initially defined by the user, the detected contours may be slightly dependent on the given centerline positions, particularly at sections with high curvature. To minimize this influence as much as possible, a final centerline is determined automatically as the midline of the detected and possibly corrected contours. The digital data are resampled and the minimum cost algorithm for contour detection is applied again. Finally, a smoothing procedure is applied to each of the detected contours and the resulting positions are corrected for pincushion distortion. Figure 4 shows the finally detected contours along the proximal portion of a left anterior descending artery.

150

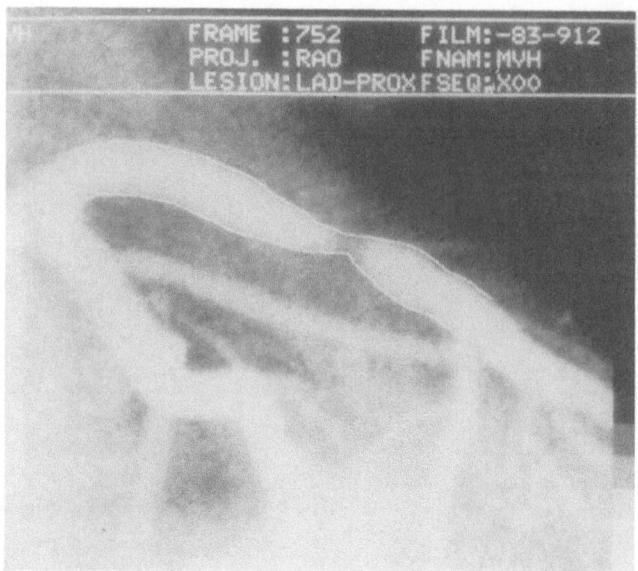

Figure 4. Automatically detected contours along the proximal portion of the LAD-artery.

Contour analysis

The diameter function D(i) of the arterial segment, calibrated in absolute milli-meters, is determined by computing the distances between corresponding con-tour points to the left and right of the centerline. From the minimal value D_m of the diameter function and the mean diameter value D_r at a user-indicated reference position, the user-defined percentage diameter (%–D) reduction is computed as

$$\%\text{–D stenosis} = (1 - \frac{D_m}{D_r}) \times 100\%$$

The mean diameter D_r is computed as the average of 11 diameter values in a symmetric region with the center at the user-defined reference position. The extent of the obstruction is determined from the diameter function D(i) on the basis of curvature analysis and expressed in millimeters.

However, the computed percentage diameter stenosis may depend heavily on the selected reference position. To minimize these variations, we have imple-mented an alternative method, denoted interpolated percentage diameter ste-nosis measurement, which is not dependent on a user-defined reference region.

The basic idea behind this technique is the computer estimation of the original diameter values over the obstructed region (reference diameter function, assum-ing there was no coronary disease present) from the actual luminal diameter

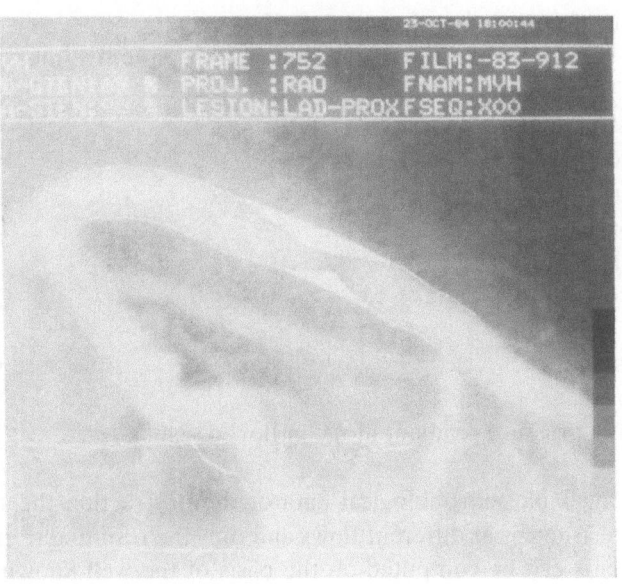

Figure 5. For the obstruction of Figure 4, the original diameter values over the obstructive region have been computed (reference diameter function, being the straight line in the diameter function). On the basis of the proximal and distal centerline segments and the computed reference diameter function, the original reference contours over the obstruction have been reconstructed. The shaded area is the 'atherosclerotic plaque'. With the reference diameter value measured at the site of minimal obstruction diameter, a percentage D-stenosis of 69% results, and a percentage area (A)-stenosis of 90%, assuming circular cross sections.

function (1–6, 10). On the basis of the proximal and distal centerline segments and the computed reference diameter function, the reference contours over the obstructed region can be reconstructed. The resulting reference contours for the arterial segment of Figure 4 are presented in Figure 5. The difference in area between the reference and the detected contours over the obstructive lesion is a measure for the 'atherosclerotic plaque' expressed in mm²; this area has been marked in Figure 5. In addition, this technique allows the assessment of the symmetry of the lesion in a given view with respect to its centerline. The symmetry measure is given as a value between 0 and 1, with 1 representing a concentric lesion and 0 the most severe case of asymmetry or eccentricity. Following this approach, the reference diameter is taken as the value of the reference diameter function at the minimal diameter position of the obstruction. Figure 5 shows the results of the interpolated technique for the obstruction of Figure 4.

In addition to the fact that the interpolated technique provides data about the area of the atherosclerotic plaque and the lesion's symmetry in a given view, there is another very practical advantage. By this technique, knowledge about the exact location of a reference, either proximal or distal to the stenosis, is not required for the analysis of repeated angiograms (8, 11).

For the example of Figure 5, the following quantitative measurements were obtained:

extent obstruction	:	11.89 mm
reference diameter	:	4.12 mm
obstruction diameter	:	1.29 mm
reference area	:	13.36 mm^2
obstruction area	:	1.31 mm^2
area atherosclerotic plaque	:	16.79 mm^2
symmetry measure	:	0.89
diameter stenosis	:	69%
area stenosis	:	90%
transstenotic pressure gradient at mean flow of 2 ml/s	:	17.6 mmHg

From the available morphological data of the obstruction the Poisseuille and turbulent resistances at different flows and thus the resulting transstenotic pressure gradients can be computed on the basis of the well-known fluid-dynamic equations (14–19, Chapter Serruys in this book).

Validation data analysis procedure

The accuracy and precision of the contour detection process have been assessed with cinefilms of nine acrylate (Perspex) models of coronary arteries with circular cross sections filled with contrast medium (3–5). These models were filmed with various settings of the quality (range 60 to 110 kV) of the X-ray system and filled with different concentrations (50% and 100%) of the contrast agent. The overall accuracy (average difference of computed results with true values) and precision (pooled standard deviation of the differences) for the percentage diameter stenosis measurements were found to be 2·00% and 2·68%, respectively, and for the absolute obstruction diameters -30μm and 90μm, respectively. These results demonstrate that the edge detection technique is highly accurate and precise.

For all studies described in this chapter, cineframes were selected at end-diastole, if possible. In cases of overlap of a segment to be analyzed with other vessels, the frame was selected at another instant in time near end-diastole. The user-determined beginning and end points of the major coronary segments were standardized according to the definitions by the American Heart Association (20). The results from the various evaluation studies were analyzed for significant differences using Student's t-test for paired values.

As a next step, the variability of repeated analyses of cineangiograms was assessed from a total of 13 end-diastolic cineframes of 13 routinely obtained coronary angiograms. These cineframes were analyzed twice by one technical analyst with a medium time interval of 28 days. A total of 13 coronary obstructions and 25 nonobstructed segments were processed.

The mean differences and standard deviations (s.d.) of the repeated measurements as well as the overall mean values of the parameters are presented in Table 1. With the exception of the measurements on the interpolated reference diameter and the mean diameter of nonobstructed segments, no significant differences were found between the repeated measurements. The s.d. of absolute measurements was less than 0.12 mm; s.d.'s of percentage diameter stenosis measurements for the user-defined and interpolated procedures were 2.74% and 3.94%, respectively.

These data show that the accuracy and the variability of the data analysis technique is excellent, despite the fact that there are many sources of variations present in the data analysis procedure. The different sources of variations and the precautions that we have taken to minimize these effects as much as possible have been listed in Table 2 and described earlier in this chapter in the context of the description of the arterial contour detection procedure.

Variability of acquisition and analysis procedures

For the interpretation of the quantitative coronary angiographic results from intervention studies, the total variability of the angiographic data acquisition *and* analysis procedures must be known. In the previous section the sources of variation and the approaches to be taken in the data analysis procedure itself have been discussed. However, the angiographic data acquisition procedure is also

Table 1. Variability in measurements of parameters of coronary arterial segments from repeated analysis of 13 cineframes.

	Overall mean value	Mean diff.	p-value	s.d. diff.
Calibration factor (mm/pixel)	0.096	0.0003	n.s.	0.002
User-defined reference (N = 13)				
Obstruction diam. (mm)	1.52	0.00	n.s.	0.10
Reference diam. (mm)	2.97	0.005	n.s.	0.12
%-D stenosis (%)	48.4	0.23	n.s.	2.74
Extent (mm)	8.42	− 0.38	n.s.	1.89
Interpolated reference (N = 13)				
Reference diam. (mm)	2.87	− 0.10	<.004	0.10
%-D stenosis (%)	47.9	− 2.08	n.s.	3.94
Nonobstructed segment (N = 25)				
Mean diam. (mm)	2.42	0.07	<.005	0.11
Length segment (mm)	17.72	0.02	n.s.	0.97

Abbreviations: %-D = percentage diameter; n.s. = nonsignificant.

Table 2. Sources of variations and approaches towards standardization in data analysis procedure.

Sources of variation	Approaches towards standardization
1. quantum noise in images.	1. spatial filtering of digital image data with a 5×5 median filter.
2. electronic noise contributions in digitizing system.	2. recursive digitization of image. (CIVICO only)
3. effects of resampling the data along scanlines through square grid of the digital image data.	3.
4. observer variations in definition of center positions within the catheter and the selected arterial segment.	4. Iterative edge detection and correction procedures.
5. possible manual corrections to the detected contours.	5.
6. selection of reference positions.	6. – Computer-defined reference position. (Interpolated technique) – for repeat studies proper documentation of analysis data on Polaroid photographs or sheet film.
7. manual definition of starting and end points in nonobstructed arterial segments for measurement of overall mean diameter.	7. use of anatomic landmarks, such as bifurcations, as much as possible.

hampered by various sources of variation (Table 3).

It will be clear that the overall variability will be dependent on the number and the qualities of the precautions taken. To assess the worst-case situation i.e. with a minimum of precautions taken, the following data were analyzed.

Worst-case variability

Out of a group of 153 patients scheduled to undergo percutaneous transluminal coronary angioplasty (PTCA), a subgroup of 26 was selected; each subject had two cineangiograms of good quality in a number of standard views that were suitable for paired analysis of the stenotic lesions (9). The first film was the

Table 3. Sources of variation in angiographic data acquisition.

1. differences in the angles and height levels of the X-ray gantry with respect to the patient at the time of repeated angiography with those used at the time of the pre-intervention study.
2. differences in vasomotor tone of the coronary arteries.
3. variations in the quality of mixing of the contrast agent with the blood.
4. angiographic quality of catheter (image contrast).
5. deviations in the size of the catheter as listed by the manufacturer from its true size.

diagnostic angiogram, while the second measurements were obtained from cin-eframes acquired immediately before the actual PTCA procedure. At the time of the angiographic investigations, no attempt was made to standardize on the inspiratory level, volume and rate of injection of the contrast agent nor on the technical characteristics of the X-ray system. More importantly, the vasomotor tone in both conditions was unknown and neglected. The median delay between the diagnostic and the PTCA angiogram was 90 days (range 1 to 250 days).

The nonsignificant mean differences in the obstruction diameters suggest that no detectable progression or regression of atherosclerotic lesions had occurred over the period of 90 days (Table 4). These paired data provide some insight in the total variability of the cineangiographic procedure and the computer analysis under worst-case circumstances, since no special care had been taken to reduce the potential sources of variability (X-ray system settings, vasomotor tone, etc.).

Under these particular conditions, the variations in absolute measurements were 0.36 mm for the obstruction diameter and 0.66 mm for the interpolated reference diameter, and in relative measurements 6.5% for the interpolated percentage diameter stenosis. As compared to the variability of the analysis procedure by itself, the total variability has now increased by a factor of 3.6 × for the obstruction diameter and by a factor of 6.6 for the interpolated reference diameter. From these data it is evident that attempts must be made to standardize the angiographic data acquisition procedure with the ultimate goal to decrease the unacceptably high variations.

Table 4. Worst-case variability in measurements of various parameters of coronary obstructions (N = 26).

	Overall mean value	Mean diff.	p-value	s.d. diff.
Obstruction diam. (mm)	1.25	0.00	n.s.	0.36
Extent (mm)	10.04	0.62	n.s.	4.34
Interpolated reference				
Reference diam. (mm)	3.72	− 0.13	n.s.	0.66
%-D stenosis (%)	66.19	− 1.92	n.s.	6.52

Abbreviations: %-D = percentage diameter: n.s. = nonsignificant.

Table 5. Approaches toward standardization in angiographic data acquisition.

1. On-line registration of X-ray system settings.
2. Administration of vasodilative drug immediately before angiographic investigation.
3. Use of iso-viscous and iso-osmolar contrast media. Administration of contrast medium by ECG-triggered injector.
4. Selection of acceptable catheter material (high angiographic image contrast and edge gradient).
5. Measurement of actual size catheter with micrometer following catheterization procedure.

The approaches that we propose for the various sources of variations of Table 3 are listed in the same order in Table 5; these will be discussed in further detail in the following sections.

Approaches towards standardization in angiographic data acquisition

On-line registration of X-ray system settings

At the Thoraxcenter a microprocessor system has been developed which collects for each angiographic investigation a number of parameters which are projected onto the patient film and printed on a lineprinter (21). Parameters describing the geometry of the X-ray gantry (Rotation of U-arm and of object, as well as distances from isocenter to focus, film and object) for a particular cinefilm run are projected onto the film immediately preceding the first angiographic image (Figure 6a), while parameters describing the selected X-ray exposure factors (kV, mA and pulse width), as well as film speed, focus, grid ratio and the radiation dose are projected onto the cinefilm immediately following the last angiographic image of this particular cinerun (Figure 6b).

A list with all these parameters and many more for the different cineruns performed during a patient study is provided on the lineprinter of the microprocessor system (Figure 7).

When a repeat angiography is scheduled the geometry of the X-ray system is re-adjusted on the basis of the available data, such that approximately the same angiographic projection is obtained. In adition, the accuracy and precision of the re-adjustments can be controlled following the study from the actual data projected onto the film and listed on the print-out. The kind of accuracy that can easily be achieved in a routine environment is presented in the section Variations in measurements with standardized protocol.

Administration of vasodilative drug immediately before angiographic investigation

One of the most important variables in the quantitative assessment of coronary arterial dimensions is the varying vasomotor tone. If no precautions are taken the vasomotor tone may even be different at the time of consecutive coronary angiographies. Yasue *et al.* have shown that there is a circadian variation in exercise capacity in patients with Prinzmetal's variant angina, among others due to the variations in vasomotor tone (22). The tone appeared to be higher in the morning than in the afternoon. They concluded that under high coronary vasomotor tone conditions, exercise can readily induce severe spasm resulting in angina pectoris. On the other hand, under low tone conditions, exercise can

```
THORAXCENTRE  ROTTERDAM    a

    CATH.LAB.    NR.  1

film  nr.        80-0618
date          30-07-1980
time             17-49-15

Calculated  distance:
        ⌐    3.9  cm  ⌐
Distance  from  Isocentre
        to  Focus             069  cm
        to  Film              019  cm
        to  Object          -  03  cm
Rotation  of  U-arm    +026  deg
Rotation  of  Object  -003  deg


    THORAXCENTRE  ROTTERDAM    b

    CATH.LAB.    NR.  1

film  nr.        80-0618
date          30-07-1980
time             17-49-25

X-ray  data:
        anode  voltage        075  kV
        anode  current       0330  mA
        pulse  time           4.0  ms
        film  speed            50  fr/s
        focus                 0.4  mm
    Grid  ratio  8           40  Lp/cm
    Radiation  dose      15.5  uR/fr
```

Figure 6. Parameters describing the geometry of the X-ray gantry (Fig 6a) and those describing the selected X-ray exposure factors for a particular angiographic procedure (Fig 6b) are projected onto the cinefilm for documentation purposes.

induce little spasm and no attacks occur except in patients with severe organic stenosis of a large coronary artery in whom only a slight degree of spasm would already occlude the artery. The examples given above make clear that the

```
FILM NR. : +80-0756      DATE: 24/11/80 THORAX CENTRUM ROTTERDAM CATH. LAB. #1
```

RUN	TIME	OBJ	PROJ	M/B	II	IID	FID	OID	ROT/B	ROT/P	MSEC	FR/SEC	kU	mA	FOC	DUR
00	12:44	LV	RAO	B	7"	025	079	- 06	-028	-001	4.0	50	078	0540	0.4	07.2
01	12:50	COR	LAO	M	7"	024	079	- 06	+047	-001	4.0	25	087	0820	0.7	05.5
02	12:51	COR	FR	M	7"	025	081	- 06	-001	-001	4.0	25	072	0780	0.7	03.9
03	12:53	COR	RAO	M	7"	027	077	- 06	-029	-005	4.0	25	071	0780	0.7	07.5
04	12:55	COR	CRC	M	7"	028	071	- 03	-029	-085	4.0	25	107	0400	0.4	06.9
05	12:56	COR	CAC	M	7"	032	078	- 03	+030	-085	4.0	25	116	0420	0.4	05.3
06	12:57	COR	CAC	M	7"	032	078	- 03	+030	-085	4.0	25	116	0410	0.4	04.4
07	13:04	COR	LAO	M	7"	031	078	- 03	+051	+002	4.0	25	087	0810	0.7	07.2
08	13:04	COR	RAO	M	7"	030	072	- 03	-031	+000	4.0	25	079	0790	0.7	05.4
09	13:07	COR	RAO	M	7"	030	072	- 03	-027	+000	4.0	25	076	0790	0.7	07.7
10	13:30	LV	RAO	B	7"	025	079	+ 04	-028	-000	1.0	50	043	0350	0.4	01.7
11	13:32	LV	RAO	B	7"	028	072	+ 11	-028	-000	1.0	50	044	0340	0.4	02.2

Figure 7. Example of print-out of parameters collected during a total of eleven cineruns performed at the time of a cardiac catheterization of a particular patient.

vasomotor tone should be controlled as much as possible in repeated angiographic studies designed to determine the effect of a given intervention on coronary dimensions.

A vasodilative drug that would be optimal in controlling the vasomotor tone of the epicardial vessel should give a quick (within 30 seconds to 1 min) and maximal response without influencing the hemodynamic state of the patient. Only nitrates and calcium antagonists satisfy these requirements. On isolated human coronary arteries the calcium antagonists may be more vasoactive than nitrates, but act more slowly (23). However, in the in vivo situation the nitrates are more vasoactive than the calcium antagonists. In a recent study by Nellessen *et al.* changes in diameter of angiographically normal coronary artery segments were investigated over a period of 30 minutes after sublingual administration of 20 mg of the calcium antagonist nifedipine (24). It was concluded that a plateau in vasodilation had not been reached at the end of the observation period, i.e. after 30 minutes. That means that it is still uncertain what the optimal time is for the angiographic investigation in terms of maximal vasodilatory effect following the oral administration of nifedipine. Rafflenbeul *et al.* demonstrated that sublingually administered nitrate and nifedipine have cumulative effects, which suggest that one should use both agents to obtain maximal vasodilation (25).

An alternative to the sublingual administration is the intracoronary injection of nitrate and/or calcium antagonist (11). This route of administration has the advantage of a very fast and complete action of the drug on the coronary vessel. Figure 8 shows the effects of repeated intracoronary administrations of nifedipine on the mean diameters of normal and poststenotic segments. A further vasodilation is observed after the 2nd administration.

A dose of 3 mg isosorbide of dinitrate (ISD) administered intracoronary has been shown to be well tolerated in clinical practice and is known to be 15× stronger than the dose of nitroglycerin necessary to obtain maximal vasodilation (27). This dose of 3 mg ISD is equivalent to a 0.3 mg intracoronary administration of nitroglycerin (28). A disadvantage of the nitroglycerin preparation is that it must be dissolved in an alcoholic solvent, since it is a lipophylic compound. Such

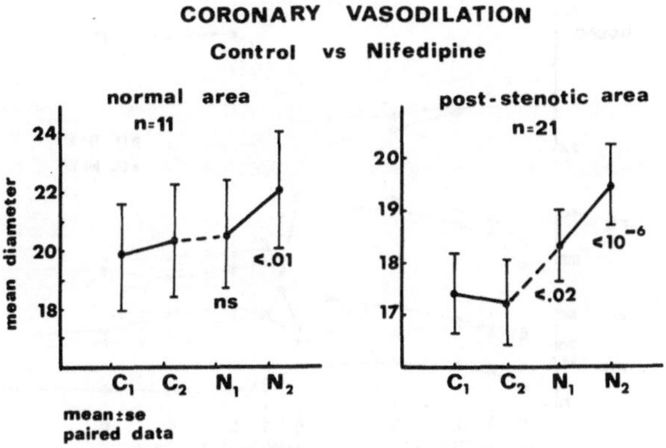

Figure 8. Effects of nifedipine administered intracoronary on the mean diameter of 11 normal and 21 poststenotic coronary segments during two control (C_1, C_2) and the two post-nifedipine (N_1, N_2) cineangiograms. The mean diameter values along the ordinate of the figures are noncalibrated values expressed in pixels. Reproduced with permission from PW Serruys *et al.* (26).

alcoholic preparations may be deleterious to the myocardium and may induce hemolysis. In addition, some of the commercial preparations of nitroglycerin contain very high levels of potassium which could provoke spasm (29).

Isosorbide of dinitrate is a hydrophylic preparation. Lablanche *et al.* have demonstrated that intracoronary and intrafemoral venous injections give identical peripheral hemodynamic and coronary changes after the first minute following administration (30, 31) (Figure 9). The effects were maximal between 2 and 4 minutes and continued after 10 minutes. The only difference was a more rapid decrease in systolic pressure after intrafemoral administration. With intracoronary injection dilation preceded the occurrence of hemodynamic effects, which is an argument for using intracoronary ISD (particularly in the treatment of spasm induced by ergometrine).

A potential advantage of the use of calcium antagonists above the nitrates is that small amounts of calcium antagonists injected intracoronary produce coronary vasodilation without any systemic effect (32, 33). On the other hand, the calcium antagonists may produce transient negative inotropic, chronotropic and dromotropic effects.

From this paragraph on coronary vasomotor tone we may conclude that the vasomotor tone should be controlled in quantitative coronary angiographic studies. The only way to achieve that is by trying to reach the ceiling of vasodilation of the vessels by means of a vasodilatory drug producing a fast and complete vasodilation without any peripheral effects. It seems that such results can be obtained most reliably by the intracoronary administration of nitrates or calcium antagonists. However, it is still unknown which of these drugs is the single most

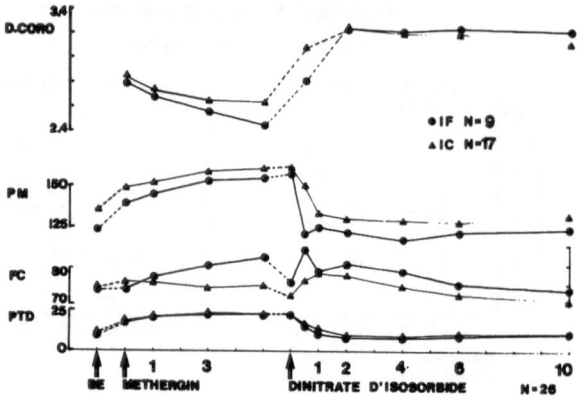

Figure 9. Intracoronary and intrafemoral venous injections of isosorbide of dinitrate give identical hemodynamic and coronary changes after the first minute following administration. The effects are maximal between 2 and 4 minutes and continue after 10 minutes. Reproduced with permission from Lablanche *et al.* (30). Abbreviations: D. CORO: diameter of coronary arterial segments in mm; FC: heart rate (beats/min); PM: systolic pressure (mmHg); PTD: end-diastolic left ventricular pressure (mmHg); IC: intracoronary group; IF: intrafemoral group; BE: baseline measurement.

potent vasodilator, and whether they should be used in combination, since they may have synergistic action.

Use of iso-viscous and iso-osmolar contrast media

Adverse effects of conventional contrast media are related to the single-valence cations, such as sodium and meglumine, to an imbalance in the ratio of sodium to calcium ions, to the high osmolality of the solutions and to their hyperviscosity. The hyperosmolality may exert its influence through the massive shifting of tissue water to the capillaries as the contrast medium flows through them, thus increasing the intravascular volume. Bentley and Henry investigating the effect of meglumine diatrizoate (Renografin-76, 1689 mOsm/liter) on animal arteries, demonstrated that the angiographic dye in concentrations not exceeding those during angiography exert potent, dose- and time-dependent vasomotor effects (34). In addition, experiments in vivo have shown that intracoronary injection of ionic, hyperosmolar, and hyperviscous contrast media produce direct myocardial depression, followed by an adrenergically mediated reflex effect that potentially could affect the vasomotor tone of the arteries (35).

To reduce these undesirable effects, much effort has been directed toward the development of new water-soluble contrast media with reduced osmolality, which are either nonionic or contain physiologic concentrations of calcium ions. These agents cause less subjective discomfort, less hemodynamic and biochemical effects, and less blood pressure and rhythm disturbances in coronary angiography. Collective studies offer experimental and clinical evidence of the advantages of the low osmolality agents in cardiac radiology (36). These improved qualities of the new angiographic dyes therefore may account for the observed decrease in variability measures, although this last hypothesis has not yet been tested.

Administration of contrast medium by ECG-triggered injector

As part of their procedures to measure the coronary flow, myocardial perfusion and coronary flow reserve from coronary angiograms, Spiller *et al.* and Vogel *et al.* have been using ECG-synchronized, power contrast medium injections to standardize the timing and flow rates of the contrast boli (37, 38). When used with an eight or nine french catheter (for example, guiding catheter for angioplasty) high flow rates can be achieved, resulting in angiograms of good quality. High flow rates can best be obtained when the contrast agent is pre-warmed to 37°C resulting in a decreased viscosity. For the left coronary artery contrast injections at a rate of 4 ml/s for a total of 7 ml have been used, and for the right coronary artery 3 ml/s for a total of 5 ml (39). Modern injectors are relatively safe in use since upper limits for the flow rate and pressure can be set; pressure rise-time is also adjustable. For quality control purposes it is advisable to register the pressure signal of the injector on paper. In our center we have employed the power injector technique in a number of clinical research studies and for the assessment of coronary flow reserve. It has been our impression that the high flow rate contributes more to image quality than the timing of the contrast administration.

Selection of acceptable catheter material

Coronary contrast catheters have been used increasingly for calibration purposes in the quantitative assessment of coronary arterial dimensions. However, to determine the accuracy of such calibration measurements from coronary cine-angiograms and the effects of catheter material, contrast filling of the catheter, and kV-setting of the X-ray source on image quality of the irradiated catheter and thus on the accuracy of the measurements, we analyzed four different catheter materials, filmed under different conditions (4). The most important results from this study will be described in this chapter; for further details the reader is referred to reference 40.

Mid-portions of the four contrast catheters were taped on a block of perspex with dimensions $10 \times 10 \times 10$ cm. Five different fillings were used for the catheters: 1) only air inside; 2) filled with water; and filled with three different concentrations of a contrast agent (Urografin-76®)* : 3) 370 mg I/cc (100% con-

---

* Schering AG, Berlin, Germany.

centration); 4) 185 mg I/cc (50% concentration); and 5) 92.5 mg I/cc (25% concentration). Each situation was filmed at four different kilovoltages, ranging from 55 to 81 kV. For calibration purposes, a cm-grid was filmed on top of the perspex block after the catheter studies had been performed.

From the analyzed portion of a contrast catheter the following parameters were measured:

1. mean diameter (mm)
2. average brightness level along centerline in catheter (B.cath)
3. average background brightness level (B.bkg), measured 10 pixels (± 0.6 mm) outside of the detected contours.
4. difference between B.cath and B.bkg, being a measure for image contrast
5. average value of the weighted sum of first and second difference functions for the left-hand side contour positions (GRAD(L))
6. average value of the weighted sum of first and second difference functions for the right-hand side contour positions (GRAD(R)).

Four catheters fabricated from different materials were used for this study:

A. woven dacron, Sones 7F catheter*
B. polyvinylchloride, Judkins 7.3F catheter* *
C. polyurethane, Femoral – Left Coronary 8F catheter* * *
D. nylon, Alvaflo 7F catheter* * * *

The true sizes of the catheters were measured with a micrometer.

Figure 10 shows the brightness distribution along a scanline across an analyzed catheter segment perpendicular to the centerline direction for each of the four catheter materials filled with 100% contrast agent and with air. In each graph the pixel positions along the scanline are plotted along the horizontal axis and the brightness levels along the vertical axis. From these eight graphs the differences in image contrast between the various materials can be appreciated, as well as the differences in the brightness distribution for a particular segment filled with 100% contrast agent or with air.

In Table 6 the true sizes of the four catheter segments, measured with a micrometer, are listed, as well as the average value and standard deviation of the values assessed with the CAAS and the average difference between the true and angiographically measured sizes. For each catheter a total of 20 measurements were available from the air and water filled catheters and from the catheters filled

---

* USCI Int., Inc., Billerica, Mass., U.S.A.
* * Cook Inc., Bloomington, IN, U.S.A.
* * * Cordis Corp., Miami, Florida, U.S.A.
* * * * Mallinckrodt GmbH, Grossostheim, West Germany.

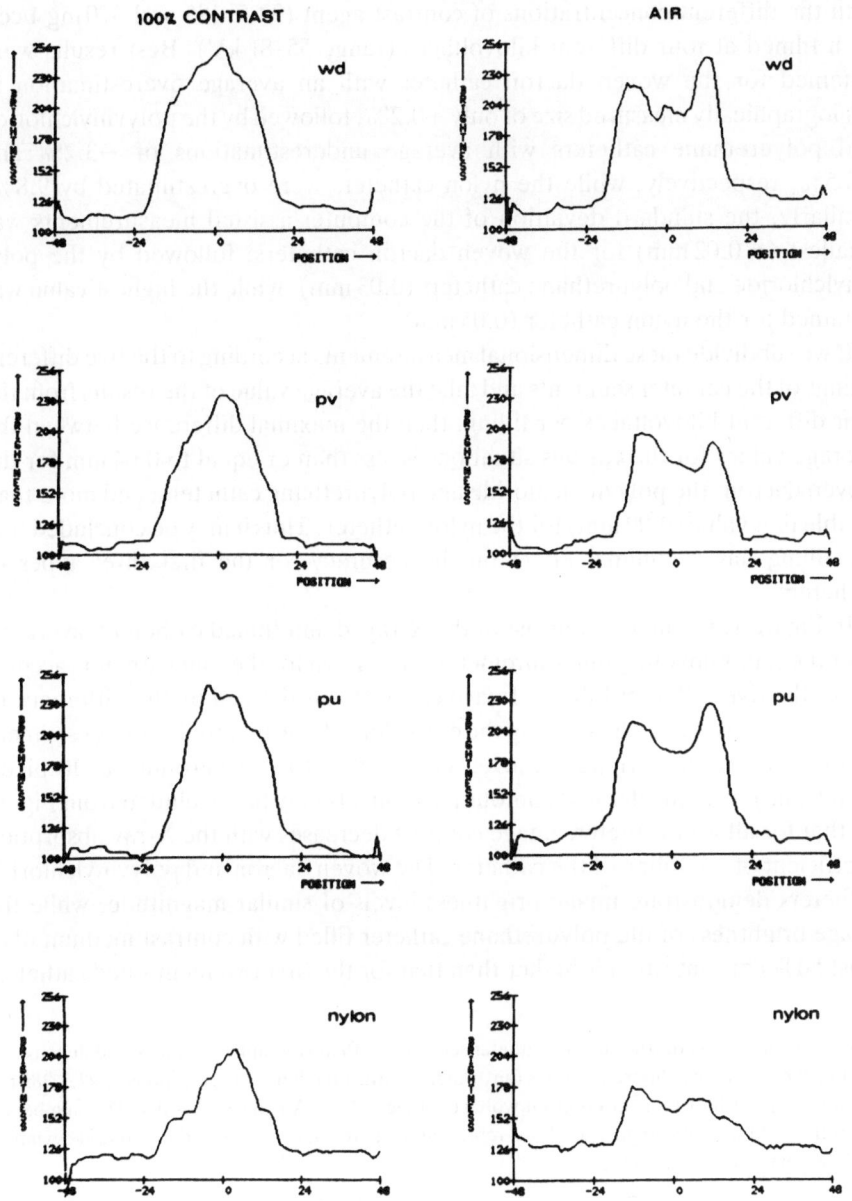

Figure 10. Examples of brightness distribution along scanlines perpendicular to the centerline directions for the four different catheters, filled with 100% contrast agent (left column) and with air (right column). The vertical order of the graphs represents the different materials (from top to bottom): woven dacron (wd), polyvinylchloride (pv), polyurethane (pu) and nylon, respectively. In each graph the pixel positions along the scanline are plotted along the horizontal axis and the brightness levels along the vertical axis.

with the different concentrations of contrast agent (92.5, 185 and 370 mg I/cc), each filmed at four different kilovoltages (range 55–81 kV). Best results were obtained for the woven dacron catheter with an average overestimation in angiographically measured size of only +0.2%, followed by the polyvinylchloride and polyurethane catheters with average underestimations of −3.2% and −3.5%, respectively, while the nylon catheters were overestimated by 9.8%. Similarly, the standard deviation of the computer-assisted measurements was smallest (= 0.02 mm) for the woven dacron catheters, followed by the polyvinylchloride and polyurethane catheters (0.03 mm), while the highest value was obtained for the nylon catheter (0.05 mm).

If we subdivide these dimensional measurements according to the five different fillings of the catheter segments and take the average value of the results from the four different kilovoltages per filling, then the maximal difference between the average values for the various situations is less than or equal to 0.04 mm for the woven dacron, the polyvinylchloride and polyurethane catheters, and more than double that value (0.09 mm) for the nylon catheter. Thus it may be concluded that the filling has a minimal effect on the accuracy for the first three types of catheters.

In Figure 11 the image contrast of the X-rayed and filmed catheters, averaged over the four kilovoltage-measurements, are shown for the four catheters according to the five different fillings. Image contrast was defined by the difference of the average brightness level along the centerline of the analyzed catheter segment and of the average brightness level measured in the background, at 10 pixels (± 0.6 mm) from the defined contour positions. It may be concluded from Figure 11, that for all four catheters image contrast decreases with the X-ray absorption coefficient of the filling of the catheter. The woven dacron and polyvinylchloride catheters demonstrate image brightness levels of similar magnitude, while the image brightness of the polyurethane catheter filled with contrast medium of at least 50% concentration is higher than that for the first two mentioned catheters

Table 6. Comparison of true sizes of catheter segments with angiographically measured dimensions, averaged over the five different fillings (air, water, contrast medium concentrations of 92.5, 185 and 370 mg I/cc), each at four different kilovoltages (range 55–81 kV) (mean ± s.d.). The numbers in parentheses in the column measured size represent the percentage values of the standard deviations with respect to the mean values.

	True size (mm)	Angiographically measured size (mm)	Average difference (%)
woven dacron	2.35	2.35 ± 0.02 (0.9%)	+0.2%
polyvinylchloride	2.44	2.36 ± 0.03 (1.3%)	−3.2%
polyurethane	2.62	2.53 ± 0.03 (1.2%)	−3.5%
nylon	2.25	2.46 ± 0.05 (2.0%)	+9.8%

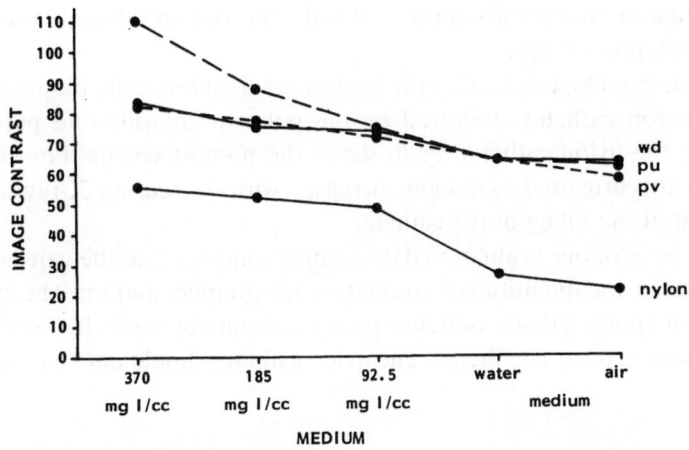

Figure 11. This graph shows image contrast for the four catheter materials as a function of the filling of the catheter. Each measurement point represents the mean value of four measurements of the catheter at four different qualities (kV-level) of the X-ray radiation.

and similar for the water and air fillings. The image contrast of the nylon catheter is significantly lower for all fillings as compared to the other three materials.

Finally, we have measured along each detected contour side the average density gradient along the contour, defined by the weighted sum of first and second difference values assessed from the edge detection algorithm; the unit of this parameter is brightness level difference per pixel. As a result, for each analyzed catheter segment, an average left gradient value (GRAD(L)) and an average right gradient value (GRAD(R)) was obtained. At the average, the differences between the GRAD(L) and GRAD(R)-values were nonsignificant. In Figure 12 the average gradient values for the four catheters, averaged over the

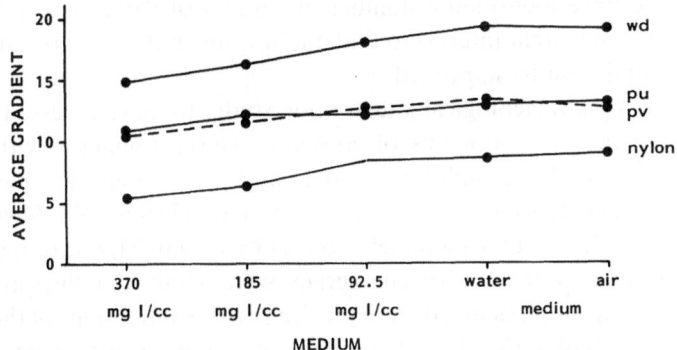

Figure 12. Average brightness gradient at the detected contour positions for the four catheter materials as a function of the filling of the catheter. Each measurement point represents the mean value of four measurements of the catheter at four different qualities (kV-level) of the X-ray radiation.

166

four kV measurements and over the left and right contour sides, are presented for the five different fillings.

It is clear from Figure 12, that the highest gradient levels are obtained with the woven dacron catheter, followed by the polyvinylchloride and polyurethane catheters; the nylon catheter again shows the poorest results. For all catheter materials the brightness gradient increases with decreasing X-ray absorption coefficient of the filling of the catheter.

On the basis of our evaluation data we may conclude that the woven dacron is most suitable for quantitative coronary angiographic studies. The polyvynyl-chloride and polyurethane catheters perform about equally well, but slightly less than the woven dacron catheter. The nylon catheter should not be used for these studies.

Measurement of actual size catheter with micrometer following catheterization procedure

It has been our experience that the size of the catheter as specified by the manufacturer often deviates from the true size, especially for disposable cathe-ters. If the manufacturer cannot guarantee narrow ranges for the size of the catheter, e.g. ± 0.05 F, it should be measured following the catheterization with a micrometer. This problem plays an even greater role for the tip of a catheter which is often hand-made and thus poorly specified; it is particularly the tip that we use most often for the calibration. For a 5.5 tip of a Sones catheter, a deviation by 0.05 F will result in an error in the computed calibration factor by 0.9 percent.

Variations in measurements with standardized protocol

Now that we have identified a number of sources of variations and proposed remedies, it is of a great interest to find out how much the poor results from the worst-case study can be improved.

As part of a pharmacological intervention study, we have assessed the 1 hour variability in the measurements of coronary arterial segments with repeated coronary angiographic examination and analysis in a group of 11 patients. Im-mediately after control cineangiographic examination in multiple views (angio 1), the first metabolite of molsidomine[R]* (Sin 1) was administered in the left main stem; 2 min. thereafter coronary angiograms were obtained in the same multiple views to study the immediate effect of the drug on the dimensions of the coronary arteries (angio 2) (41). One hour later these angiograms were repeated to assess the long-term effect of the drug (angio 3). A fourth angiographic procedure

* Cassella, Frankfurt am Main, Germany.

(angio 4) was carried out after a second intracoronary administration of the drug to determine whether further dilatation could be achieved. For this study, a nonionic contrast medium (iohexol*) was administered. The spatial positions of the X-ray source and image intensifier with respect to the patient and the voltage (kV) and current (mA) of the X-ray generator were acquired on-line with each angiographic procedure. Great care was taken to ensure that identical positions were used in the corresponding views.

By comparing the arterial dimensions from angio's 2 and 4, we can assess the overall variability, when standardization of the angiographic procedure is attempted (including 'control' of the vasomotor tone). Each analyzed cineframe was separately calibrated on the basis of the displayed contrast catheter. A total of 16 coronary obstructions were analyzed, as well as 90 nonobstructed segments.

The results on the variability in X-ray gantry settings between the angio's 2 and 4 are presented in Table 7. The angular variability, computed from the absolute differences of angular settings, was less than 4.2 degrees and the variability in the various positions of image intensifier and X-ray source less than 3.0 cm. There were no significant differences between the repeated X-ray system settings. These results show that the X-ray system settings can be reproduced quite accurately in routine clinical practice.

The mean differences in the measured parameters from angio's 2 and 4 were all nonsignificant (Table 8). The standard deviation of the differences for the obstruction diameter now equals 0.22 mm, for the interpolated reference diameter 0.15 mm and for the interpolated percentage diameter stenosis 7.23%.

From Tables 1, 4 and 8, the mean differences and standard deviations of the differences in the obstruction and interpolated reference diameters, as well as in the interpolated percentage diameter stenosis, have been summarized in Table 9 for repeated analysis, and the best-controlled and worst-case angiographic studies.

The mean differences in absolute diameters were below 0.13 mm in all studies.

Table 7. Variability in X-ray gantry settings with repeated cineangiographic studies (N = 25).

	Overall mean value	Mean diff.	p-value	s.d. diff.
Rotation U-arm (degrees)	31.2	0.3	n.s.	4.2
Rotation pat./C-arm (degrees)	26.4	0.3	n.s.	2.2
Isocenter-Image Intensifier distance (cm) (IID)	22.6	1.1	n.s.	3.0
Focus-Isocenter distance (cm) (FID)	72.8	− 0.3	n.s.	0.8
Object-Isocenter distance (cm) (OID)	5.3	0.2	n.s.	1.4

* Omnipaque®, Nyegård, Oslo, Norway.

Table 8. Variabilities in measurements of various parameters of coronary arterial segments from repeated coronary angiographic studies and analysis in best controlled situation. Angiograms 2 and 4 were performed immediately following administration of a vasodilatory drug. Time between angio's 2 and 4 was approximately 1 hour (see text).

	Overall mean	angio 4–2		
		Mean diff.	p-value	s.d. diff.
Calibration factor	0.094	− 0.001	n.s.	0.002
(mm/pixel) (N = 25)				
User-defined Reference (N = 16)				
Obstruction diam. (mm)	2.13	0.00	n.s.	0.22
Reference diam. (mm)	3.57	0.06	n.s.	0.28
%-D stenosis (%)	41.3	0.75	n.s.	8.09
Extent (mm)	6.28	− 0.15	n.s.	2.03
Interpolated reference (N = 14)				
Reference diam. (mm)	3.32	0.05	n.s.	0.15
%-D stenosis (%)	38.1	1.21	n.s.	7.23
Nonobstructed segments (N = 90)				
Mean diam. (mm)	3.05	0.07	n.s.	0.24
Length segment (mm)	14.03	− 0.03	n.s.	1.02

The variability in obstruction diameter for these three types of studies ranged from 0.10 mm for the repeated analysis only to 0.36 mm for the worst-case angiographic study. Likewise, the variability in the interpolated reference diameter was smallest for the repeated analysis and largest for the worst-case study (0.66 mm). The worst-case study clearly demonstrates that the variability in absolute dimensions increase if no special care is taken to reduce the potential sources of variation.

The variabilities in the interpolated percentage diameter reduction were smallest for the repeated analysis study and 84% and 65% higher for the best-

Table 9. Summary of the differences (mean and s.d.) in the absolute diameter measurements and interpolated percentage diameter stenosis for repeated analysis, and the best-controlled and worst-case angiographic studies.

	Mean diff.			s.d. diff.		
	Repeated analysis	Best contr.	Worst case	Repeated analysis	Best contr.	Worst case
Obstruction diam. (mm)	0.00	0.00	0.00	0.00	0.22	0.36
Interp. ref. diam. (mm)	− 0.10	0.05	− 0.13	0.10	0.15	0.66
Interp. %-D sten. (%)	− 2.08	1.21	− 1.92	3.94	7.23	6.52

controlled and worst-case angiographic studies, respectively. The mean differences were all less than 2.08%.

The data from Table 9 thus make clear that the variabilities in the obstruction diameters with repeated angiographic studies and analyses were 2.2 to 3.6 times greater than those from repeated analyses only, and 1.5 to 6.6 times greater for the interpolated reference diameters. This was caused by the sources of variation in the data acquisition procedure described above. Alderman *et al.* (42) found an increase in variability in absolute sizes with an angiographic study compared with repeated analysis only by a factor of 3; we found an increase by a factor of 1.5 to 2.2. In their study identical calibration factors, computed from the spatial positions of the image intensifier and X-ray source with respect to the patient, were used for the initial and repeat angiographic studies. This means that their actual variations in arterial size would be greater than the ones reported, if the calibration factor was also assessed repeatedly from the catheter as was done in our study.

Conclusions

We have developed and validated extensively a procedure for the quantitative analysis of coronary cineangiograms that can be applied on a routine basis. This procedure is based on an accurate, automated method for the contour detection of arterial segments. Various absolute and relative dimensional parameters are derived from the diameter data. From our validation data the following conclusions may be drawn.

1. Arterial dimensions can be assessed with high accuracy and reproducibility from coronary cineangiograms.
2. Variabilities in the measurement of arterial dimensions increase with repeated angiography.
3. Variabilities increase further if no special care is taken to reduce potential error sources.
4. Angiographic and biological changes are sources of major concern.
5. Further attempts towards standardization of angiographic procedure are seriously needed.

Acknowledgements

The authors wish to thank M.J. Kanters-Stam and S.M. Spierdijk for their secretarial assistance with the preparation of this manuscript.

References

1. Reiber JHC, Gerbrands JJ, Booman F, Troost GJ, Boer A den, Slager CJ, Schuurbiers JCH: Objective characterization of coronary obstructions from monoplane cineangiograms and three-dimensional reconstruction of an arterial segment from two orthogonal views. In: Applications of computers in medicine. MD Schwartz (Ed.) IEEE Cat. No. TH0095-0, 1982: 93–100.
2. Kooijman CJ, Reiber JHC, Gerbrands JJ, Schuurbiers JCH, Slager C, Boer A den, Serruys PW: Computer-aided quantitation of the severity of coronary obstructions from single view cineangiograms. First IEEE Comp. Society Intern. Symp. on Medical Imaging and Image Interpretation. IEEE Cat. No. 82 CH1804-4, 1982: 59–64.
3. Reiber JHC, Kooijman CJ, Slager CJ, Gerbrands JJ, Schuurbiers JCH, Boer A den, Wijns W, Serruys PW, Hugenholtz PG: Coronary artery dimensions from cineangiograms; methodology and validation of a computer-assisted analysis procedure. IEEE Trans. Medical Imaging MI-3, 1984: 131–141.
4. Reiber JHC, Serruys PW, Kooijman CJ, Wijns W, Slager CJ, Gerbrands JJ, Schuurbiers JCH, Boer A den, Hugenholtz PG: Assessment of short-, medium-, and long-term variations in arterial dimensions from computer-assisted quantitation of coronary cineangiograms. Circulation 71, 1985: 280–288.
5. Reiber JHC, Serruys PW, Slager CJ: Quantitative coronary and left ventricular cineangiography. Martinus Nijhoff Publishers, 1986.
6. Reiber JHC, Kooijman CJ, Slager CJ, Ree EJB van, Kalberg RJN, Tijdens FO, Plas J van der, Frankenhuyzen J van, Claessen WCH: Taking a quantitative approach to cine-angiogram analysis. Diagnostic Imaging, April 1985: 87–89.
7. Serruys PW, Booman F, Troost GJ, Reiber JHC, Gerbrands JJ, Brand M van den, Cherrier F, Hugenholtz PG: Computerized quantitative coronary angiography applied to percutaneous transluminal coronary angioplasty: advantages and limitations. In: Transluminal Coronary Angioplasty and Intracoronary Thrombolysis. M Kaltenbach, A Gruentzig, K Rentrop, WD Bussmann (Eds.). Springer-Verlag, Berlin, 1982: 110–124.
8. Serruys PW, Wijns W, Brand M van den, Ribeiro V, Fioretti P, Simoons ML, Kooijman CJ, Reiber JHC, Hugenholtz PG: Is transluminal coronary angioplasty mandatory after successful thrombolysis? A quantitative coronary angiographic study. Brit Heart J 50, 1983: 257–265.
9. Wijns W, Serruys PW, Brand M van den, Suryapranata H, Kooijman CJ, Reiber JHC, Hugenholtz PG: Progression to complete coronary obstruction without myocardial infarction in patients who are candidates for percutaneous transluminal angioplasty: a 90-day angiographic follow-up. In: Prognosis of Coronary Heart Disease. Progression of Coronary Arteriosclerosis. H. Roskamm (Ed.). Springer-Verlag, Berlin/Heidelberg/New York/Tokyo, 1983: 190–195.
10. Wijns W, Serruys PW, Reiber JHC, Brand M van den, Simoons ML, Kooijman CJ, Balakumaran K, Hugenholtz PG: Quantitative angiography of the left anterior descending coronary artery: correlations with pressure gradient and results of exercise thallium scintigraphy. Circulation 71, 1985: 273–279.
11. Serruys PW, Hooghoudt TEH, Reiber JHC, Slager C, Brower RW, Hugenholtz PG: Influence of intracoronary nifedipine on left ventricular function, coronary vasomotility, and myocardial oxygen consumption. Brit Heart J 49, 1983: 427–441.
12. Serruys PW, Lablanche JM, Reiber JHC, Bertrand ME, Hugenholtz PG: Contribution of dynamic vascular wall thickening to luminal narrowing during coronary arterial vasomotion. Z. Kardiol. 72, 1983: 116–123.
13. Arntzenius AC, Kromhout D, Barth JD, Reiber JHC, Bruschke AVG, Buis B, Gent CM van, Kempen-Voogd N, Strikwerda S, Velde E.A. van der: Diet, Lipoproteins, and the progression of coronary atherosclerosis. The Leiden Intervention Trial. N. Engl. J. Med. 312, 1985: 805–811.
14. McMahon MM, Brown BG, Cukingnan R, Rolett EL, Bolson E, Frimer M, Dodge HT: Quantitative coronary angiography: measurement of the 'critical' stenosis in patients with unsta-

ble angina and single-vessel disease without collaterals. Circulation 60, 1979: 106–113.

15. Kirkeeide R, Wüsten B, Gottwik M: Computer assisted evaluation of angiographic findings. In: Thrombose and Atherogenese. Pathophysiologie und Therapie der arteriellen Verschluss-krankheit. K. Breddin (Ed.), Verlag Gerhard Witzstrock, Baden-Baden/Köln/New York, 1981: 414–417.

16. Brown BG, Bolson EL, Dodge HT: Arteriographic assessment of coronary atherosclerosis. Review of current methods, their limitations and clinical applications. Arteriosclerosis 2, 1982: 2–15.

17. Gould KL, Kelley KO: Physiological significance of coronary flow velocity and changing stenosis geometry during coronary vasodilation in awake dogs. Circ. Res. 50, 1982: 695–704.

18. Gottwik MG, Siebes M, Kirkeeide R, Schaper W: Hämodynamik von Koronarstenosen. Z. Kardiol. 73 (Suppl. 2), 1984: 47–54.

19. Siebes M, Lenzen H, Gottwik M, Schlepper M: Influence of geometric errors in quantitative angiography on the evaluation of stenotic hemodynamics. Comp. Cardiol. 1983: 385–388.

20. Austen WG, Edwards JE, Frye RL, Gensini GG, Gott VL, Griffith LSC, McGoon DC, Murphy ML, Roe BB: A reporting system on patients evaluated for coronary artery disease. Report of the Ad Hoc Committee for Grading of Coronary Artery Disease, Council on Cardiovascular Surgery. Dalles, 1975. American Heart Association, 1975. Circulation 51–2, no. 4, 1975: 7–40.

21. Boer A. den: A microprocessor system for on-line registration of the X-ray system settings. Internal report, Thoraxcenter, 1982.

22. Yasue H, Omote S, Takizawa A, Nagao M, Miwa K, Tanaka S: Circadian variation of exercise capacity in patients with Prinzmetal's variant angina: role of exercise-induced coronary arterial spasm. Circulation 59: 1979: 938–948.

23. Ginsburg R: The isolated human epicardial coronary artery. Am J Cardiol 52, 1983: 61A–66A.

24. Nellessen U, Rafflenbeul W, Daniel W, Hecker H. Reil G-H, Raude E, Lichtlen P: Dilation of human epicardial coronary arteries after sublingual nifedipine and its relationship to blood levels. In: Proc 6th Intern. Adalat® Symp. PR Lichtlen (Ed.). Excerpta Medica, Amsterdam (in press).

25. Rafflenbeul W, Lichtlen PR: Release of residual vascular tone in coronary artery stenoses with nifedipine and glyceryl trinitrate. In: Proc 5th Intern Adalat® Symp. New Therapy of Ischaemic Heart Disease and Hypertension. M. Kaltenbach, HN Neufeld (Eds). Excerpta Medica, Amsterdam/Oxford/Princeton, 1983: 300–308.

26. Serruys PW, Booman F, Steward R, Michels R, Reiber JHC, Hugenholtz PG: Unstable angina pectoris and coronary arterial vasomotion: which role for nifedipine? In: Unstable Angina Pectoris. W. Rafflenbeul, PR Lichtlen, R Balcon (Eds). Georg Thieme Verlag, Stuttgart/New York, 1981: 103–120.

27. Feldman RL, Marx JD, Pepine CJ, Conti CR: Analysis of coronary responses to various doses of intracoronary nitroglycerin. Circulation 66, 1982: 321–327.

28. Strauer BE: Isosorbide dinitrate: its action on myocardial contractility in comparison with nitroglycerin. Int J Clin Pharmacol 8, 1973: 30–36.

29. Webb SC, Canepa-Anson R, Rickards AF, Poole-Wilson PA: High potassium concentration in a parenteral preparation of glyceryl trinitrate. Need for caution if given by intracoronary injection. Br Heart J 50, 1983: 395–396.

30. Lablanche JM, Delforge MR, Tilmant PY, Thieuleux FA, Bertrand ME: Effects hémodynamiques et coronaires du dinitrate d'isosorbide: Comparaison entre les voies d'injection intracoronaire et intraveineuse. Arch Mal Coeur 75, 1982: 303–316.

31. Lablanche JM, Delforge MR, Tilmant PY, Thieuleux FA, Bertrand ME: Action coronarodilatatrice de l'isosorbide dinitrate injectable. La Nouvelle Presse Médicale 11, 1982: 2057–2061.

32. Kaltenbach M, Schultz W, Kober G: Effects of nifedipine after intravenous and intracoronary administration. Am J Cardiol 44, 1979: 832–838.

33. Serruys PW, Brower RW, Katen HJ ten, Bom AM, Hugenholtz PG:Regional wall motion from radiopaque markers after intravenous and intracoronary injections of nifedipine. Circulation 63, 1981: 584–591.

34. Bentley K, Henry PD: Spasmogenic effect of angiographic dye on normal and atherosclerotic arteries. Circulation 62 (Suppl III), 1980: III–218 (Abstract).

35. Higgins CB, Schmidt W: Direct and reflex myocardial effects of intracoronary administered contrast materials in the anesthetized and conscious dog: comparison of standard and newer contrast materials. Invest. Radiol. 13, 1978: 205–216.

36. Cumberland DC: Low-osmolality contrast media in cardiac radiology. Invest Radiol 19, 1984: S301–S305.

37. Spiller P, Schmiel FK, Pölitz B, Block M, Fermor U, Hackbarth W, Jehle J, Körfer R, Pannek H: Measurement of systolic and diastolic flow rates in coronary artery system by X-ray densitometry. Circulation 68, 1983: 337–347.

38. Vogel RA, Bates ER, O'Neil WW, Aueron FM, Meier B, Gruentzig AR: Coronary flow reserve measured during cardiac catheterization. Arch Intern Med 144, 1984: 1773–1776.

39. LeGrand V, Aueron FM, Bates ER, O'Neil WW, Hodgson JMcB, Mancini GBJ, Vogel RA: Reversibility of coronary collaterals and alteration in regional coronary flow reserve after successful angioplasty. Am J Cardiol 54, 1984: 453–454.

40. Reiber JHC, Kooijman CJ, Boer A den, Serruys PW: Assessment of dimensions and image quality of coronary contrast catheters from cineangiograms. Cath and Cardiov. Diagn 11, 1985: 521–531.

41. Schultz W, Wendt T, Scherer D, Kober G: Diameter changes of epicardial coronary arteries and coronary stenoses after intracoronary application of SIN 1, a molsidomine metabolite. Z Kardiol 72, 1983: 404–409.

42. Alderman EL, Berte LE, Harrison DC, Sanders W: Quantitation of coronary artery dimensions using digital image processing. In: Digital Radiography. WR Brody (Ed.) SPIE 314, 1982: 273–278.

Part III: Can we measure coronary blood flow from contrast injection?

Determination of coronary blood flow and myocardial perfusion by digital image processing

Paul Spiller and F.-K. Schmiel

Summary

The application of digital subtraction angiography for the measurement of coronary blood flow and myocardial perfusion is described. The angiographic images are transformed into a video signal and digitized by means of an A/D converter (conversion rate: 10 MHz, gray scale resolution: 8 bits = 256 levels). The digitized images are buffered as a matrix (256 lines, 512 pixels/line) in a fast semiconductor memory and transferred via a DMA-interface to a computer system (PDP-11). Following processing by a software program the resulting images are retransferred to the buffer memory and displayed on a TV-monitor via a D/A converter.

Flow measurements are performed by subtracting two consecutive frames of the coronary angiogram. The essential information of the resulting difference image is the position of the front of the contrast medium. By processing a sequence of such difference images the propagation of the front can be visualized. The velocities of coronary blood flow can be determined quantitatively from the front displacement-versus-time plot.

To assess the hemodynamic relevance of coronary artery stenoses flow measurements during hyperemia are necessary. The prerequisite for such evaluation is that the flow increases to the same extent in different nonstenosed branches of the same vessel. This was proven by flow measurements before and after Dipyridamole: flow rates increased by the same percentage.

The opacification of the myocardium by contrast medium injected into the coronary arteries if visualized by subtraction of nonopacified mask images from the opacified images acquired during the same phase of the cardiac cycle. The washin and washout phase of the contrast medium can be seen on the difference images. By integration of the brightness levels a densogram can be determined, describing functionally the passage of the contrast medium through the myocardium. We found a close correlation between the risetime of the densograms and the qualitatively evaluated Tl-scintigrams at rest for the same patients. Thus, we suggest that the rise-time be a quantitative measure of myocardial perfusion.

Introduction

To date digital image processing is frequently and routinely used by many radiologists for angiographic imaging of peripheral arteries and by some cardiologists to delineate the left ventricle by intravenous injection of contrast medium. The evaluation of the coronary arteries and the myocardium by digital angiography, however, continues to remain a topic of research. The purpose of this chapter is to discuss some aspects regarding the acquisition and quantitative analysis of angiographic image series for the measurement of coronary blood flow as well as of myocardial perfusion.

Earlier studies with analog devices have shown that flow rates in coronary arteries can be determined on the basis of the propagation of injected contrast material. The principle of the measurement is based upon the calculation of the transit time from density-time curves (densograms) assessed at two positions over the artery, thereby defining a fixed distance. The measurements reveal a flow pattern typical for coronary arteries and have a good reproducibility (1).

However, despite these promising results, flow measurements with analog devices are hampered by considerable problems.

Firstly, the short measurement sections result in short transit times with resulting relatively large errors in flow measurements. Secondly, the propagation of contrast medium in the arteries and vessel motion are superimposed. Thirdly, the scatter of the measurements cannot be assessed as flow rates are determined from only two measuring points. These difficulties in the measurement of coronary flow can be reduced by employing digital techniques.

Until 1980 the assessment of myocardial perfusion by X-ray techniques was an aim for the future. Since then, the rapid developments in digital computer techniques for image acquisition and processing have enabled us not only to visualize the opacification of the myocardium but to obtain quantitative information, as well. Which of the appearance-, rise- or washout-times assessed from the density-time curves is the best indicator of myocardial perfusion, however, remains an unanswered question. For that reason several groups are working towards the improvement and validation of functional parameters to quantify regional and global myocardial perfusion (2, 3).

Principle of digital measurements of coronary flow and myocardial perfusion

By digital subtraction of two consecutive cineframes of a cinecoronary angiogram the exact position of the front of the contrast medium can be localized on each single frame. The difference is zero in all parts of the images where the density information remained unchanged; that means, the difference image basically reveals only those structures which are caused by the displacement of the front.

Myocardial perfusion is evaluated from the passage of the contrast medium

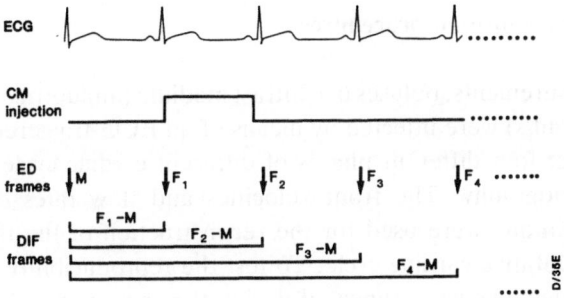

Figure 1. Scheme of image subtraction. A mask image M from the last cycle before the injection of contrast medium (rectangular pulse) is subtracted from the opacified images $F_1, F_2, F_3, \ldots$ resulting in a sequence of difference images (F_i–M, etc.).

through the myocardium. Prior condition for visualization is the elimination of background structures, i.e. lung tissue, ribs and the diaphragm. This is achieved by digital subtraction of a mask image taken before the injection of the contrast medium from contrast images selected from the same phase in the cardiac cycle.

The procedure for digital imaging of myocardial perfusion is shown schematically in Figure 1. The last image at the R-wave immediately before the injection of the contrast medium is taken as a mask M. If this mask is subtracted from the R-wave triggered opacified images F_i, a sequence of difference images F_i–M is obtained, demonstrating the passage of the contrast medium at end diastole. This procedure can be applied not only on R-wave synchronized images, but on all other images of the cardiac cycle, provided the images F_i and the mask M are taken from the same phase in the cardiac cycle.

Digital image processing system

The hardware of the image processing system consists of a PDP 11/10 computer plus peripherals (Fig. 2). The video converted cinecoronary angiograms are digitized by a fast analog-to-digital converter.

As the sampling rate of the A/D-converter is much higher than the transfer rate of 1 megacycles per second of the PDP 11/10 computer system, the digitized pixels from the total image are buffered as a matrix in a fast semiconductor memory. The matrix is composed of 256 lines with 512 pixels each. The total range of brightness levels is linearly divided into 256 steps. After an entire frame has been scanned, the image is transferred to the computer system. Following the digitization of two frames the difference matrix can be computed by the processor and returned to the image memory. Its content can be plotted or displayed onto a TV-monitor via a digital-to-analog converter.

Angiographic acquisition procedures

For flow measurements, boluses of contrast medium (amidotricoate, 1.0 to 1.5 ml, flow rate 4–5 ml/s) were injected by means of an ECG-triggered power injector during at least four different phases of different cardiac cycles during routine coronary angiography. The front velocities and flow rates obtained by this sampling technique were used for the reconstruction of the flow pattern of a single representative cardiac cycle. To test the reproducibility of the measurements, the injections were repeated during the same phase. The intervals between single bolus injections were at least 30 s.

The passages of the contrast boluses were recorded by means of a biplane X-ray angiography system simultaneously in right and left anterior oblique projections on 35 mm cinefilm (100 frames/s, 70–85 kV, 270 mA). A projection angle was chosen such that superimposition of different branches of the vessel did not occur. During the measurements the patient's ECG, the cine synchronizing pulses necessary to relate the recorded parameters to the single cineframes in both projections, and the signal of the contrast medium injector were recorded continuously. Before and after each injection the pressure in the ostium of the coronary artery was measured via the injection catheter.

For perfusion measurements, boluses of 4 ml contrast medium were injected (flow rate 4 ml/s). The start of injection was triggered on the R-wave of the ECG 2.5 s after the beginning of the angiographic investigation. The angiograms were recorded on cinefilm in right and left anterior oblique projections (50 frames/s) for at least 15 s. During the acquisition the same parameters as described for the flow measurements were recorded. The reproducibility was tested by repeated injections.

The intervals between single bolus injections were about 5 min. The patients had to hold their breath in deep inspiration during the angiographic investigations.

Quantitative evaluation of the cinefilms

The cineangiograms were projected via a light-stabilized projection head onto a video camera (Figure 2). The analog video signals were digizited, processed by the computer system and displayed on a TV-monitor. To measure coronary flow, the front velocities of the contrast medium in two different branches of the left coronary artery were determined from displacement-time plots during systole and diastole. The diameter and the distances covered by the bolus fronts were measured biplane from the cineangiographic frames with the appropriate magnification factors (4).

In Figure 3 the procedure of digital image subtraction for flow measurements is demonstrated. In the upper part two consecutive single frames of a cineangio-

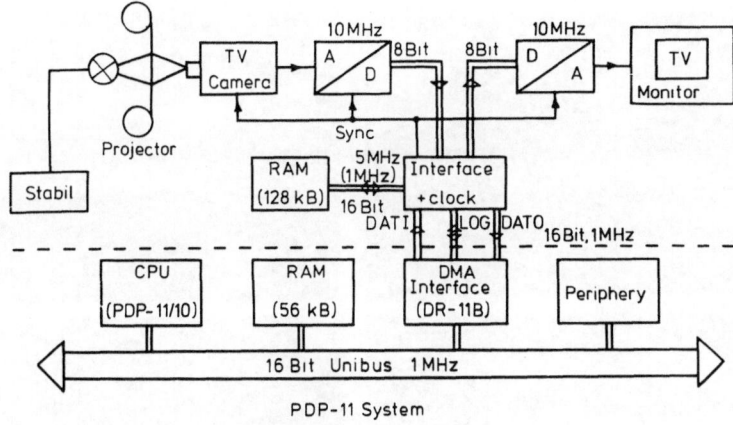

PDP-11 System

Figure 2. Hardware diagram of the digital image processing system. For further details see text.

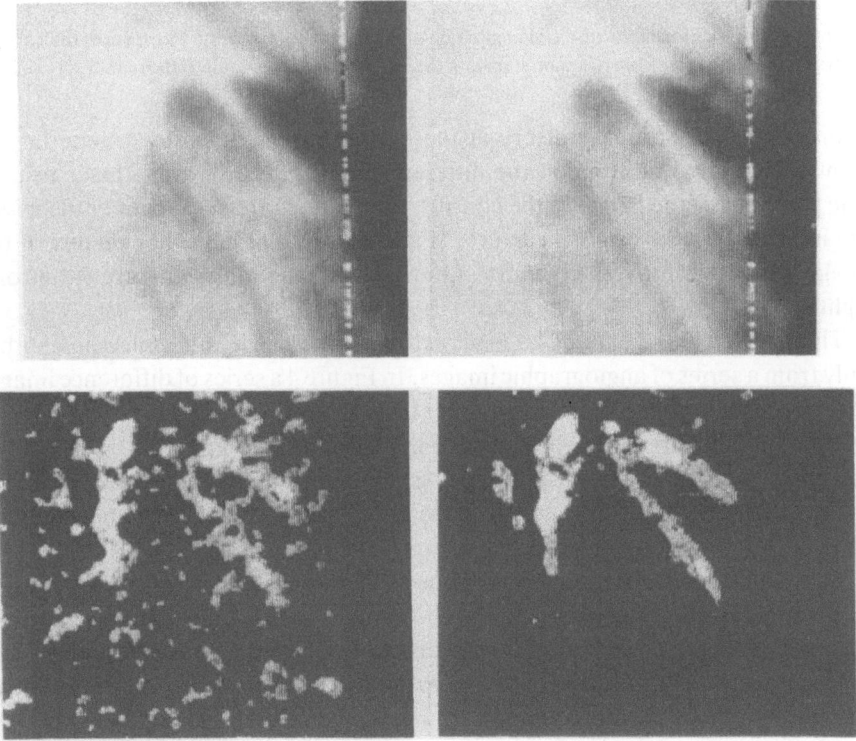

Figure 3. Upper part: two consecutive frames of a cineangiogram of the left coronary artery. *Lower part:* resulting difference image (left), and same image after filtering and smoothing (right).

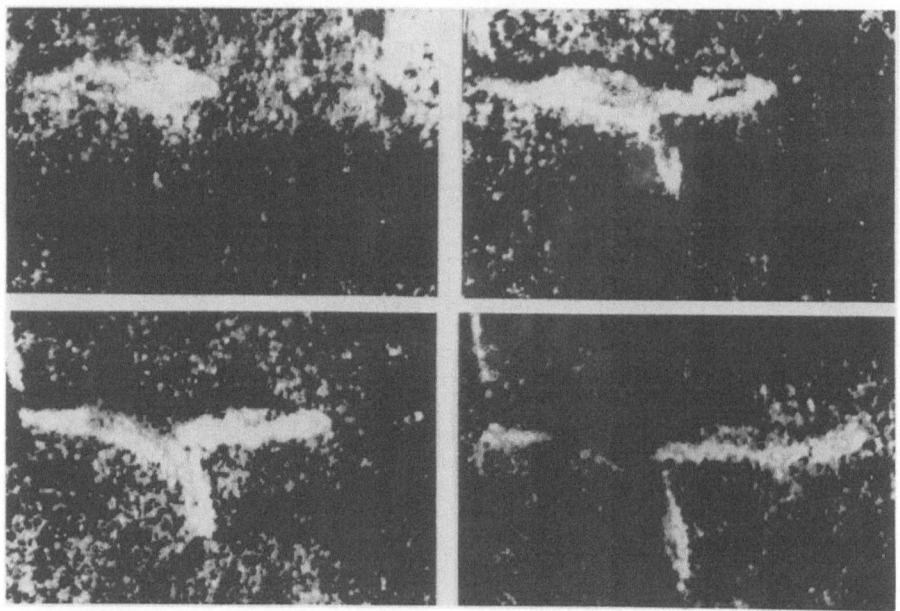

Figure 4. Difference images from a cineangiogram of the left coronary artery. The front of the bolus of contrast medium moves from the main stem into the left anterior descending and circumflex branches.

gram of the left coronary artery at the early filling with contrast material are shown. By digital subtraction the difference image of these two frames results. The positions of the fronts of the contrast medium in three branches of the vessel are indicated by the bright structures (Figure 3 bottom, left). The quality of the image can be improved by digital filtering and smoothing (Figure 3 bottom, right).

The flow of blood cannot be assessed from one single difference image, but only from a series of angiographic images. In Figure 4 a series of difference images is depicted. The contrast medium moves from the main stem into the left anterior descending and circumflex branches of the left coronary artery.

That means that the flow of the contrast medium – or in other words – the flow of blood opacified by the contrast medium, can be visualized and analyzed qualitatively from angiographic series in a functional sense.

For quantitative determinations of flow velocities from such series the propagation of the front is measured frame-to-frame. The travelled distances at time increments of 10 ms are plotted as a displacement-time curve (Figure 5). The diagram shows that the velocity of propagation remains nearly constant during the measurement period of about 150 ms. In contrast to analog videodensitometric techniques the velocity is determined not just from one distance and one transit time, but from a complete displacement-time plot. The average flow velocity can be determined by fitting a linear function through the measurement

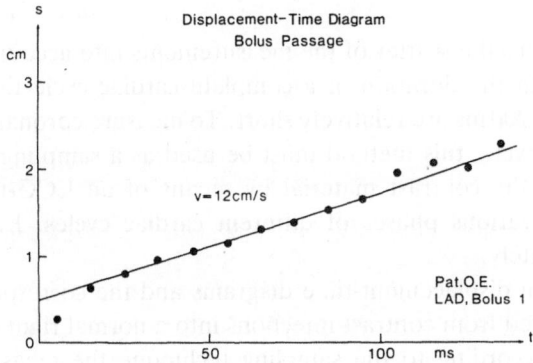

Figure 5. Displacement-time diagram assessed from a series of difference images. The displacement s of the contrast bolus is plotted versus time t. The velocity v is determined from the slope of the line.

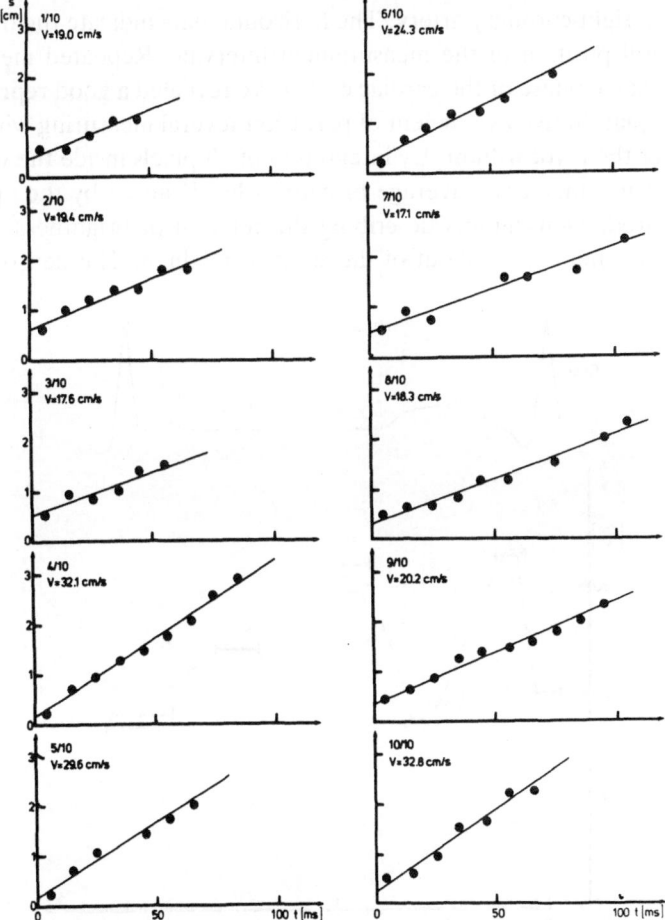

Figure 6. Displacement-time diagrams and corresponding flow velocities determined from ten bolus injections into the right coronary artery. The measurements cover different phases of a cardiac cycle (sampling technique).

182

points, which takes the scatter of the measurements into account.

Compared with the duration of a complete cardiac cycle the measurement periods of 100 to 200 ms are relatively short. To measure coronary flow throughout a complete cycle, this method must be used as a sampling technique. We therefore inject the contrast material by means of an ECG-triggered power injector during various phases of different cardiac cycles. Each injection is evaluated separately.

In Figure 6 ten displacement-time diagrams and the corresponding flow velocities determined from contrast injections into a normal right coronary artery are depicted. According to the sampling technique the measurements cover different phases of the cardiac cycle (4).

The values of the flow velocities can be used to reconstruct the flow curve of a single representative cardiac cycle. Figure 7 demonstrates the typical phasic flow pattern of a right coronary artery. The horizontal bars indicate the duration and the temporal position of the measurement intervals. Repeated measurements during the same phase of the cardiac cycle have revealed a good reproducibility.

For the quantitative assessment of perfusion several measuring windows were placed over the myocardium. By integration of all pixels inside the windows for each difference image the average brightness level caused by the opacification was measured. Densograms describing the relation of brightness versus time reveal the washin and washout of the contrast medium. The densograms were

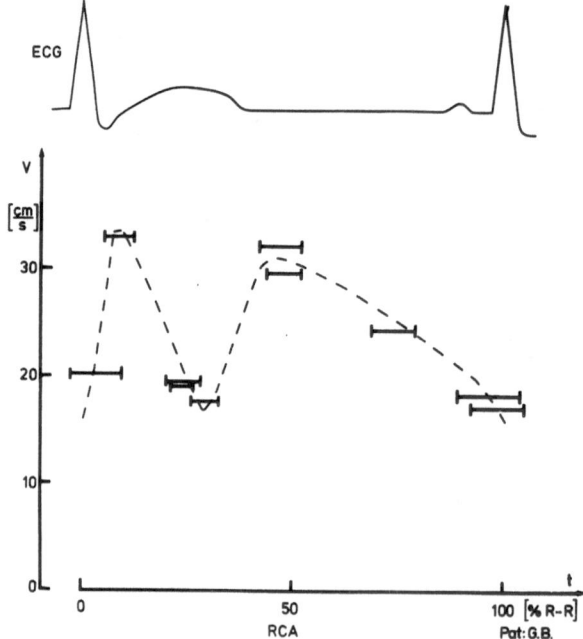

Figure 7. Flow values measured in a right coronary artery. The horizontal bars depict the flow velocity (v) and the time interval of measurement, calibrated in % of the R–R-interval of the patient's ECG.

analyzed by measuring the rise-time, i.e. the time interval between the beginning and the point of maximal value of the curve. To improve the accuracy of the measurement six densograms at different phases throughout the cardiac cycle were evaluated. The mean rise-time was calculated by averaging these values, excluding those outside of the standard error of the mean of the six measured rise-times. In each patient four different measuring windows were analyzed in the left anterior oblique projection of the cinefilm.

Results

Measurements of coronary flow

Ultimate goal of coronary blood flow measurements is the determination of the functional significance of coronary artery lesions in a quantitative manner. To assess the severity of moderate stenoses which do not limit resting coronary flow, measurements during hyperemia are necessary. Prerequisites for these evaluations are identical flow velocities at rest and nearly the same flow increases during hyperemia in different branches of the coronary vessels.

The validity of the first condition could be proven in several patient studies. In Figure 8 an example of the increase in flow by Dipyridamole i.v. is depicted.

Flow values before (solid lines) and after (dashed lines) Dipyridamole administration determined during four different phases of the cardiac cycle are shown. In this case flow increased after Dipyridamole during systole and diastole by about 50 percent. Figure 9 summarizes coronary blood flow measurements performed simultaneously in the left anterior descending and circumflex

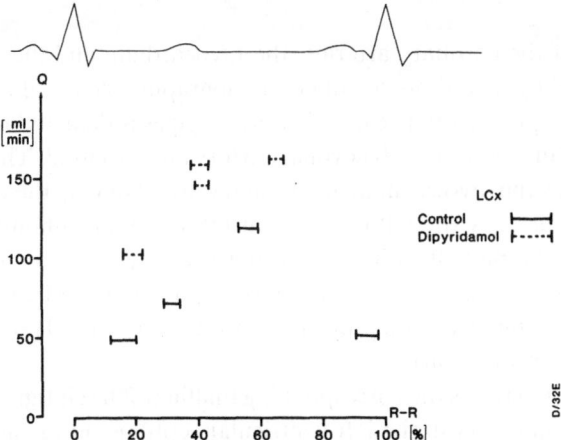

Figure 8. Flow values before (solid lines) and after (dashed lines) Dipyridamole administration in a circumflex branch of a normal left coronary artery. Systolic and diastolic flows increase after Dipyridamole.

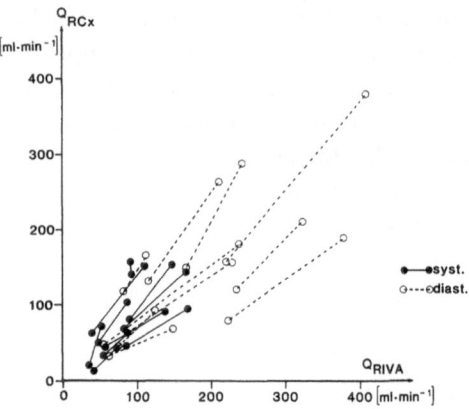

Figure 9. Summary of flow measurements performed simultaneously in the left anterior descending (abscissa) and circumflex branches (ordinate) of the left coronary artery. Both flow values are characterized by only one point. The lines connect corresponding values before and after Dipyridamole. The flow rates in almost all of these normal vessels increase by the same percentage.

branches of normal left coronary arteries. In this presentation both flow values are characterized by only one point. The lines connect corresponding values before and after Dipyridamole. It is evident that on average the flow rates in these normal vessels increase by the same percentage. That means that the prerequisites for flow measurements in patients with coronary artery disease have been met.

Measurements of myocardial perfusion

Visualization of the coronary arteries, the myocardium and the coronary veins can be achieved by digital processing of angiographic scenes of about 15 s duration. As an example a sequence of difference images is depicted in Figure 10. At first only the branches of the left coronary artery are opacified. Then the contrast medium perfuses the myocardium and is then washed out via the coronary veins. All regions perfused by the left coronary artery are homogenously opacified.

In contrast to this patient with normally perfused myocardium, Figure 11 shows a sequence of images which characterize an occlusion of the left anterior descending artery with an unperfused septum and a normally perfused posterior wall (left anterior oblique projection).

Figure 12 demonstrates the corresponding thallium-201 scintigram at rest with a marked perfusion defect in the left ventricular septum and the apex.

For quantitative measurement of perfusion measuring windows were positioned over the myocardium. By integration of all pixels inside a window for each difference image the average brightness level, being a measure for opacification,

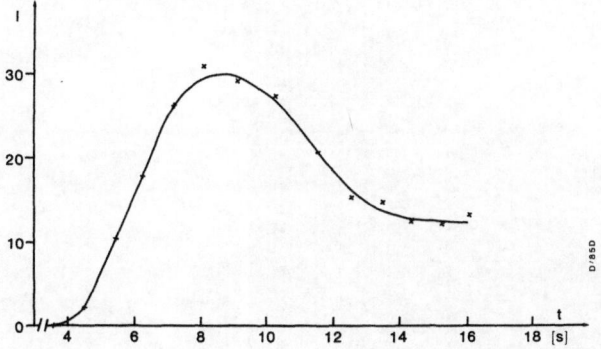

Figure 13. Densogram (density-time curve) demonstrating myocardial perfusion. Each measurement point depicts the average brightness level within a measuring window in a difference image representing contrast opacification.

was assessed as a function of time. In Figure 13 the washin and washout phases of the contrast medium can readily be appreciated. Obviously, the washout phase of this densogram cannot be described by an exponential decay, i.e. perfusion cannot be determined from this curve in a similar manner as from indicator dilution curves. Even after a period of 16 s the opacification does not reach the baseline, but remains at a plateau.

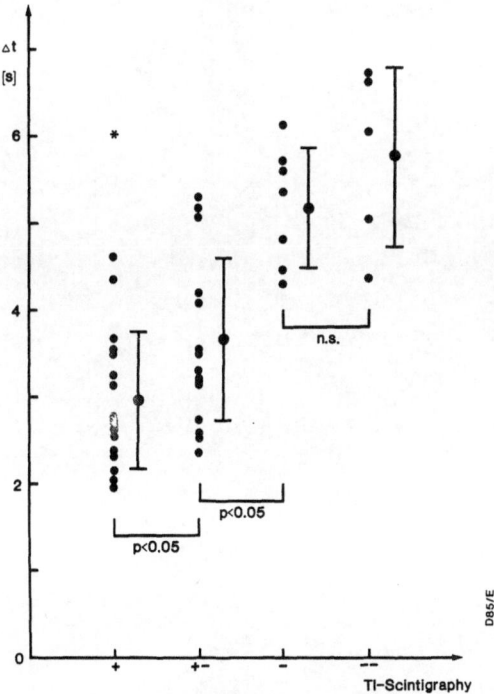

Figure 14. Correlation of the rise-times (Δ t) of myocardial densograms with qualitative evaluations of thallium-201 scintigrams at rest. (+ normal, + − slightly reduced, − markedly reduced perfusion; − −perfusion defect or scar) For further details see text.

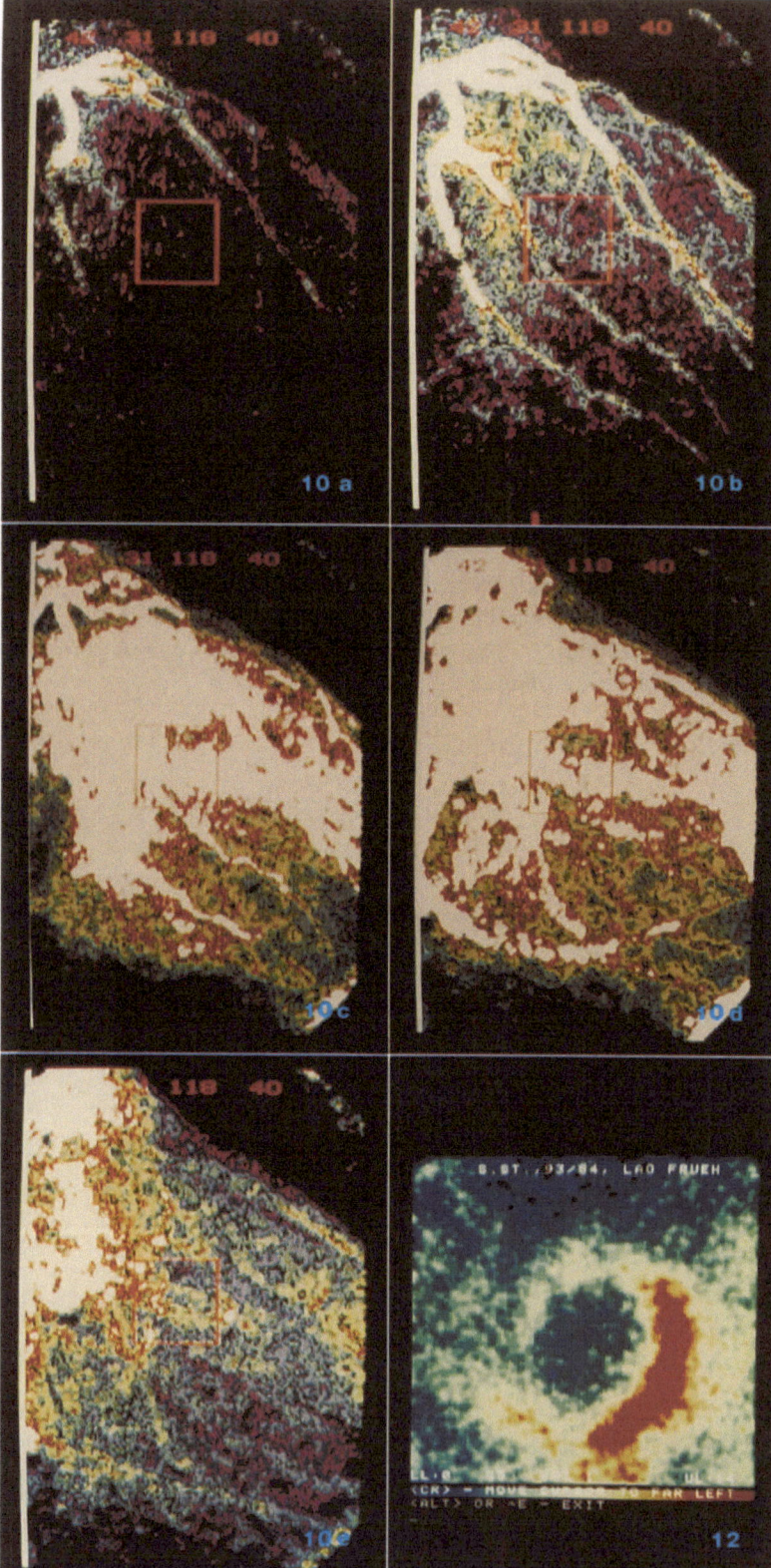

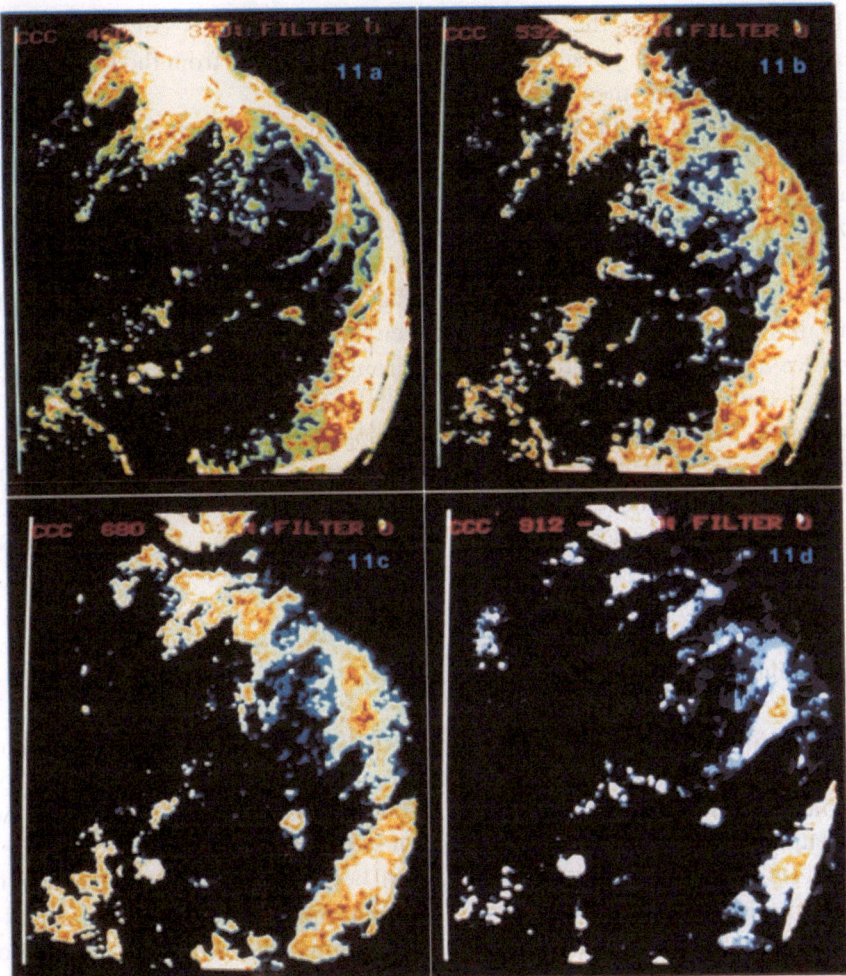

Figure 11. Sequence of difference images demonstrating myocardial perfusion. Due to occlusion of the left anterior descending coronary artery only the posterior wall of the left ventricle is normally perfused (same patient as in Figure 12).

←

Figure 10. Sequence of difference images demonstrating myocardial perfusion. From the first three panels a–c the washin phase (opacification of the coronary arteries and maximum opacification of the myocardium) can be seen, whereas the last two panels d and e show the washout phase (opacification of the coronary veins).

Figure 12. Thallium-201 scintigram of a left ventricle at rest with a perfusion defect in the septal and apical regions (left anterior oblique projection).

If we assume, that the duration of the washin phase is correlated to the perfusion, it might be possible to determine the perfusion from the leading slope of the densogram by measuring the rise-time.

It seems to be difficult, if not impossible, to prove in patients that the rise-time of the densograms is a measure of myocardial perfusion. In Figure 14 the rise-time was correlated to qualitative results of thallium scintigraphy at rest. The perfusion determined from the scintigrams was classified into four groups: + normal, + − slightly reduced, − markedly reduced, and − − perfusion defect or scar. The rise-times of the four groups were on average 3.0, 3.7, 5.2 and 5.8 s respectively. The differences in the rise-times between the four groups were statistically significant except between the − and − − groups. There is only one measurement point − depicted by the asterix − which falls out of range. In this case the prolonged, pathological rise-time of the densogram was combined with a normal scintigram. The reason for this discrepancy became obvious from the coronary angiogram which showed a right proponderant coronary artery perfusing the apex of the left ventricle. As we evaluated only the injection of contrast medium into the left coronary artery, we measured an artificially prolonged rise-time.

Discussion

The greatest advantage of the digital versus analog technique is the higher accuracy that can be achieved for measuring coronary blood flow. It results from the fact that the flow velocities are determined from a plot instead of only two measurement values. The method was validated by comparison with photodensitometry. There was no systematic deviation between values determined by both methods; that means that on the basis of the determination of the front velocity of the contrast medium by digital subtraction techniques the coronary blood flow measurements overestimate the true values by about 20%, similar to that of video- or photodensitometric evaluations.

The main difficulty in determining coronary flow − the motion of the vessels −, however, remains a problem. Since the motion is superimposed upon the propagation of the bolus of contrast medium, it has to be taken into account. Until today, the images have to be reregistered manually according to the apparent vessel motion. Assessment of the degree of motion and the diameters of the vessels by semi-automatic means can be expected by software techniques. Such developments are necessary to shorten the time-consuming analysis of angiographic scenes and seem to be a requirement for routine clinical application.

The aim of our first series of measurements in patients with normal coronary arteries was to establish the basis for determinations of coronary blood flow in patients with coronary artery disease. Figure 9 shows that the relative increases in flow induced by Dipyridamole in the left anterior descending and circumflex branches of these normal left coronary arteries were nearly identical in almost all patients. If one assumes that the flow reserve is limited in stenotic arteries, a striking difference in flow increase after Dipyridamole i. v. between normal and stenotic branches of the same coronary artery can be expected.

According to the results from Gould *et al.* in dogs with implanted Doppler flow velocity transducers and from our own studies, the increase in flow velocity after coronary vasodilatation does not represent the true augmentation of the volume flow as the vessel diameter increases as well (5).

Several groups have shown that the myocardium can be visualized by injection of contrast medium using digital image subtraction (2, 3, 6). The principle is based on the elimination of intervening background structures from the contrast image by subtraction of a nonopacified mask image which must be congruent with respect to the background structures (Figure 1). Normal perfusion is characterized by homogenous washin and washout of the contrast medium, reduced perfusion by inhomogenities. These images are comparable to thallium scintigrams at rest.

Considerable problems arise, however, from the attempt to assess perfusion quantitatively. From earlier studies it is known that coronary blood flow and myocardial perfusion are strikingly influenced by the contrast medium injected (7, 8). Following an injection of a small bolus of amidotricoate coronary flow increases by about 30 percent, while the duration of the flow increase lasts at least 19 s.

That means that these effects have to be taken into account in perfusion measurements by means of contrast opacification of the myocardium.

Therefore, in our measurements the time period between two contrast injections was usually 5 min. It must be mentioned, however, that even after this rather long time lag the mask images before the second injection were not identical to those of the preceding contrast scene. A possible explanation may be that after injection only a portion of the contrast medium passes the myocardium and appears immediately in the coronary vein system. Another portion seems to remain in the extra- and intracellular spaces of the tissue (9–11).

In pharmocokinetic studies Langemann showed that one hour after injection 25 percent of the concentration of amidotricoat in blood could be found in heart muscle (10).

Whether different shapes of the density-time curves determined over the myocardium (Figures 15 and 16) reflect normal or abnormal contrast medium washout, still remains an open question. Unexplained, too, is the fact that densograms of the same patient derived from different myocardial regions are similar.

Because of the variations of the densograms during the washout phase, we measured the rise-time in an attempt to quantify myocardial perfusion. The correlation of this quantitative term with the results of qualitative evaluations of thallium scintigrams proved that the rise-time is a measure of perfusion (Figure 14). Repeated determinations revealed a good reproducibility (Figure 17). While

190

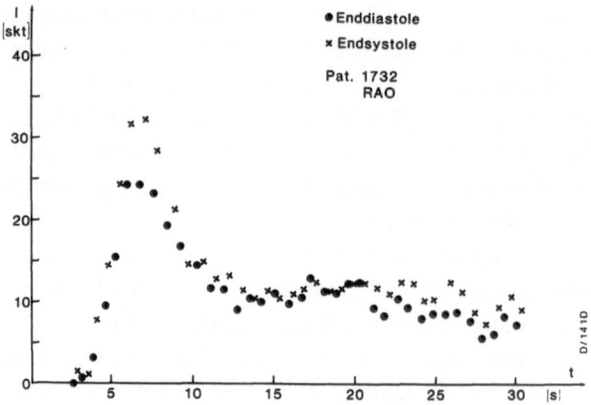

Figure 15. Densogram with one peak density and a prolonged washout phase.

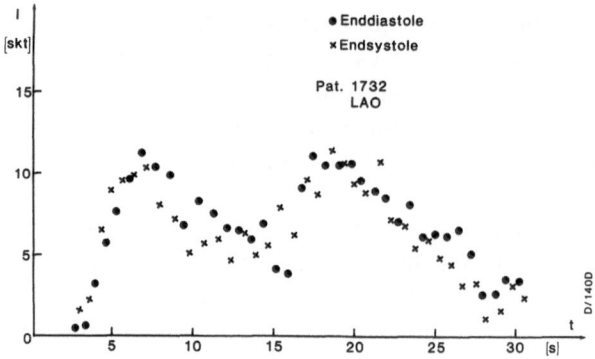

Figure 16. Densogram with two peak densities.

Nivatpumin *et al.* propose parameters from the washout phase, Vogel *et al.*, also determine a parameter, the appearance time, from the washin phase (2).

Which of these terms is the best indicator of myocardial perfusion can only be assessed from extensive experimental studies. Two problems of the analysis of density-time curves from the myocardium, however, can only be reduced but not solved: 1) the poor resolution in time resulting from the heart motion can be decreased by averaging several values of the derived parameters; and 2) the superimposition of different myocardial walls can be minimized by using several angiographic projections.

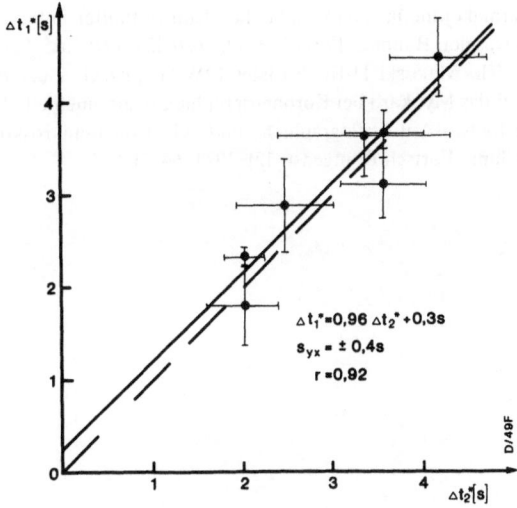

Figure 17. Correlation of the two independent determinations of the mean rise-time. The dots represent the mean value of six measurements. The bars characterize the standard deviations. The mean values of the rise-times are closely correlated.

References

1. Spiller P, Schmiel FK, Pölitz B, Block M, Fermor U, Hackbarth W, Jehle J, Körfer R, Pannek H: Measurement of systolic and diastolic flow rates in the coronary artery system by X-ray densitometry. Circulation 68, 1983: 337–347.
2. Vogel R, LeFree M, Bates E, O'Neill W, Foster R, Kirlin P, Smith D, Pitt B: Application of digital techniques to selective coronary arteriography: Use of myocardial contrast appearence time to measure coronary flow reserve. Am Heart J 107, 1984: 153–163.
3. Whiting JS, Nivatpumin Th, Pfaff M, Vas R, Drury K, Diamond G, Swan HJC, Forrester JS: Assessing the coronary circulation by digital angiography: Bypass graft and myocardial perfusion imaging. In: Digital Imaging in Cardiovascular Radiology, PH Heintzen, R Brennecke (Eds.), Georg Thieme Verlag, Stuttgart, New York, 1983: 205–212.
4. Spiller P, Jehle J, Pölitz B, Schmiel FK: A digital X-ray image processing system for measurement of phasic blood flow in coronary arteries. Comp Cardiol 1982: 223–226.
5. Gould, KL, Kelley KO: Physiological significance of coronary flow velocity and changing stenosis geometry during coronary vasodilation in awake dogs. Circ Res 50, 1982: 695–704.
6. Spiller PFK, Schmiel M, Haude M, Jehle J, Lösse B, Pölitz B: Messung der Myokardperfusion mittels digitaler Bildverarbeitung. In: Digitale Radiographie, HE Riemann and J Kollath (Eds.). Konstanz, 1985.
7. Bussmann W–D, Rutishauser W, Noseda G, Preter B, Meier W: Influence of a new contrast medium (Metrizoate) on coronary blood flow. In: Roentgen-, Cine- and Videodensitometry, PH Heintzen (Ed.), Georg Thieme Verlag, Stuttgart, 1971: 133–139.
8. Hackbarth W, Bircks W, Pölitz B, Körfer R, Schmiel FK, Spiller P: Vergleich videodensitometrischer und elektromagnetischer Flussmessungen in aortokoronaren Bypassgefässen. Fortsch Röntgenstr 132, 1980: 554–560.
9. Dean PB: The influence of concentration and dose upon the extravascular distribution of intra-arterially injected meglumine diatrizoate. Fortsch Röntgenstr 127, 1977: 63–68.

10. Lagemann K: Pharmakokinetik angiographischer Kontrastmittel unter besonderer Berücksichtigung des extravasalen Raumes. Fortsch Röntgenstr 123, 1975: 515–521.

11. Löhr E, Göbbeler Th, Makoski H-Br, Strötges MW, Popitz G: Über die Einwirkung von Konstrastmitteln auf das Myokard bei Koronarographien (experimentelle Untersuchungen des Elektrolyt-Stoffwechsels, Autoradiographien und elektronen-mikroskopische Autoradiographien), 1. Mitteilung. Fortsch Röntgenstr 121, 1974: 64–71.

Densitometric assessment of coronary blood velocity and flow in man from coronary angiography: possibilities and problems

Rüdiger Simon, I. Amende, G. Herrmann, W. Quante and P.R. Lichtlen

Summary

A roentgen videodensitometric technique is described that has been developed and used in our laboratories to assess regional coronary artery hemodynamics during routine coronary angiography. The mean travelling time of the contrast bolus (rapid bolus injection of 2–3 cc Urografin 76%) between two sampling sites on the coronary artery is derived by logarithmic videodensitometry from tape-stored video-angiograms. True spatial length and average cross section of the vessel between sampling sites are obtained by morphometric techniques from concomitant biplane cineangiograms, using a multisegmental model. From dimensions and travelling time, mean blood velocity and flow through the vessel are calculated.

Experience with more than 200 measurements has proven, that the procedure on the patient is short, simple, and safe. Replicate determinations have demonstrated a sufficient reproducibility for travelling time ($r = 0.94$), as well as for arterial dimensions ($r = 0.96$). Mean blood velocity in the mid parts of coronary arteries was found to range from 2 to 22 cm/sec under resting conditions.

Blood velocity in aortocoronary venous bypass grafts varied from 4 to 33 cm/ sec, and blood flow ranged from 15 to 170 ml/min. Velocity as well as flow did not correlate with the arterial cross section or the absence or presence of obstructions in the vessel under study, indicating that coronary function cannot be predicted from coronary dimensions.

We conclude that densitometry is advantageous since it can provide an estimate of regional coronary function from routine coronary angiography. At the present time, however, only blood velocity can be assessed in absolute terms for unbranched and branched vessels, whereas flow in absolute terms can only be given for unbranched vessels.

Introduction

The analysis of coronary angiograms is routinely restricted to coronary morphology. It has long been shown, however, that coronary angiography can provide more than just anatomical information. When the contrast agent that is injected for the visualization of the coronary vessels, is regarded as an indicator and indicator dilution principles are applied, functional parameters such as blood velocity and flow in single coronary arteries can be derived.

More than 10 years ago, roentgen cine- and videodensitometric techniques have been described for the measurement of blood flow in the coronary circulation from coronary angiograms (1–3). Based on these concepts, an integrated videodensitometric system has been developed in our laboratories, that has undergone continuous improvement and today allows densitometric measurements from routine diagnostic coronary angiography.

System and methods

Our X-ray system allows the acquisition of biplane 35 mm cineangiograms simultaneously with undisturbed (flickerless) video recordings (plumbicon TV camera) at 50 frames/sec during synchronized and stabilized pulsed radiation. For densitometric measurements, a projection is chosen such that the vessel under study is positioned as parallel as possible to the input screen of the image intensifier in one plane. As an example, Figure 1 shows a bypass graft to the left anterior descending coronary artery in a right anterior oblique projection. A motor-driven, crescent-shaped copper filter mounted within the housing of the X-ray tube, is adjusted to the border of the heart to obtain a more homogeneous background. The patient is advised to hold his breath at mid-inspiration, and a bolus injection of 2 to 3 cc of contrast medium (Urografin 76%) is performed at the coronary ostial site, using a simple hand-held injector (Cordis). This angiographic scene (lasting 12 to 15 sec) is stored on video tape together with the ECG of the patient for later densitometric evaluation.

Simultaneously, biplane cineangiograms are taken in orthogonal projections for a morphometric assessment of vessel dimensions. A grid of small metal spheres attached to the input screen of the image intensifier and recorded on film and videotape, allows compensation for image distortion (pincushion effect) and enables the localization of corresponding sites in video and cine images. An overall calibration factor is derived by comparing the measured dimensions of a 2 cm metal sphere that is filmed at the site of the vessel after the angiographic procedure, with its known dimensions.

As all contrast medium does not enter the vessel under study in most instances, the Stewart-Hamilton principle for flow determination does not apply. Blood flow is therefore derived by a combined densitometric and morphometric

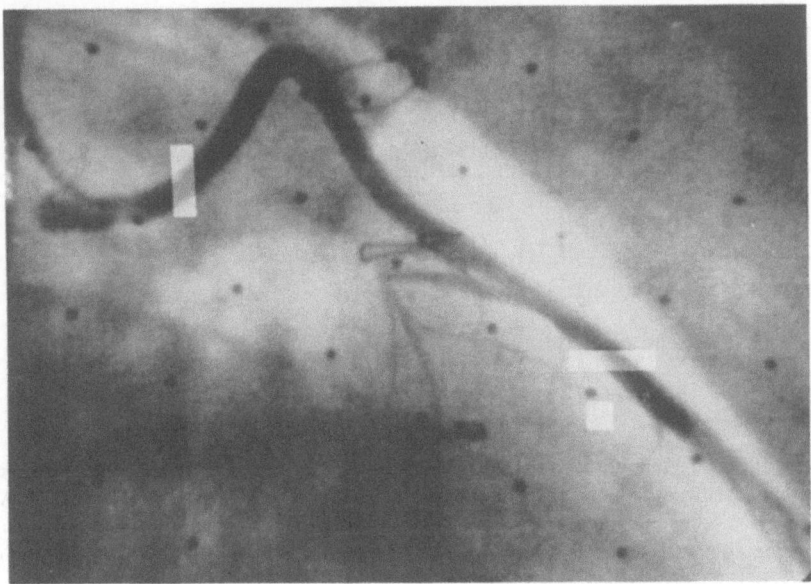

Figure 1. Aortocoronary venous bypass graft to a left anterior descending artery in RAO projection, with densitometric measuring windows and calibration grid superimposed (see text).

method, that requires the assessment of the velocity of the contrast bolus and the length and the volume of the vessel between two distinct measuring sites (1, 2). A diagram of our system is shown in Figure 2. When the tape is replayed, two sampling fields (windows, see Figure 1), are positioned in the TV-image over proximal and distal sites of the vessel. These windows are provided by a contour unit coupled to a microcomputer and x/y digitizing pen, and may have any desired size and shape. The electronic circuitry of the 2-channel videodensitometer performs high-fidelity logarithmic conversion and subsequent integration of all image intensities within each window in a dynamic frame-by-frame manner. Radiation scatter and veiling glare in the image intensifier are taken into account by automatic subtraction of a preset fraction of the video voltage (black level) for each image point before logarithmic conversion (4).

The brightness information from a third window that is positioned adjacent to the vessel over the myocardium, controls an automated gain control circuitry (AGC) in the densitometer input and compensates for undesired shifts in radiation intensity, as well as for the accumulation of contrast medium in the myocardial background (5). The output signal of each densitometer channel is a contrast dilution curve (densogram) that is proportional to the dynamic contents of contrast medium within the part of the coronary artery covered by the sampling window. These densograms are fed into a small microcomputer (CBM 8032) via a 10 bit analog-to-digital converter. The original densograms are superimposed by cyclic undulations due to the movement of the heart (see Figure 3, upper part). A

196

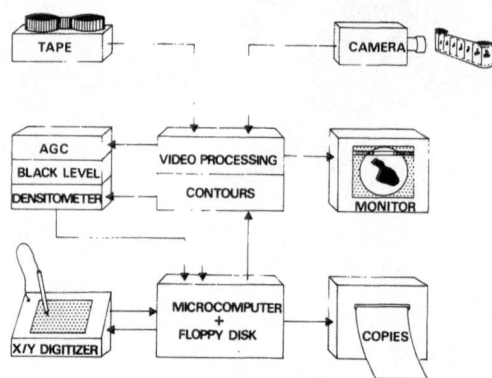

Figure 2. Block diagram of the system for videodensitometric and morphometric analysis of cine-angiograms. AGC: Automated gain control circuitry in the densitometer input. Black level: Automated black level compensation (see text). The densitometer includes logarithmic conversion and subsequent integration of all video voltages within a sampling window for 2 independent channels.

computer routine subtracts these cyclic undulations in a beat-per-beat fashion, using the R-wave of the ECG as reference. From the resulting compensated densograms, the program calculates the travelling time of the contrast bolus between the sampling sites. Since hand injections are used, we cannot neglect a possible influence of the injection on the shape of the densograms. We therefore use as many points on the curves as possible and derive travelling time as the time

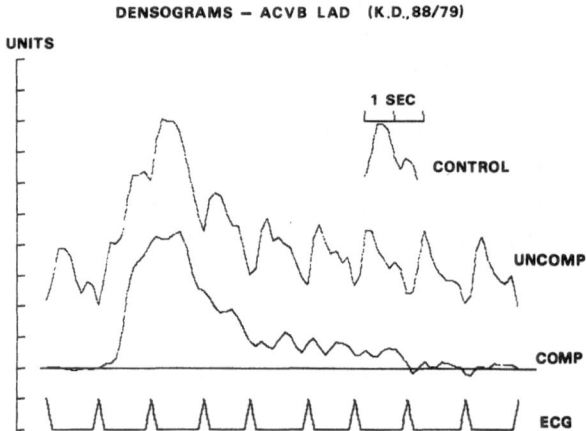

Figure 3. Densogram from proximal window in Figure 1. *Upper curve:* Original densogram (uncomp). *Lower curve:* Computer processed densogram (comp) after beat-to-beat subtraction of densitometric data of a representative heart cycle derived from several beats before contrast injection (control). *Bottom:* Computer-stored QRS-complex of the ECG used for compensation of mean cycle length to actual cycle length.

CORONARY DIMENSIONS FROM BIPLANE ANGIOGRAPHY

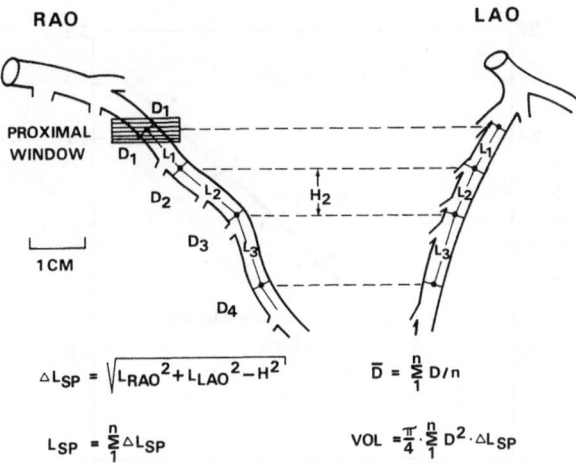

$$\Delta L_{SP} = \sqrt{L_{RAO}^2 + L_{LAO}^2 - H^2}$$

$$\bar{D} = \sum_{1}^{n} D/n$$

$$L_{SP} = \sum_{1}^{n} \Delta L_{SP}$$

$$VOL = \frac{\pi}{4} \cdot \sum_{1}^{n} D^2 \cdot \Delta L_{SP}$$

Figure 4. Determination of coronary artery dimensions from biplane cineangiography in orthogonal projections. The computer program adjusts both projections to identical scaling factors and divides the vessel between the proximal and distal (not shown) windows into approximately 20 segments. Total length between windows (L_{SP}) is approximated as the sum of segmental lengths (ΔL_{SP}). Total volume (vol) is derived by summing up segmental volumes.

interval between the individual transit times of both curves, where transit time T for each densogram is defined as:

$$T = \frac{\int t \cdot c(t) \cdot dt}{\int c(t) \cdot dt}$$

according to the concepts of classical indicator theory (6).

Vessel dimensions are derived from the 35 mm biplane cineangiograms. Tracings of the vessel are fed into the microcomputer via the x/y digitizer and the vessel is divided into at least 20 corresponding equidistant segments in both projections. For each segment, spatial length and volume are calculated according to the principles outlined in Figure 4, and total length and volume of the vessel between the windows are obtained as the sum of segmental values, respectively.

Finally, mean blood velocity is derived as spatial length divided by travelling time, and mean blood flow is obtained as vessel volume between sampling sites divided by travelling time.

Reproducibility and accuracy

The reproducibilities of both videodensitometric and morphometric measurements were studied in 15 patients. For two subsequent contrast injections (inter-

198

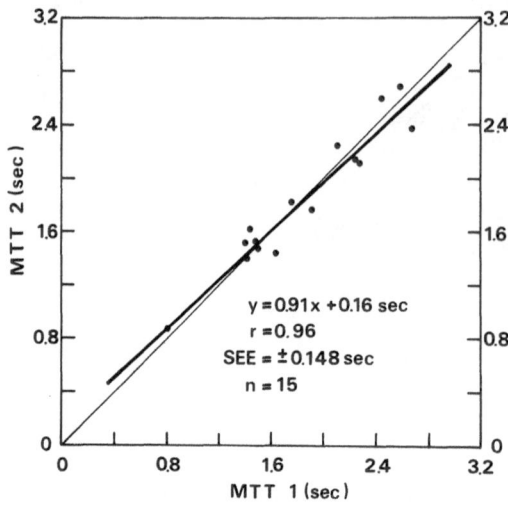

Figure 5. Replicate determinations of bolus travelling time in 15 native LAD arteries. MTT 1: First measurement. MTT 2: repeated assessment 2 minutes later.

val two minutes) into the left coronary artery, a good correlation for replicate determinations of travelling times as well as luminal diameters of the left anterior descending artery were obtained (Figures 5 and 6). Since the position of the sampling windows was kept constant for both measurements, reproducibility for travelling time also applies to blood velocity. These data also confirm that alterations in coronary hemodynamics after small intracoronary contrast injections have subsided within two minutes, in accordance with previous studies using different techniques (7).

The reliability and the accuracy of the underlying principles have been proven previously. Rutishauser and coworkers as well as Smith and coworkers have used similar techniques and reported excellent correlations between densitometric and electromagnetic flow measurements in coronary vessels in animals (1, 2). Spiller and coworkers have demonstrated comparable results in patients for flow measurements in vein grafts during bypass surgery (8). Their results, however, may not apply to the different condition of a conscious patient during clinical heart catheterization. Furthermore, they have been obtained in unbranched vein grafts, and may not apply to branched coronary arteries.

Since there is no independent technique available for the assessment of regional coronary artery flow in humans, we have attempted to validate our method in 24 patients by comparing changes in blood flow due to interventions, measured simultaneously by densitometry and the coronary sinus thermodilution technique (9). Seventeen of these patients had normal coronary arteries and normal cardiac

REPLICATE DIAMETER DETERMINATIONS
IN 15 NATIVE CORONARY ARTERIES (LAD)

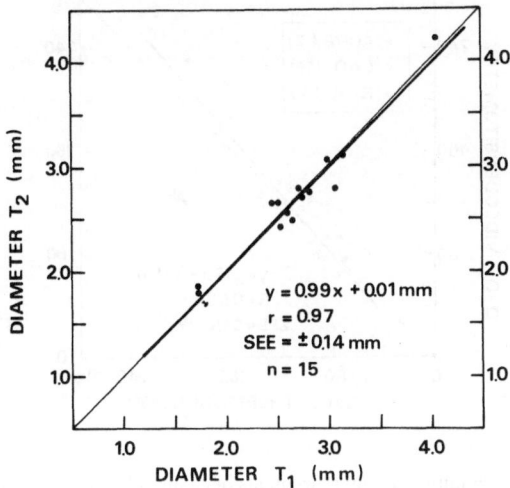

Figure 6. Replicate determinations of coronary diameters from biplane cineangiograms (concomitant with travelling time measurements in Figure 5). Diameter T_1: First measurement. Diameter T_2: Vessel diameter at repeated assessment, 2 minutes later.

function. Seven patients had had bypass surgery for single vessel disease: all of them showed a patent bypass graft that supplied a proximally occluded LAD; the other coronaries were normal. Alterations in coronary blood flow were induced by sublingual administration of nitroglycerin (0.8 mg) or nifedipine (20 mg), or an intravenous infusion of 0.5 mg/kg dipyridamole in these patients, and changes were assumed to be uniform on the arterial and the venous side of the coronary circulation. As demonstrated in Figure 7, a sufficient correlation was obtained between both techniques indicating that changes in coronary blood flow are reflected accurately by videodensitometry in unbranched as well as in branched coronary vessels.

Clinical experience

Overall, more than 200 measurements have been performed in patients. Some of these results have been published previously (10).

Bypass grafts

Figure 8 presents mean blood velocity and flow through 36 aortocoronary venous

200

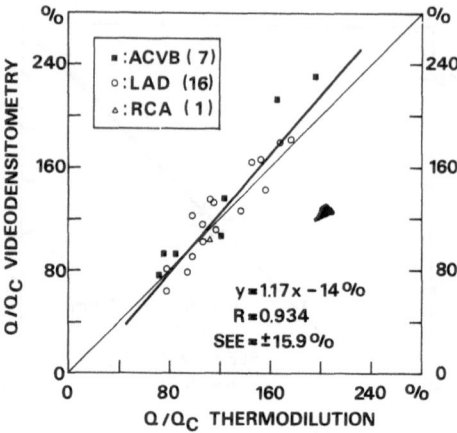

Figure 7. Comparison of simultaneous measurements of changes in blood flow by videodensitometry and the coronary sinus thermodilution method. Flow (Q) values are expressed as percentage of the control flow (Q$_c$). Different symbols refer to the densitometric measurements on 16 native left anterior descending arteries (LAD), 7 bypass grafts to the LAD (ACVB), and 1 native right coronary artery (RCA).

BYPASS GRAFT DIAMETER, VELOCITY (V) AND FLOW (Q) IN 36 PATIENTS

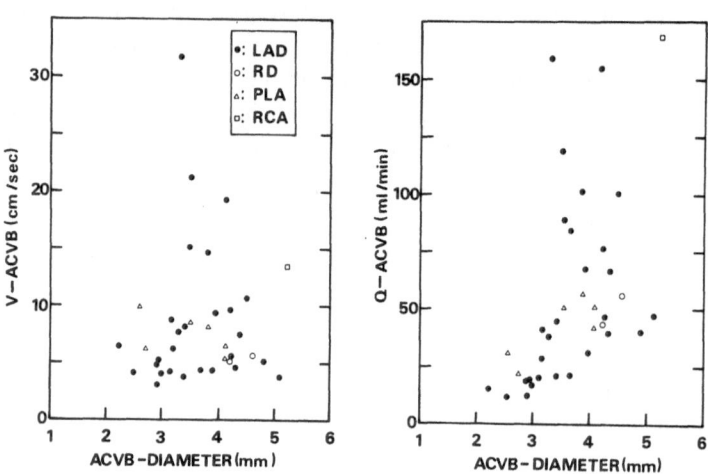

Figure 8. Relations between mean blood velocity and flow with average graft diameter in 36 nonobstructed venous bypass grafts. Different symbols refer to grafts to the LAD, to diagonal branches (RD), to marginal branches of the left circumflex artery (PLA), or to the right coronary artery (RCA).

bypass grafts with respect to luminal bypass diameter in 36 patients under resting conditions. Blood flow >70 ml/min or blood velocity >10 cm/sec were observed only in grafts to the LAD and the RCA, but not in grafts to diagonal or marginal circumflex branches. The overall results were comparable to those obtained with similar techniques in previous studies (2, 3). Blood velocity was found to be independent of the luminal size of the bypass. Blood flow through the graft did not show an overall correlation to bypass diameter, although there was a tendency to lower flow rates in vein grafts below 3 mm in diameter (Figure 8). It is of interest, however, that a significant inverse linear relationship was found between graft lumen and total regional coronary resistance in the area supplied by the graft, calculated as mean aortic pressure/bypass flow ($r = -0.63$, $p<0.001$), indicating that the bypass may adapt to the needs of the supplied region in the postoperative state (for details see (10)).

Native coronary arteries

Hemodynamics, average vessel diameter and mean blood velocity between the sampling windows in the LAD obtained by videodensitometry in 30 patients, matched for normal and obstructed vessels, are summarized in Table 1. Under resting conditions, no differences were found in diseased and undiseased arteries. It is evident, that blood flow in the LAD could not be derived in absolute terms by a simple comparison of arterial volume and contrast travelling time between two sampling sites, as used in the bypass grafts. Since one or more branchings between the sampling windows had to be included in the native LAD, flow through the side branches would have been neglected. A theoretical solution would be to derive flow as measured blood velocity multiplied by the luminal cross section of the artery at the proximal entry side, i.e. at the proximal sampling

Table 1. Hemodynamics, diameter, velocity and flow in 30 LAD arteries with and without obstructions.

	N	HR min^{-1}	AOP mmHg	Mean DLAD mm	Prox DLAD mm	Velocity cm/sec	Flow ml/min
Normal LAD	14	73±12	92±14	2.9±0.7	4.1±0.5	6.5±5.1	52.1±38.8
Stenosis <75%	6	80±17	99±11	2.9±0.7	3.9±0.8	5.4±3.1	37.3±19.8
Stenosis ≥75%	10	75±14	93± 9	2.7±0.4	3.8±0.6	5.2±3.2	39.7±38.4

HR: heart rate. AOP: mean aortic pressure. Mean DLAD: mean LAD diameter between sampling windows. Prox DLAD: LAD diameter at proximal window. Differences between groups were not statistically significant. Flow values calculated as: velocity × prox DLAD^2/4 × π × 60.

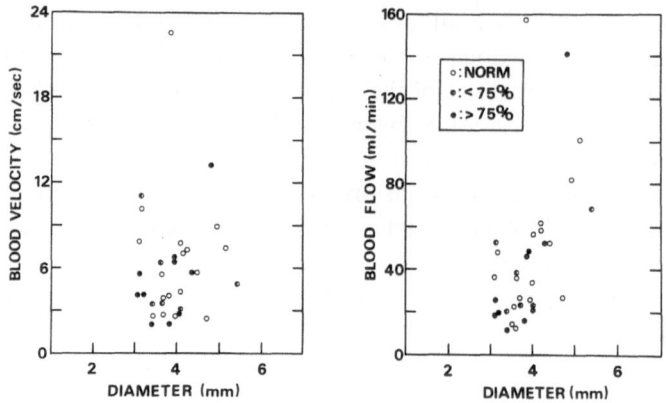

PROXIMAL DIAMETER, BLOOD VELOCITY AND ESTIMATED FLOW IN 33 SINGLE CORONARY ARTERIES IN MAN, ASSESSED BY VIDEODENSITOMETRY
30 LAD, 2 MARGINAL BRANCHES (CX), 1 RCA

Figure 9. Relations between mean blood velocity and calculated blood flow with vessel diameter within the proximal sampling window in 33 native coronary arteries. Open circles: Nonobstructed vessels. Half-closed circles: Arteries obstructed <75% in diameter. Closed circles: Obstructions >75% of vessel diameter.

window. Blood velocity and blood flow values estimated according to this principle in 33 branched coronary arteries have been plotted as a function of the luminal diameter of the artery at the proximal sampling window (Figure 9). Velocity as well as flow did not correlate with the diameter of the vessel. For the 30 left anterior descending arteries included in Figure 9, mean LAD flow values estimated according to this principle and matched for nonobstructed and obstructed arteries, are shown in the table. A comparison with the known results from independent methods suggests that this densitometric principle slightly underestimates regional flow. Thermodilution measurements in the great cardiac vein, for example, have revealed values between 50 and 80 ml/min for mean blood flow in the LAD region (9, 11). This discrepancy is most probably due to the fact that densitometry is likely to underestimate blood velocity in branched vessels. Since the total cross section of the stem and the side branches of a coronary artery increases after each branching (12), a successive drop in blood velocity towards peripheral sites is to be anticipated. Accordingly, we found an inverse correlation between measured blood velocity and the spatial distance between the sampling windows in measurements on 27 native LAD vessels in patients (Figure 10).

These data suggest that it is not possible to determine flow in absolute terms by any simple densitometric approach in branched coronary arteries. Nevertheless, the technique can be used to estimate changes in regional blood flow after interventions in unbranched as well as branched vessels, as described above.

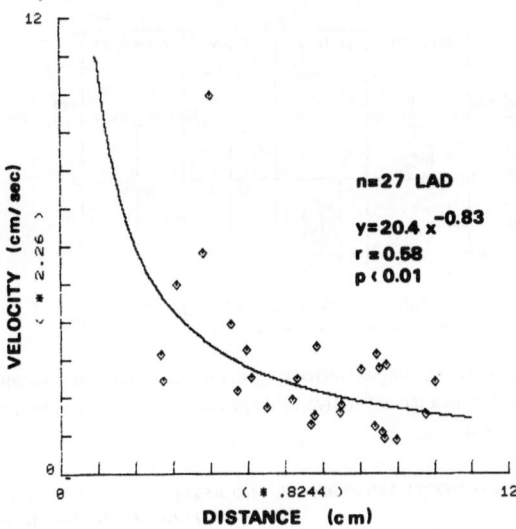

Figure 10. Blood velocities in the native LAD in 27 patients with regard to the (spatial) distance of the measuring windows on the vessel. Proximal window was defined in all cases at the origin of the LAD from the left coronary artery. Abscissa: Window distance in multiples of 0.824 cm. Ordinate: Velocity in multiples of 2.26 cm/sec.

Drug interventions

Finally, some results of vasodilator drug studies are presented. We have used the densitometric technique to investigate the effects of the vasodilator drugs nitroglycerin and nifedipine on regional hemodynamics in native coronary arteries as well as in venous bypass grafts. Measurements were performed before and 3 to 5 minutes after 0.8 mg sublingual nitroglycerin and before and 8 minutes after sublingual 10 mg nifedipine. In 9 native left anterior descending arteries (8 without and 1 with an obstruction >75% diameter stenosis), nitroglycerin increased vessel diameter by 14%, blood velocity fell by 25%, whereas flow and regional resistance remained unchanged (Figure 11). In 12 bypass grafts (Figure 12) blood velocity as well as flow fell by 14% and 12%, respectively, whereas the graft diameter was unchanged by nitroglycerin. After nifedipine, the diameter of native coronary arteries (8 LAD, 1 RCA, Figure 13) also increased slightly (+7%). In contrast to nitroglycerin, however, nifedipine increased flow (+17%) and decreased regional coronary resistance (−14%), whereas blood velocity remained unchanged. In 8 bypass grafts (Figure 14), blood velocity (+47%) as well as flow (+32%) increased, whereas graft diameter did not change significantly.

These data demonstrate that these drugs, that are widely used in the treatment of coronary disease, have different actions on coronary artery hemodynamics.

CHANGES IN CORONARY HEMODYNAMICS AFTER 0.8MG S.L. NITROGLYCERIN

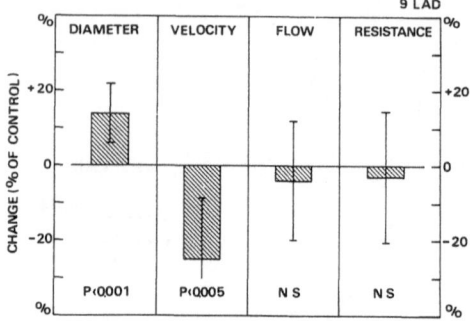

Figure 11. Effects of 0.8 mg of sublingual nitroglycerin on artery diameter, mean blood velocity, mean blood flow, and regional resistance in 9 native LAD arteries, given in percentage changes from control values. Mean values ± s.d.

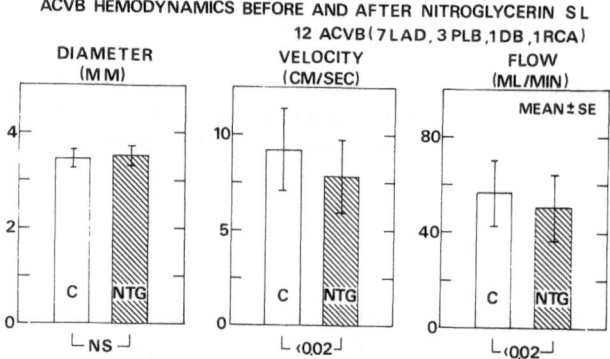

Figure 12. Effects of 0.8 mg of sublingual nitroglycerin on luminal diameter, mean blood velocity and flow in 12 aortocoronary vein grafts. Mean values ± s.d.

CHANGES IN CORONARY HEMODYNAMICS AFTER 10MG S.L. NIFEDIPINE

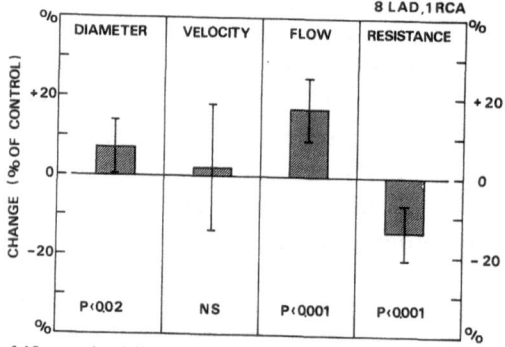

Figure 13. Effects of 10 mg of sublingual nifedipine on artery diameter, mean blood velocity, mean blood flow, and regional resistance in 8 native LAD and 1 RCA arteries, given as percentage changes from control values before nifedipine. Mean values ± s.d.

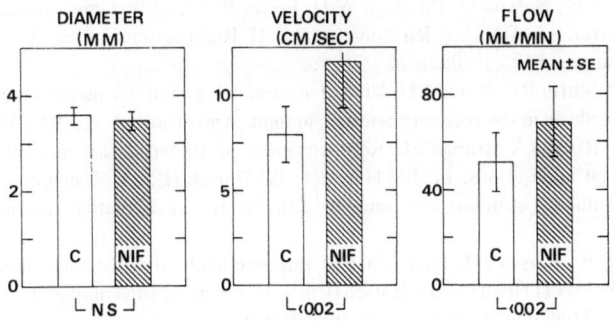

Figure 14. Effects of 10 mg of sublingual nifedipine on luminal diameter, mean blood velocity, and flow in 8 aortocoronary vein grafts, given in percentage changes from control values.

Sublingual nitroglycerin dilates the epicardial arteries, but does not change or may slightly decrease coronary arterial blood flow. In contrast, sublingual nifedipine acts on epicardial as well as on resistance vessels and can increase flow in native arteries and in bypass grafts, which may be of interest in the treatment of coronary artery disease and angina pectoris.

Summary and comment

In our experience, densitometry offers a unique possibility for the measurement of regional hemodynamics in coronary arteries. Experience with more than 200 measurements in patients has proven that the procedure on the patient is short, simple, and safe. Under certain conditions, routine coronary angiography can be analyzed by videodensitometric techniques, thus reducing hazards and investigation time for patient and investigator. Since our method uses standard X-ray equipment and conventional radiopaque indicators and techniques, the implementation during clinical heart catheterization is facilitated considerably.

According to the simple basic principles outlined above, measurements of blood flow and velocity are possible in unbranched parts of the coronary circulation, and changes in flow can be estimated in unbranched and branched vessels. The method therefore seems to be especially suitable for intervention studies, e.g. the assessment of regional coronary artery hemodynamics before and after drug administration.

So far, a technique to estimate flow in absolute terms in branched coronary arteries does not seem to be at hand. Digital imaging techniques, that have elicited a new interest in contrast densitometry, may perhaps in the future provide a new approach to this still unsolved problem.

References

1. Rutishauser W, Noseda G, Bussman W-D, Preter B: Blood flow measurement through single coronary arteries by Röntgen densitometry. Part II: Right coronary artery flow in conscious man. Am J Roentgenol 109, 1970: 21–24.

2. Smith HC, Sturm RE, Wood EH: Videodensitometric system for measurement of vessel blood flow, particularly in the coronary arteries, in man. Am J Cardiol, 32, 1973: 144–150.

3. Smith HC, Robb RA, Ritman EL: Röntgen videodensitometric assessment of myocardial blood flow: clinical applications. In: PH Heintzen, HJ Bürsch (Eds.), Röntgen-videotechniques for dynamic studies of structure and function of the heart and circulation. Thieme Stuttgart, 1978: 39–48.

4. Brennecke R, Bürsch JH, Heintzen PH: Improvements in videodensitometric measurement techniques. In: PH Heintzen, JH Bürsch (Eds.). Röntgen-videotechniques for dynamic studies of structure and function of the heart and circulation. Georg Thieme-Verlag, Stuttgart, 1978: 15–22.

5. Simon R, Ziegler K, Grimm J: Videodensitometer mit automatischer Regelung des Video-ingangs. Biomedizinische Technik, 24, 1979: 156–157.

6. Zierler KL: Theoretical basis of indicator-dilution methods for measuring flow and volume. Circ Research 1962, 10, 393–408.

7. Bassan M, Ganz W, Marcus HS, Swan HJC: The effect of intracoronary injection of contrast medium upon coronary blood flow. Circulation 51, 1975: 442–445.

8. Spiller P, Schmiel FK, Pölitz B, Block M, Fermor K, Hackbarth W, Jehle J, Körfer R, Pannek H: Measurement of systolic and diastolic flow rates in the coronary artery system by X-ray densi-tometry. Circulation 68, 1983: 337–347.

9. Ganz W, Tamura K, Marcus HS, Donoso R, Yoshida S, Swan HJC: Measurement of coronary sinus blood flow by continuous thermodilution in man. Circulation, 44, 1971: 181–195.

10. Simon R, Amende I, Oelert H, Hetzer R, Borst HG, Lichtlen PR: Blood velocity, flow, and dimensions of aortocoronary venous bypass grafts in the postoperative state. Circulation 66, 1981: I-34–I-39.

11. Pepine CJ, Mehta J, Webster WW Jr, Nicholas WW: In vivo validation of a thermodilution method to determine regional left ventricular blood flow in patients with coronary disease. Circulation 58, 1978: 795–802.

12. Rafflenbeul W, Lichtlen P: Quantitative Koronarangiographie: Das Druckmessverhältnis sich verzweigender Koronararterien. Zeitschr. Kardiologie 69, 1970: 235 (Abstract).

Part IV: Coronary obstruction and its physiologic significance

Assessment of stenosis severity

K. Lance Gould and R.L. Kirkeeide

Summary

Visual interpretations of coronary arteriograms are marked by such great inter-observer and intraobserver variability that comparison of arteriograms from different subjects, or at different times in the same subject, are of limited value for assessing severity, changes in severity or functional significance of coronary artery stenosis. The universal use of percent diameter narrowing as a clinical measure of severity ignores other geometric characteristics of stenoses such as length, absolute diameter, multiple lesions in series or eccentric narrowings which may be worse in one view as compared to another view. Accordingly, we have developed an approach for analyzing coronary artery stenoses in both anatomic and functional terms. In this chapter an overview of the functional and anatomic approaches for quantifying severity of coronary artery stenoses is presented, their validation and equivalence outlined and the remaining problems to be solved indicated.

Our quantitative analysis of coronary arteriograms requires high quality orthogonal X-rays processed in two different ways. In the first, the entire region of interest on the arteriogram is digitized with the borders of the arteriogram identified automatically utilizing an edge detection method in computer software without visual interpretation. In the second approach, the stenosis of interest is analyzed by integrating the optical density diametrically across the long axis of the artery image. The arterial cross-sectional areas measured by both techniques are automatically compared for each segment of the artery. The border recognition technique is accurate with a $\pm 0.1\,$mm error for lesions that are not crescentic in shape to less than $0.5\,$mm diameter. However, for crescentic shaped lesions, border recognition is inadequate because the atheromatous mass may project into the arterial lumen within the limits of the X-ray borders. For crescentic lesions the integrated density technique is more accurate since the optical density across the artery reflects displacement of contrast media by a crescentic atheroma projecting into the lumen of the artery. Therefore, where the border recognition and integrated density technique do not agree, the integrated density method is used for determining the severity of the stenosis. The dimensions determined by these automated techniques are then incorporated into validated fluid dynamic equations in order to predict the functional, pressure-flow effects of the stenosis as well as coronary flow reserve. Our results demonstrate that our automated, quantitated coronary arteriographic analysis predicts pressure-flow characteristics or coronary flow reserve as a single measure of stenosis severity reflecting all the integrated, combined effects of the geometric characteristics of the lesion including absolute diameter, percent stenosis, length and shape. Our results further demonstrate that consideration of a single dimension alone such as percent diameter narrowing or absolute diameter alone do not correlate or predict with coronary flow reserve measured independently by flow meter.

Introduction

The functional significance of coronary artery stenoses derives from their effects on coronary blood flow. Assessing their functional significance from arteriograms is difficult, in part, because of the variety of shapes they present. Stenoses may be long, short, segmental, diffuse, symmetric, asymmetric and/or tapering. No single anatomic criterion or measurement can describe their appearance or account for this variety of shapes having hemodynamic effects. Consequently, the concept of coronary flow reserve as a functional measure of stenosis severity was initially proposed by Gould in 1974 on the basis of empirical observations and was subsequently developed as a physiologic diagnostic method (1–12). Because the measurement of percent diameter narrowing was the accepted standard for describing stenosis severity at that time, the concept of coronary flow reserve was initially demonstrated by relating the fall in coronary flow reserve to percent diameter narrowing for experimental coronary stenoses having relatively uniform length and absolute diameter. Many others have confirmed these findings and showed the effects of changing specific geometric dimensions of a stenosis on coronary flow reserve (13–21). We have also demonstrated the validity of quantitative coronary arteriography for predicting the functional pressure-flow characteristics of stenoses if *all* the dimensions of the lesion are taken into account, including percent diameter narrowing, absolute diameter, length and asymmetry of the stenosis (22).

Recent reports (23–25) have described a poor correlation between coronary flow reserve and percent diameter narrowing in human coronary artery disease and have proposed absolute diameter as a better measure of stenosis severity. However, these studies did not use biplane arteriographic views or did not utilize complete fluid dynamic equations accounting for all the geometric dimensions of the stenoses. Therefore, the use of absolute stenosis diameter as a measure of severity remains moot. Their results confirm, however, previous publications indicating that percent diameter narrowing alone is not a satisfactory measure of stenosis severity (1–14, 26).

There are several reasons for defining the relation between coronary flow reserve and stenosis geometry. Bomberger *et al.* (27) have demonstrated that experimental stenoses over a prolonged period of time may undergo 'molding' in-vivo whereby lesions may change dimensions. A stenosis may become longer with worsening absolute diameter but less severe percent diameter narrowing, or may become more or less, eccentric, or may become more severe in one part but less severe in another part. Assessment of severity or changing severity therefore requires some measurement reflecting all the dimensions of a stenosis.

Even with complete quantitative coronary arteriography (28), description of altered geometry is difficult if the stenosis dimensions change in opposite directions. In order to obtain an integrated, single measure of stenosis severity, Brown *et al.* (28) initially developed quantitative coronary arteriography to calculate stenosis resistance from all dimensions based upon fluid dynamic equations. Although Brown has demonstrated the value of quantitative arteriography for clinical research (29, 30, 31), calculated resistance is difficult to relate to common physiologic measurements of pressure and flow. Therefore, Gould *et al.* (4, 12, 22) used the pressure gradient-flow relations of a stenosis, either directly measured or derived from quantitative coronary arteriography, as a means of quantifying severity in more physiologic terms. In either case, the use of stenosis resistance or of pressure-flow relations are oriented towards fluid dynamics and are somewhat alien to physiology and medicine. Their use, therefore, is not easily assimilated into a clinical or into a standard physiologically oriented research laboratory.

Consequently, we have proposed coronary flow reserve as a single measure of stenosis severity which is conceptually more physiologically oriented and more easily measured in the physiology laboratory by flow meter or radiolabeled microspheres (1–12). With current development of positron emission tomography into a practical and affordable clinical method for assessing perfusion, the noninvasive determination of coronary flow reserve in man now also appears feasible. Although our initial studies beginning some years ago indicated the potential value of measuring coronary flow reserve, there has only recently been a rigorous, systematic theoretical or experimental proof to date that coronary flow reserve reflects the effects of all the combined, integrated dimensions of a tapering coronary artery stenosis in vivo (40).

Accordingly, the approach to this problem requires consideration of two different basic concepts about how stenosis severity is quantified: anatomically and functionally. The *anatomic* severity of a coronary lesion is measured in geometric terms, i.e., percent narrowing, absolute diameter, length, and shape. Quantitative coronary arteriography delineates these dimensions which are then used to calculate the functional or pressure-flow characteristics according to theoretical fluid dynamic equations. The *functional* severity of a stenosis is described in physiologic terms, i.e., by directly measured coronary blood flow, pressure gradient or distal perfusion pressure, and coronary flow reserve from which certain deductions about geometric severity can be made.

Both the anatomic and functional approaches to quantifying severity are derived from, or related to, fluid dynamics of flow in narrowed tubes. In theory, therefore, the two approaches should be interchangeable and equivalent both mathematically and experimentally. The purpose here is to provide an overview of functional and anatomic approaches for quantifying severity of coronary artery stenoses, to outline their validation in the literature and to indicate the remaining problems.

Anatomic imaging of the coronary arteries

Visual interpretations of coronary arteriograms are marked by such great inter-observer and intraobserver variability that comparison of arteriograms from different subjects, or at different times in the same subject, are of limited value for assessing severity, changes in severity, or functional significance of coronary artery stenoses. The universal use of relative percent diameter narrowing as a clinical measure of severity ignores other geometric characteristics of stenoses such as length, absolute diameter, multiple lesions in series or eccentric narrowings which may be worse in one view as compared to another view.

Quantitative coronary arteriography was originally proposed by Brown *et al.* (28) and subsequently validated in-vivo by Gould *et al.* (22, 32). It requires high quality coronary arteriograms taken in two views angled at 90° to each other. Significant errors appear with deviation from orthogonal views (33, 34). The X-ray images may then be processed in two different ways. In the first, the images are optically magnified onto a digitizing tablet with the borders of the artery traced by hand and thereby digitized for computer processing (22, 28–31). There is some subjectivity in tracing the arterial borders visually. In the second approach, the entire region of interest on the arteriogram is digitized with the borders of the artery identified automatically by computer software without visual interpretation (35–40). In our laboratory this automated computer technique utilizes an edge detection method as well as analysis of the integrated optical density (gray scale) diametrically across the artery image. The cross-sectional areas measured by both techniques are automatically compared for each segment of the artery. Disagreements between the two methods may occur, especially for eccentric lesions in which the border recognition technique using orthogonal biplane views is not as accurate as the densitometry technique (39, 40), or in cases where other optically dense structures (catheters, other vessels, etc.) are superimposed on the arterial segment of interest. In the latter circumstance, the diameter is best determined by the automated border recognition approach. An example of the arteriogram is shown in Figure 1 and of an auto-

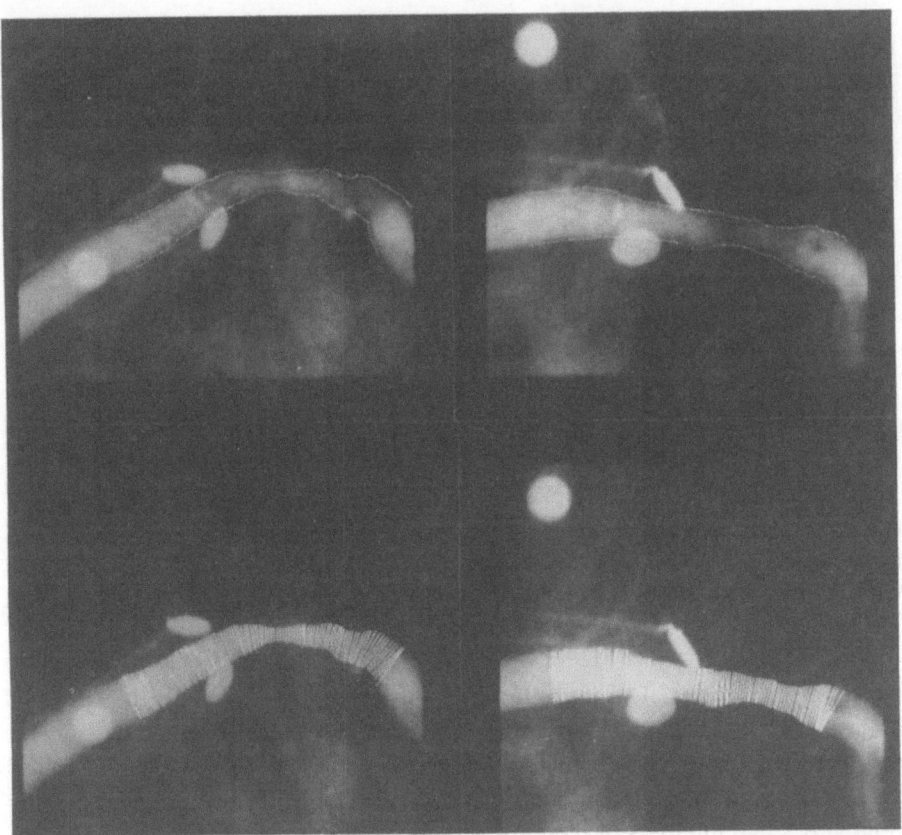

Figure 1. A biplane angiogram of a coronary stenosis taken in two perpendicular views. The automatic border recognition program identifies the edges of the artery and measures the diameters from which the geometric characteristics of stenosis are determined.

mated analysis in Figure 2 showing the arterial borders identified automatically. Also shown are the diameters of the artery measured at increments along the long axis of the stenosis for purposes of computing the various geometric dimensions of the lesion.

After the borders of the opacified artery on the arteriogram are identified, the stenosis is analyzed by quantitatively adding the exit losses to the integrated viscous losses along the length of the stenosis. The final computer print-out gives the measured dimensions and predicted pressure drop for a given coronary flow as well as the pressure gradient-flow relation (12, 22). It should be emphasized that quantitative arteriography cannot predict the actual flow or the actual gradient unless flow is independently measured. Since that is not possible in man, it predicts the pressure gradient – flow relation, i.e., the range of gradients, for a range of flows. The automated technique is accurate to 0.1 mm (39, 40) for

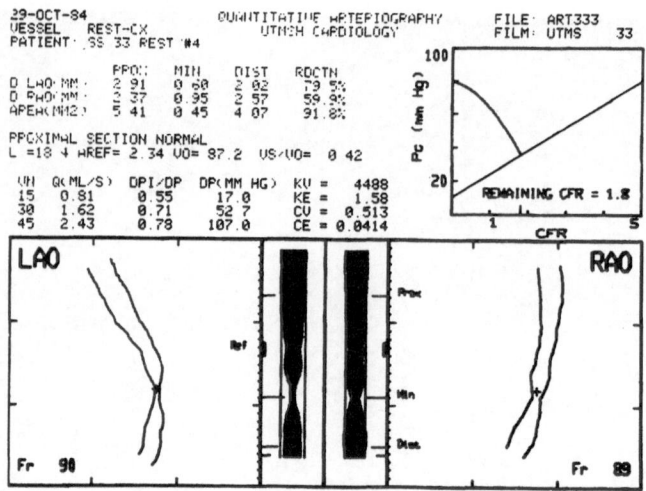

Figure 2. Computer printout of X-ray analysis showing the dimensions of the stenosis, the predicted pressure gradients for a given range of coronary flow and a graph indicating the X-ray predicted coronary flow reserve (in the upper right corner of the printout) derived from all stenosis dimensions of length, absolute diameter, relative percent narrowing and asymmetry.

absolute dimensions. The reproducibility of any given dimension utilizing this approach is remarkably good with approximately ± 2% to 3% variation on sequential repeated X-ray images of the same stenosis (12, 22). As demonstrated by Brown *et al.* (41) such geometric accuracy allows intervention studies using relatively small numbers of patients in randomized therapeutic trials. Quantitative coronary arteriography is therefore of great value in determining progression or regression of coronary disease.

Functional analysis of coronary artery stenosis

Pressure gradient-flow relation

The functional severity of a coronary artery narrowing may also be defined by the relation of pressure gradient to flow, measured directly by implanted instruments without knowledge of anatomic geometry (4). Coronary artery stenosis not only reduces the maximum increase in coronary flow but also causes a reduction in distal coronary perfusion pressure due to pressure losses across the stenosis. The upper panel of Figure 3 shows a normal coronary artery with the expected increase in flow after a vasodilatory stimulus (42). Aortic and distal coronary artery pressures show no significant difference or gradient in the absence of a stenosis. However, in the lower panel, coronary stenosis restricts the increase in coronary flow and causes a pressure loss or gradient with lowered distal coronary

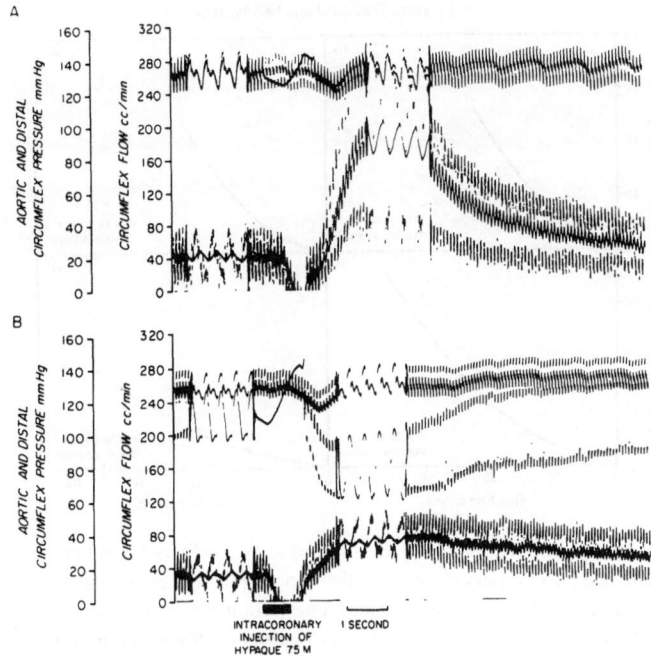

Figure 3. Recordings of coronary flow, proximal and distal coronary pressures in a normal coronary artery (upper panel) and in a stenotic coronary artery (lower panel). Resting coronary blood flow is equal in the two arteries but the increase in flow seen after a coronary vasodilator or stress fails to increase in the presence of a stenosis. Normally flow will increase three to five times demonstrating a coronary flow reserve of up to five. The coronary flow reserve of the stenotic coronary artery is greatly reduced, as shown in the lower panel. At rest there is a pressure gradient of approximately 30 mmHg between the aorta and the distal coronary artery caused by the stenosis. Following a vasodilatory stimuli, coronary flow increases slightly in the stenotic artery with a marked increase in the pressure gradient. Flow increases appropriately in the normal coronary artery with no pressure gradient. Thus, the small increase in coronary flow through the stenotic artery was associated with a large increase in the pressure gradient and fall in distal coronary perfusion pressure. Reproduced from Lipscomb and Gould (1975).

perfusion pressure. There is a direct correlation between the degree of flow increase and the increase in the pressure gradient across the stenosis.

Thus, coronary vascular bed vasodilatation may cause only a modest increase in total arterial coronary flow, but a large fall in distal coronary perfusion pressure (2, 3) with attendant fall in subendocardial perfusion (8, 43, 44). The quantitative relation between coronary blood flow and the pressure gradient across the stenosis during diastole is a hemodynamic measure of stenosis severity, as shown in Figure 4. In the absence of a stenosis, there is a mild, (5 to 8 mmHg) gradient at maximum flows following administration of a potent coronary vasodilator. In the presence of a stenosis, the pressure gradient-flow relation becomes much steeper, with a higher pressure gradient for any given flow. With a severe

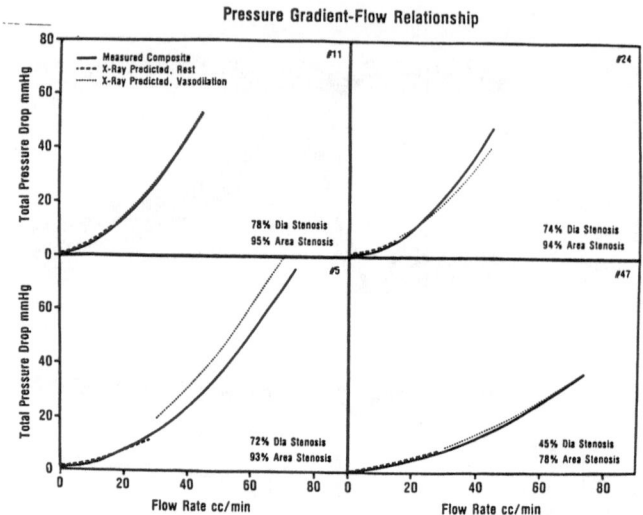

Figure 4. Relations of diastolic pressure gradient and coronary blood flow for mild to severe coronary stenoses. With an increase in coronary blood flow, the stenosis pressure gradient increases. The X-ray predicted pressure gradient-flow relations (dashed lines) compare to those directly measured by implanted catheter and flow meters in a dog model of coronary stenosis (solid lines). The steeper curves are associated with the more severe stenoses. Reproduced from Gould *et al.* (1982).

coronary stenosis, this relation becomes very steep, with a large increase in pressure gradient for a small increase in coronary flow caused by distal arteriolar vasodilation. This pressure gradient-flow relation acquired during diastole characterizes the functional severity of coronary artery stenoses in hemodynamic terms rather than in terms of anatomic geometry (4, 11, 12, 22).

For a fixed stenosis, the pressure gradient increases in a curvilinear relation to flow according to quadratic fluid dynamic equations (4, 11, 12, 22). For anatomic analysis of angiograms, X-ray geometry is used to determine the viscous and inertial coefficients of the fluid dynamic equations from geometric dimensions. In functional or hemodynamic analysis, many simultaneous pressure gradients and coronary flows are directly measured over a wide range from low to high coronary flows. The values of the coefficients are then determined by an iterative process of finding the quadratic equation best fitting the directly measured pressure flow data (4, 12, 22). This approach is suitable only for experimental animals in which direct pressure flow measurements can be made by implanted instruments.

Coronary flow reserve

An essential concept relating stenosis anatomy to its functional effects is that of coronary flow reserve. It is defined as the ratio of maximum coronary flow after a

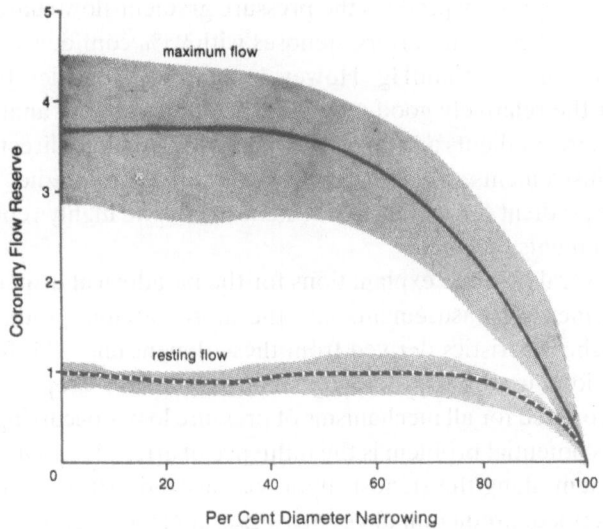

Figure 5. Coronary flow reserve is reduced at 40–50% diameter narrowing (solid line) whereas resting flow is not impaired until 80–85% diameter narrowing. Reproduced from Gould *et al.* (1974).

maximal vasodilatory stimulus to resting flow, as first described experimentally by Gould *et al.* (1) and explained in fluid dynamic terms by Young *et al.* (45–48) and Mates (14). The concept is demonstrated in Figure 5. Under resting conditions, coronary blood flow in an artery doesn't change until a relatively tight stenosis of 80–85% diameter narrowing. However, coronary flow reserve is impaired at 40–50% diameter narrowing, whereas flow in a normal artery increases three to four times in response to a vasodilatory stimulus such as pharmacologic coronary vasodilators, a brief coronary occlusion or physical stress.

The normal three to four-fold relative increase after a vasodilatory stimulus identifies a coronary flow reserve of three to four. Coronary artery narrowing limits this coronary flow reserve to an extent that is proportional to the severity of the stenosis. This approach to evaluating coronary stenoses has been shown practical experimentally and clinically (5–10, 23–25). For a stimulus which normally increases coronary flow to five or six times baseline levels, coronary flow reserve becomes impaired with mild stenoses 3 to 12 mm long of an approximately 30% to 40% diameter narrowing of a 3 mm diameter artery.

Relation between anatomic and functional characteristics of coronary stenosis

We have experimentally validated the basic theory and X-ray techniques of quantitative coronary arteriography applied in vivo to tapering, narrowed coronary arteries (22). In that study analysis of anatomic geometry on coronary arteriograms appropriately predicts the pressure gradient-flow characteristics or functional effects of coronary artery stenoses with 95% confidence intervals for individual values of ± 18.5 mmHg. However, there was considerable scatter of the data about the relatively good overall correlation between anatomic, X-ray predicted pressure gradients at a given flow compared to those directly measured by implanted instruments. This scatter makes it diffcult to predict accurately a given pressure gradient for an individual stenosis despite highly repeatable geometric measurements.

There are several possible explanations for the paradoxical disparity between repeatable geometric measurements and the more variable predictions of the pressure flow characteristics derived from these dimensions. The first reason is that the equations used for predicting stenosis pressure drop may not have sufficiently accounted for all mechanisms of pressure losses occurring in vivo. An example of this potential problem is the influence of arterial velocity profiles and their development along the stenosis upon viscous and exit pressure losses. As previously described, prediction of viscous losses along the stenosis was based on the assumption of fully-developed, laminar flow conditions (parabolically-shaped velocity profiles) existing from the proximal end of the stenosis to the minimal area section. The expansion pressure losses were predicted on the basis of a one-dimensional flow through an abrupt expansion (the velocity profiles being everywhere flat from the minimal area section to the normal artery section distal to the stenosis). There is an obvious contradiction in these two assumptions which needs to be resolved.

Theoretically, neither of the assumptions is likely to be true. Redevelopment of an initially fully-developed flow following an abrupt change in flow geometry, such as the abrupt contraction, requires a finite length to occur. For flow conditions similar to those in coronary arteries, the required distance for flow development, the entrance length, is on the order of 5–25 local arterial diameters depending on the coronary flowrate. Intrastenotic flow for most coronary stenoses is therefore likely to be underdeveloped with parabolically shaped velocity profiles being approached only with very long stenoses, under resting flow conditions. For such flow conditions, viscous losses across coronary stenoses would be greater than that predicted by the presently used equations (48, 49) as would the inertial expansion losses as previously hypothesized (14, 49). Entrance losses, previously assumed to be negligible in quantitative arteriography, are related to the issue of flow profile effects since entrance geometry may profoundly affect flow profiles in the stenotic segment and therefore influence exit losses as well. Thus, entrance effects are likely to be significant on theoretical grounds but have not been accounted for in quantitative arteriography to date.

The second of the major possible reasons for the scatter in predicted versus directly measured results is uncertainty in border recognition of the artery on arteriograms. The border of an opacified artery on X-ray demonstrates a penumbra or border zone of less radiodensity between the more radiodense central lumen of the artery and the radiolucent area external to the artery (12, 22, 33, 38–40, 50). This edge unsharpness or penumbra zone is due to two radiographic effects: the progressive decrease in contrast media depth as the lumen edge is approached from the lumen center (subject unsharpness) and the finite resolving capabilities of the X-ray imaging system. A satisfactory overall correlation between predicted vs. measured pressure gradients was obtained in our laboratory only when the arterial border was drawn by visual estimate in the center of this penumbral zone. Normally, with relatively round cross-sections the border zone constitutes 10 to 15% of a 3 mm diameter coronary artery. However, at a stenosis, particularly as eccentricity increases, this zone may become relatively large. Border recognition consequently becomes more uncertain. Since hemodynamic effects are proportional to the diameter of the stenosis raised to the fourth power, a small uncertainty in border definition may introduce a large uncertainty into the hemodynamic effects calculated from X-ray measured dimensions. The degree of this uncertainty in border definition and the extent of associated uncertainty in resulting hemodynamic predictions has not been described by formal error analysis.

Automated border recognition programs offer a promising solution to reducing these uncertainties when combined with densitometric analysis of the arterial X-ray image. The combination of the border recognition and density techniques is particularly useful because background corrected radiodensity is integrated across the artery image (including the entire border zone) to yield a measure of vessel cross-sectional area independent of its sectional shape (38–40, 51–54). They also eliminate the human error in visual interpretation of the penumbra.

As discussed subsequently in more detail, another promising approach using quantitative arteriography expresses stenosis severity in terms of impairment of coronary flow reserve (40) rather than the pressure gradient-flow relation which is difficult to apply practically. However, the limits of uncertainty for all of these new techniques have not been systematically defined. It is important to emphasize that even with these limitations, quantitative arteriographic measurements as previously described (12, 22, 28) are objective, allow statistical analysis, provide several orders of magnitude more accuracy than previous visual estimates of stenosis severity and may also be used to predict coronary flow reserve from X-ray angiographic studies (40).

In addition to the above major issues discussed, a number of more minor questions frequently arise. Can quantitative coronary arteriography account for diffuse coronary artery disease in which there is no discrete single lesion? Since the equations include absolute dimensions, they are applicable to this circumstance with length being whatever length of artery the observer wants to analyze, even the entire artery. In that case viscous friction, as accounted for in the first term of these equations, would cause the major pressure loss since length would be large and the second term, reflecting exit pressure loss, would be fairly small in the absence of a discrete lesion. As a variation of this same question, the combined effects of multiple stenoses in series can be accounted for by appropriate fluid dynamic analysis (2, 55).

The final complication of applying quantitative arteriography is due to dynamically changing stenosis first described by Gould *et al.* experimentally (4, 11, 12) developed further by Walinsky *et al.* (56), Schwartz *et al.* (57), Santamore *et al.* (58) and observed by Brown *et al.* in humans (30, 31, 59). A significant proportion of human coronary stenoses have some part of the arterial wall sufficiently intact and flexible, that vasomotion of the stenotic segment may occur (60) or of the artery on either side of the stenosis. Both types of vasomotion alter stenosis geometry sufficiently to change its functional characteristics. The appropriate fluid dynamic equations are still applicable as long as the altered geometry is used (12). A flexible-walled, very severe coronary stenosis may also behave as a pressure-dependent flow regulator, like a Starling resistor (61) which is a more complex problem not yet fully described.

Isolated measurement of one dimension of a stenosis

Quantitation of arterial stenosis in vivo has been sufficiently complex and poorly understood in terms of basic theory, physiologic-hemodynamic effects, experimental preparation and imaging technology that a number of studies have utilized indices or approximate estimates of severity. The old issue of the relative value of percent diameter narrowing versus absolute diameter narrowing is an example of controversy based upon approximations or incomplete analysis and lack of perspective into the multiple facets of the fluid dynamics or physiology involved.

The limitations of percent diameter narrowing compared to absolute diameter was proposed as long as 20 years ago (62) with the discussion continuing to our own analysis integrating both approaches with fluid dynamic principles (11). The issue frequently resurfaces, possibly in part due to lack of considering all the aspects of the problem based on complete fluid dynamic equations. For example, Collins *et al.* (63), White *et al.* (23), Harrison *et al.* (24) and Marcus (25, 64), reconfirmed previous reports on the limitations of percent diameter narrowing as a measure of stenosis severity by comparison to coronary flow reserve. They concluded that absolute diameter is a more important measure of severity. A generally applicable description of stenosis severity requires both absolute diameter and relative percent narrowing in addition to length, absolute diameter of the normal artery and blood viscosity. In any given circumstance one of these factors may be the dominant contributor to total pressure loss. For example, for mild diffuse narrowing with no discrete stenosis, absolute diameter and length of the diffusely involved segment might be the most important geometry. On the other hand, for a short orifice like stenosis, percent diameter narrowing might be most important. Most lesions are between these extremes. Their studies, however, do reemphasize the importance of functional assessment of stenosis severity using coronary flow reserve as we originally proposed.

Unfortunately, there are problems with coronary flow reserve as well (65, 66). The maximum flow achievable with vasodilatory stimulus, the resting blood flow and their ratio (coronary flow reserve) are reasonably variable between individual subjects and perhaps in the same individual at different times, depending on a number of factors unrelated to presence or severity of stenosis, such as adrenergic tone, presence of hypertrophy, perfusion pressure, and type stimulus for increasing flow. Relative perfusion reserve (67), as might be quantitatively measured using positron perfusion tracers (20, 67–69), may eliminate some of this variability since part of the heart serves as an internal control area for the rest of the heart. The optimal stimulus for increasing coronary flow has also not been worked out and is likely different for different individuals. One would anticipate that the type of stimulus for maximizing coronary flow in an unsteady 70-year-old would be different than for a 40-year-old athletic individual. Thus, the type of stimulus and normal responses have to be identified.

The problem of assessing severity is hindered by the lack of a readily applied gold standard. The correlation of angiographic dimensions with postmortem measurements suggest that angiographic measurements are only qualitative (70–73), and Marcus *et al.* (25) report that the postmortem exam of the undistended coronary artery overestimates severity. Because of the issue of arterial distensibility and geometric changes, an important test of an angiographic system is an X-ray phantom consisting of contrast filled tubes of varying diameters immersed in a scattering media (38, 39). Metal phantoms such as machined brass rods which are commonly used, are inappropriate because they lack the graded decrease in depth of contrast along the radius of an opacified artery (50). For validation studies of quantitative arteriography there are only two approaches – appropriate X-ray phantoms and in-vivo testing by comparison to direct measurements of pressure-flow characteristics or coronary flow reserve.

Conclusions

Since our first introduction of the concept (1) we are evolving toward the viewpoint that maximum myocardial perfusion, or coronary flow reserve, may, per se, be the best integrated, single measure of stenosis severity reflecting all its combined geometric and fluid dynamic characteristics. As indicated earlier, the measurement of coronary flow reserve also reflects, or is affected by, diffuse narrowing where the entire artery is smaller than it would normally be relative to the size of its distal vascular bed.

The concept of coronary flow reserve as a single integrated measure of all the geometric dimensions of a stenosis is illustrated conceptually in Figure 6. This figure is derived from previously validated, standard fluid dynamic equations relating pressure gradient across the stenosis to coronary flow and stenosis

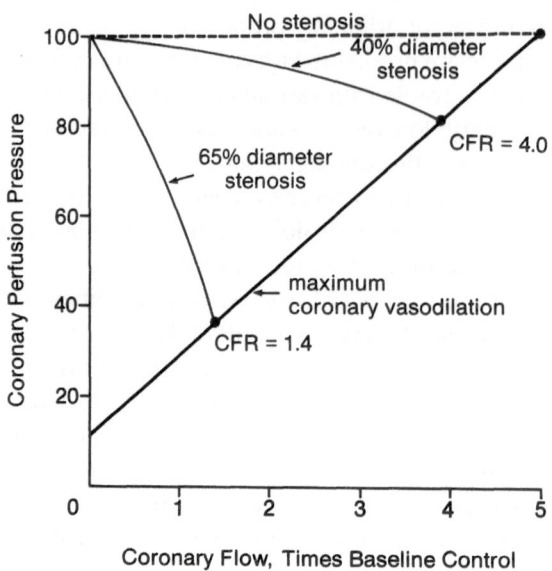

Figure 6. Relation of coronary perfusion pressure to coronary flow reserve and severity of stenosis. A 20% reduction in coronary flow reserve from five to four is associated with a 40% diameter narrowing. A more severe reduction of coronary flow reserve from five to 1.4 is associated with a more severe 65% diameter narrowing. The dashed line shows the normal increase in flow in the absence of a stenosis to five times baseline levels. From Kirkeeide *et al.* (1984).

dimensions (40). For a given aortic pressure, the distal coronary pressure (vertical axis and shown by the downward curved line), can then be related to coronary flow, here expressed as a ratio to resting flow levels or in terms of coronary flow reserve (40). The rising straight line plots the normal, experimentally observed, relation between coronary perfusion pressure and flow under conditions of maximal coronary vasodilation in the absence of a stenosis, as previously reported (44). It shows the maximum possible flow in the artery in the absence of a stenosis at a given perfusion pressure under conditions of maximum coronary vasodilation. The intersection of this straight line with the vertical axis gives the coronary pressure at zero flow.

The schematic of Figure 6 shows theoretically how coronary flow reserve is related to, or might be predicted from stenosis dimensions by quantitative arteriography. The downward curving line, representing the distal coronary perfusion pressure – flow relation can be predicted from stenosis dimensions for any measured blood pressure. The point at which the downward curving line, showing the distal pressure-flow relation for the stenosis, intersects the rising linear line showing the maximum normal flow at a given perfusion pressure, gives the coronary flow reserve for that stenosis. For example, for a normal, nonstenotic coronary artery with a coronary flow reserve of five, the perfusion pressure under these circumstances would be normal, shown as 100 mmHg for purposes of illustration. A 40% diameter stenosis 3 to 12 mm long in a normally 3 mm diameter artery would reduce this coronary flow reserve to approximately four in association with a pressure gradient across the stenosis that reduced the distal perfusion pressure to 80 mmHg. Although it is a powerful conceptual approach with preliminary experimental support (40), validation of this approach will require more work in order to avoid the pitfalls of focusing on a single facet of the problem.

We have previously documented the necessity of accounting for all stenosis dimensions which affect hemodynamic severity of stenoses (38–40), confirmed by others (23–25, 64). Percent diameter narrowing correlates poorly with directly measured or arteriographically determined coronary flow reserve as described above, taking into account all stenosis dimensions of length, absolute diameter, relative percent narrowing and asymmetry. Thus, percent diameter narrowing is virtually useless as a reference standard for measuring stenosis severity. For example, a 60% diameter narrowing is associated with a range of arteriographically determined coronary flow reserves from 1.5 to 4.5, based on all stenosis dimensions. Since the defects seen on perfusion images during pharmacologic stress are related to coronary flow reserve, those defects do not relate to percent diameter narrowing. Therefore, we no longer utilize percent diameter narrowing alone as the reference gold standard for determining physiologic significance or sensitivity and specificity of imaging techniques for diagnosing coronary artery disease.

Percent area reduction also correlates poorly with arteriographically determined coronary flow reserve based on all dimensions. For example, an 80% area reduction is associated with an arteriographically determined coronary flow reserve ranging from 2 to 4.5, depending on the absolute dimensions. We therefore have also rejected area reduction alone as a reference gold standard. Minimum absolute cross sectional lumen area of the stenosis has been previously suggested as a better measure of stenosis severity than percent narrowing (25, 26). However, minimum absolute lumen area of the stenosis also correlates poorly with arteriographically determined coronary flow reserve based on all stenosis dimensions. The correlation is poor because the effect of a given absolute minimum area will depend on the absolute diameter of the normal proximal artery and its length. A given stenosis cross-sectional area does not impair coronary flow reserve of a normally small vessel but will reduce coronary flow reserve of a large artery. For example, an absolute stenosis minimum area of 1 mm^2 may be associated with a coronary flow reserve ranging from 1.5 to 4.5 depending on the diameter of the normal artery as well as the length of the stenosis. We have therefore rejected absolute cross sectional lumen area of the stenosis as a reference gold standard of stenosis severity. Thus, coronary flow reserve is a single integrated measurement of severity, accounting for all stenosis dimensions of length, absolute diameter, relative percent narrowing and asymmetry (40). It may be directly measured or determined arteriographically based on all stenosis dimensions of absolute diameter, relative percent narrowing, integrated length effects and asymmetry.

Arteriographically determined coronary flow reserve is theoretically and experimentally closely related to the relative distribution of a perfusion tracer in the heart during maximal coronary vasodilation. Accordingly, clinical coronary arteriograms in our laboratory are quantitatively analyzed by a completely automated technique utilizing simultaneously both border recognition algorithms and integrated, arterial cross-sectional densitometry to obtain all geometric dimensions of the stenosis with an accuracy of ± 0.1 mm for diameters less than 0.5 mm (38, 39) and a reproducibility of 2–3% (12, 22). The program also predicts the pressure-flow characteristics (12, 22) and coronary flow reserve of the stenosis (40) based on precise geometric dimensions as validated in vivo by direct flowmeter-pressure measurements in instrumented dogs. For determining the sensitivity and specificity of rest-stress positron imaging for diagnosis of coronary artery disease, significant disease was defined as an arteriographically determined coronary flow reserve of less than 3.0 for any stenosis in one or more major proximal coronary arteries. Optimal coronary vasodilation was achieved using intravenous dipyridamole combined with hand grip stress (5–10). Since N-13 ammonia, previously described as a perfusion imaging agent (9, 10) requires a cyclotron, a more readily obtainable radionuclide, Rb-82, from a ^{82}Sr-^{82}Rb generator was injected intravenously as a perfusion indicator (74) at rest and during coronary vasodilation. Simultaneous multislice tomography of the entire heart was carried out using the state-of-the-art University of Texas positron camera (75–80).

The preliminary results of blinded reading of images indicate that our protocol, consisting of intravenous dipyridamole combined with hand grip stress, and positron tomography of the entire heart using the University of Texas positron camera, has a sensitivity and specificity of between 95% to 100% for identifying significant coronary artery disease. These results indicate that X-ray determined coronary flow reserve is a single measure of stenosis severity, taking into account all its geometric dimensions and correlates with perfusion defects seen by state-of-the-art positron imaging.

References

1. Gould KL, Lipscomb K, Hamilton GW: Physiologic basis for assessing critical coronary stenosis. Instantaneous flow response and regional distribution during coronary hyperemia as measures of coronary flow reserve. Am J Cardiol 33, 1974: 87–94.
2. Gould KL, Lipscomb K: Effects of coronary stenoses on coronary flow reserve and resistance. Am J Cardiol 34, 1974: 48–55.
3. Gould KL, Lipscomb K, Calvert C: Compensatory changes of the distal coronary vascular bed during progressive coronary constriction. Circulation 51, 1975: 1085–1094.
4. Gould KL: Pressure-flow characteristics of coronary stenoses in unsedated dogs at rest and during coronary vasodilation. Circ Res 43, 1978: 242–253.

5. Gould KL: Noninvasive assessment of coronary stenoses by myocardial perfusion imaging during pharmacologic coronary vasodilation. I. Physiologic basis and experimental validation. Am J Cardiol 41, 1978: 267–278.

6. Gould KL, Westcott RJ, Albro PC, Hamilton GW: Noninvasive assessment of coronary stenoses by myocardial perfusion imaging during pharmacologic coronary vasodilatation. II. Clinical methodology and feasibility. Am J Cardiol 41, 1978: 279–287.

7. Albro PC, Gould KL, Westcott RJ, Hamilton GW, Ritchie JL, Williams DL: Noninvasive assessment of coronary stenoses by myocardial imaging during pharmacologic coronary vasodilatation. III. Clinical trial. Am J Cardiol 42, 1978: 751–760.

8. Gould KL: Assessment of coronary stenoses with myocardial perfusion imaging during pharmacologic coronary vasodilatation. IV. Limits of detection of stenosis with idealized experimental cross-sectional myocardial imaging. Am J Cardiol 42, 1978: 761–768.

9. Gould KL, Schelbert HR, Phelps ME, Hoffman EJ: Noninvasive assessment of coronary stenoses with myocardial perfusion imaging during pharmacologic coronary vasodilatation. V. Detection of 47 percent diameter coronary stenosis with intravenous Nitrogen-13 ammonia and emission-computed tomography in intact dogs. Am J Cardiol 43, 1979: 200–208.

10. Schelbert HR, Wisenberg G, Phelps ME, Gould KL, Henze E, Hoffman EJ, Gomes A, Kuhl DE: Noninvasive assessment of coronary stenoses by myocardial imaging during pharmacologic coronary vasodilation. VI. Detection of coronary artery disease in human beings with intravenous N-13 ammonia and positron computed tomography. Am J Card 49, 1982: 1197–1207.

11. Gould KL: Dynamic coronary stenosis. Am J Cardiol 45, 1980: 286–292.

12. Gould KL, Kelley KO: Physiological significance of coronary flow velocity and changing stenosis geometry during coronary vasodilation in awake dogs. Circ Res 50, 1982: 695–704.

13. Young DF, Cholvin NR, Kirkeeide RL, Roth AC: Hemodynamics of arterial stenoses at elevated flow rates. Circ Res 41, 1977: 99–107.

14. Mates RE, Gupta RL, Bell AC, Klocke FJ: Fluid dynamics of coronary artery stenosis. Circ Res 42, 1978: 152–162.

15. Roth AC, Young DF, Cholvin NR: Effect of collateral and peripheral resistance on blood flow through arterial stenoses. J Biomechanics 9, 1976: 367–375.

16. Elzinga WE, Skinner DB: Hemodynamic characteristics of critical stenosis in canine coronary arteries. J Thoracic Cardiov Surgery 69, 1975: 217–222.

17. Hillis WS, Friesinger GC: Reactive hyperemia: An index of the significance of coronary stenoses. Am Heart J 92, 1976: 737–740.

18. Feldman RL, Nichols WW, Pepine CJ, Conti CR: Hemodynamic significance of the length of a coronary arterial narrowing. Am J Cardiol 41, 1978: 865–871.

19. Folts JD, Gallagher K, Rowe GG: Hemodynamic effects of controlled degrees of coronary artery stenosis in short-term and long-term studies in dogs. J Thoracic and Cardiov Surg 73, 1977: 722–727.

20. Mullani NA, Gould KL: First pass measurements of regional blood flow with external detectors. J Nucl Med 24, 1983: 577–581.

21. Hoffman JIE: Maximal coronary flow and the concept of coronary vascular reserve. Circulation 70, 1984: 153–159.

22. Gould KL, Kelley KO, Bolson EL: Experimental validation of quantitative coronary arteriography for determining pressure-flow characteristics of coronary stenosis. Circulation 66, 1982: 930–937.

23. White CW, Wright CB, Doty DB, Hiratzka LF, Eastham CL, Harrison DG, Marcus ML: Does visual interpretation of the coronary arteriogram predict the physiologic importance of a coronary stenosis? N Eng J Med 310, 1984: 819–824.

24. Harrison DG, White CW, Hiratzka LF, Doty DB, Barnes DH, Eastham CL, Marcus ML: The value of lesion cross-sectional area determined by quantitative coronary angiography in assessing the physiologic significance of proximal left anterior descending coronary arterial stenoses. Circulation 69, 1984: 1111–1119.

25. Marcus ML, Armstrong ML, Heistad DD, Eastham CL, Mark AL: Comparison of three methods of evaluating coronary obstructive lesions: Postmortem arteriography, pathologic examination and measurement of regional myocardial perfusion during maximal vasodilation. Am J Cardiol 49, 1982: 1699–1706.

26. Fiddian RV, Byar D, Edwards EA: Factors affecting flow through a stenosed vessel. Arch Surg 88, 1964: 83–90.

27. Bomberger RA, Zarins CK, Glagov S: Resident research award. Subcritical arterial stenosis enhances distal atherosclerosis. J Surg Research 30, 1981: 205–212.

28. Brown BG, Bolson E, Frimer M, Dodge HT: Quantitative coronary arteriography. Estimation of dimensions, hemodynamic resistance, and atheroma mass of coronary artery lesions using the arteriogram and digital computation. Circulation 55, 1977: 329–337.

29. McMahon MM, Brown BG, Cukingnan R, Rolett EL, Bolson E, Frimer M, Dodge HT: Quantitative coronary angiography: Measurement of the 'critical' stenosis in patients with unstable angina and single-vessel disease without collaterals. Circulation 60, 1979: 106–113.

30. Brown BG, Bolson E, Petersen RB, Pierce CD, Dodge HT: The mechanisms of nitroglycerin action: Stenosis vasodilatation as a major component of the drug response. Circulation 64, 1981: 1089–1097.

31. Brown BG, Lee AB, Bolson EL, Dodge HT: Reflex constriction of significant coronary stenosis as a mechanism contributing to ischemic left ventricular dysfunction during isometric exercise. Circulation 70, 1984: 18–24.

32. Gould KL, Lee D, Lovgren K: Techniques for arteriography and hydraulic analysis of coronary stenoses in unsedated dogs. Am J Physiol 235, 1978: H350–H356.

33. Spears JR, Sandor T, Baim DS, Paulin S: The minimum error in estimating coronary luminal cross-sectional area from cineangiographic diameter measurements. Cath and Cardiov Diagn 9, 1983: 119–128.

34. Spears JR, Sandor T, Als AV, Malagold M, Markis JE, Grossman W, Serur JR, Paulin S: Computerized image analysis for quantitative measurement of vessel diameter from cineangiograms. Circulation 68, 1983: 453–461.

35. Sanders WJ, Alderman EL, Harrison DC: Coronary artery quantitation using digital imaging processing techniques. Comp Cardiol 1979: 15–20.

36. Reiber JHC, Serruys PW, Kooijman CJ, Wijns W, Slager CJ, Gerbrands JJ, Schuurbiers JCH, Boer A den, Hugenholtz PG: Assessment of short-, medium-, and long-term variations in arterial dimensions for computer-assisted quantitation of coronary cineangiograms. Circulation 71, 1985: 280–288.

37. Selzer RH, Blankenhorn DH: The identification of the variation of atherosclerosis plaques by invasive and non-invasive methods. In: Atherosclerosis clinical evaluation and therapy. GC Lenzis and Descovich (Eds.) MTP Press Limited, Boston, 1982: 453–465.

38. Kirkeeide RL, Fung P, Smalling RW, Gould KL: Automated evaluation of vessel diameter from arteriograms. Comp Cardiol 1982: 215–218.

39. Kirkeeide RL, Smalling RW, Gould KL: Automated measurement of artery diameter from arteriograms. Circulation 66, 1982: II–325 (Abstract).

40. Kirkeeide RL, Parsel L, Gould KL: Prediction of coronary flow reserve of stenotic coronary arteries by quantitative arteriography. Circulation 70, 1984: II–250 (Abstract).

41. Brown BG, Bolson EL, Dodge HT: Arteriographic assessment of coronary atherosclerosis. Review of current methods, their limitations, and clinical applications. Arteriosclerosis 2, 1982: 2–15.

42. Lipscomb K, Gould KL: Mechanism of the effect of coronary artery stenosis on coronary flow in the dog. Am Heart J 89, 1975: 60–67.

43. Weintraub WS, Hattori S, Agarwal JB, Bodenheimer MM, Banka VS, Helfant RH: The relationship between myocardial blood flow and contraction by myocardial layer in the canine left ventricle during ischemia. Circ Res 48, 1981: 430–438.

44. Bache RJ, Schwartz JS: Effect of perfusion pressure distal to a coronary stenosis on transmural myocardial blood flow. Circulation 65, 1982: 928–935.
45. Young DF, Cholvin NR, Roth AC: Pressure drop across artificially induced stenoses in the femoral arteries of dogs. Circ Res 36, 1975: 735–743.
46. Young DF, Tsai FY: Flow characteristics in models of arterial stenoses. I. Steady flow. J Biomechanics 6, 1973: 395–410.
47. Young DF, Tsai FY: Flow characteristics in models of arterial stenoses. II. Unsteady flow. J Biomechanics 6, 1973: 547–559.
48. Seeley BD, Yound DF: Effect of geometry on pressure losses across models of arterial stenoses. J Biomechanics 9, 1976: 439–448.
49. Lipscomb K, Hooten S: Effect of stenotic dimensions and blood flow on the hemodynamic significance of model coronary arterial stenoses. Am J Cardiol 42, 1978: 781–792.
50. Siebes M, Gottwik M, Schlepper M: Qualitative and quantitative experimental studies on the evaluation of model coronary arteries from angiograms. Comp Cardiol 1982: 211–214.
51. Rutishauser W: Equipment for cinedensitometry from 35–mm film. In: Roentgen-, Cine-, and Videodensitometry. P.H. Heintzen (Ed). Georg Thieme Verlag, Stuttgart, 1971: 68–73.
52. Crawford DW, Brooks SH, Selzer RH, Barndt Jr R, Beckenback ES, Blankenhorn DH: Computer densitometry for angiographic assessment of arterial cholesterol content and gross pathology in human atherosclerosis. J Lab Clin Med 89, 1977: 378–392.
53. Nichols AB, Gabrieli CFO, Fenoglio JJ, Esser PD: Quantification of relative coronary arterial stenosis by cinevideodensitometric analysis of coronary arteriograms. Circ 69, 1984: 512–522.
54. Serruys PW, Reiber JHC, Wijns W, Brand M van den, Kooijman CJ, Katen HJ ten, Hugenholtz PG: Assessment of percutaneous transluminal coronary angioplasty by quantitative coronary angiography: Diameter versus densitometric area measurements. Am J Cardiol 54, 1984: 482–488.
55. Talukder N, Karayannacos PE, Nerem RM, Vasko JS: An experimental study of the fluid dynamics of multiple noncritical stenoses. J Biochemical Engineering, 1977: 74–82.
56. Walinsky P, Santamore WP, Weiner L, Brest AN: Dynamic changes in the haemodynamic severity of coronary artery stenosis in a canine model. Cardiov Res 13, 1979: 113–118.
57. Schwartz JS, Carlyle PF, Cohn JN: Effect of dilation of the distal coronary bed on flow and resistance in severely stenotic coronary arteries in the dog. Am J Cardiol 43, 1979: 219–224.
58. Santamore WP, Walinsky P: Altered coronary flow responses to vasoactive drugs in the presence of coronary arterial stenosis in the dog. Am J Cardiol 45, 1980: 276–285.
59. Brown BG, Josephson MA, Petersen RB, Pierce CD, Wong M, Hecht HS, Bolson E, Dodge HT: Intravenous dipyridamole combined with isometric handgrip for near maximal acute increase in coronary flow in patients with coronary artery disease. Am J Cardiol 48, 1981: 1077–1085.
60. Logan SE: On the fluid mechanics of human coronary artery stenosis. IEEE Trans on Biom Eng BME-22, 1975: 327–334.
61. Gould KL: Collapsing coronary stenosis – a Starling resistor. Int J Cardiol 2, 1982: 39–42.
62. Fiddian RV, Byar D, Edwards EA: Factors affecting flow through a stenosed vessel. Archives of Surgery 88, 1964: 105–112.
63. Collins SM, Skorton DJ, Harrison DG, White CW, Eastham CL, Hiratzka LF, Doty DB, Marcus ML: Quantitative computer-based videodensitometry and the physiological significance of a coronary stenosis. Comp Cardiol 1982: 219–222.
64. Marcus M, Wright C, Doty D, Eastham C, Laughlin D, Krumm P, Fastenow C, Brody M: Measurements of coronary velocity and reactive hyperemia in the coronary circulation of humans. Circ Res 49, 1981: 877–891.
65. Gewirtz H, Williams DO, Most AS: Quantitative assessment of the effects of a fixed 50% coronary artery stenosis on regional myocardial flow reserve and transmural distribution of blood flow. J Am Coll Cardiol 1, 1983: 1273–1280.
66. Hoffman JIE: Maximal coronary flow and the concept of coronary vascular reserve. Circulation 70, 1984: 153–159.

67. Mullani NA: Myocardial perfusion with rubidium-82: III. Theory relating severity of coronary stenosis to perfusion deficit. J Nucl Med 25, 1984: 1190–1196.
68. Mullani NA, Goldstein RA, Gould KL, Marani SK, Fisher DJ, O'Brien Jr HA, Loberg MD: Myocardial perfusion with Rubidium-82: I. Measurement of extraction fraction and flow with external detectors. J Nucl Med 24, 1983: 898–906.
69. Goldstein RA, Mullani NA, Marani SK, Fisher DJ, Gould KL, O'Brien Jr HA: Myocardial perfusion with rubidium-82: II. Effects of metabolic and pharmacologic interventions. J Nucl Med 24, 1983: 907–915.
70. Vlodaver Z, Frech R, Van Tassel RA, Edwards JE: Correlation of the antemortem coronary arteriogram and the postmortem specimen. Circulation 47, 1973: 162–169.
71. Grondin CM, Dyrda I, Pasternac A, Campeau L, Bourassa MG, Lespérance J: Discrepancies between cineangiographic and postmortem findings in patients with coronary artery disease and recent myocardial revascularization. Circulation 49, 1974: 703–708.
72. Gallagher KP, Folts JD, Rowe GG: Comparison of coronary arteriograms with direct measurements of stenosed coronary arteries in dogs. Am Heart J 95, 1978: 338–347.
73. Hutchins GM, Bulkley BH, Ridolfi RL, Griffith LSC, Lohr FT, Piasio MA: Correlation of coronary arteriograms and left ventriculograms with postmortem studies. Circulation 56, 1977: 32–37.
74. Yano Y, Budinger TF, Chiang G, O'Brien HA, Grant PM: Evaluation and application of alumina-based RB-82 generators charged with high levels of SR-82/85. J Nucl Med 20, 1979: 961–966.
75. Mullani NA, Ficke DC, Hartz R, Markham J, Wong WH: System design of fast PET scanners utilizing time-of-flight. IEEE Trans Nucl Sci NS-28, 1981: 104–108.
76. Philippe EA, Mullani N, Wong W, Hartz R: Real-time image reconstruction for time-of-flight positron emission tomography (TOFPET). IEEE Trans Nucl Sci NS-29, 1982: 524–528.
77. Mullani N, Wong W, Hartz R, Philippe E, Yerian K: Sensitivity improvement of TOFPET by the utilization of the inter-slice coincidences. IEEE Trans Nucl Sci NS-29, 1982: 479–483.
78. Wong W-H, Mullani NA, Phillipe EA, Hartz R, Gould KL: Image improvement and design optimization of the Time-of Flight PET. J Nucl Med 24, 1983: 52–60.
79. Mullani NA, Gaeta J, Yerian K, Wong WH, Hartz RK, Philippe EA, Bristow D, Gould KL: Dynamic imaging with high resolution time-of-flight PET Camera – TOFPET I. IEEE Trans Nucl Sci NS-31, 1984: 609–613.
80. Wong W-H, Mullani NA, Wardworth G, Hartz RK, Bristow D: Characteristics of small barium fluoride (BaF$_2$) scintillator for high intrinsic resolution time-of-flight positron emission tomography. IEEE Trans Nucl Sci NS-31, 1984: 381–386.

Effects of coronary atherosclerosis on coronary reserve

Melvin L. Marcus, D.G. Harrison, C.W. White and L.F. Hiratzka

Summary

To assess the physiologic significance of coronary obstructions in patients at the time of open-heart surgery we have studied coronary reactive hyperemic responses to a 20-second coronary occlusion. Coronary blood flow velocity was measured with a single crystal pulsed-Doppler probe coupled to the surface coronary vessel with a small suction cup. Our studies have demonstrated that normal vessels supplying a normal myocardium increase coronary blood flow velocity 5–6 fold following release of a 20-second coronary occlusion. Furthermore, patients with severe coronary obstructions (greater than 90% diameter narrowing) have markedly blunted reactive hyperemic responses (i.e. less than a two-fold increase in coronary blood flow velocity following release of a 20-second coronary occlusion). In patients with obstructions of intermediate severity (10–90% diameter narrowing) the relationship between percent stenosis and the reactive hyperemic response was poor. In other studies, we have shown that the measurement of absolute cross-sectional area of a lesion with quantitative coronary angiographic techniques allows a better separation of patients with normal and abnormal coronary reserve than the use of percent stenosis. These studies emphasize the futility of utilizing percent stenosis to assess the physiologic significance of coronary obstructions in patients with atherosclerosis, particularly when the coronary obstructive lesions are of intermediate severity (10–90% diameter stenosis).

Introduction

Studies employing coronary angiography performed over the past 25 years have contributed immensely to our understanding of the pathophysiology and natural history of coronary atherosclerosis. In addition, the interpretation of the coronary arteriogram has served as an important guide to therapeutic decisions such as the need for bypass surgery or angioplasty. Nonetheless, the coronary arteriogram is far from a perfect diagnostic procedure. There is substantial intra- and interobserver variability (1) in the interpretation of the angiogram. Also, the ability to assess the physiological significance of individual coronary obstructions from visual interpretation of the angiogram has come into serious question (2–3).

In this brief review we will present data which seriously challenge the notion that percent stenosis of a lesion on a coronary arteriogram 'standard-of-the-day' is a satisfactory method of assessing the physiologic significance of individual coronary obstructive lesions. In addition, we will briefly discuss some new sophisticated approaches to assessing the physiologic significance of individual coronary obstructions in patients.

Assessing coronary reserve in individual coronary vessels by measuring coronary reactive hyperemic responses during open-heart surgery

We have developed a method of assessing coronary reserve in individual coronary vessels which employed a pulsed-Doppler flow probe applied to coronary vessels with a suction cup (4). This approach has several advantages. First, the single crystal Doppler probe can be placed on the anterior surface of the heart at the time of open-heart surgery without dissection of the coronary vessel. As a consequence, the measurements of coronary blood flow velocity can be obtained without subjecting the patient to any significant risk. Second, extensive animal studies have shown that changes in coronary blood flow velocity measured with the Doppler system correlate closely with changes in coronary flow (see Figure 1). Furthermore, coronary reactive hyperemic responses measured with the Doppler system are nearly identical to coronary reactive hyperemic responses obtained with an electromagnetic flowmeter (see Figure 2). Third, with the Doppler system we have defined the quantitative characteristics of coronary reactive hyperemia in man. Transient coronary occlusions which range in duration from 1–20 seconds produce progressively greater coronary reactive hyperemic responses (Figure 3). The maximal dilator response which is elicited with occlusions of 20 seconds in duration or longer serves as an excellent index of coronary reserve in the individual vessel being examined. Fourth, we have shown that age (5), gender (6) or the vessel studied (right coronary artery versus left coronary artery) (6) do not influence the magnitude of the coronary reactive hyperemic response.

Although the coronary reactive hyperemic response is a valuable index of coronary reserve it is only valid if mean aortic pressure is in the physiologic range (7), coronary collaterals in the perfusion field of the vessel being occluded do not exist, substantial cardiac hypertrophy is absent (8) and the myocardium perfused by the vessel being examined is viable and functioning reasonably well. In our studies, data were only included if the confounding factors noted above were either adequate (mean aortic pressure) or absent (coronary collaterals, ventricular hypertrophy and myocardial infarction on impaired ventricular function).

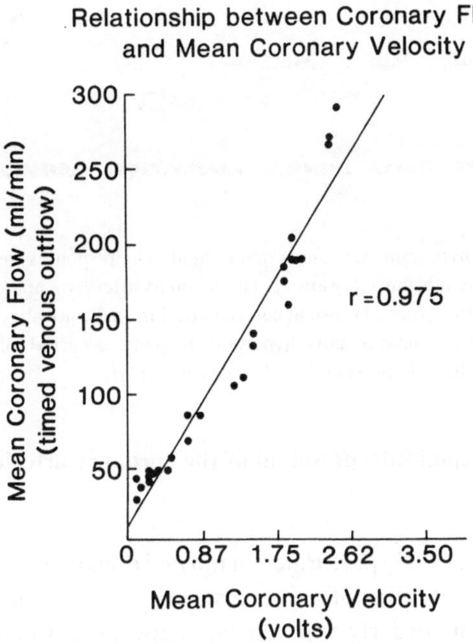

Relationship between Coronary Flow and Mean Coronary Velocity

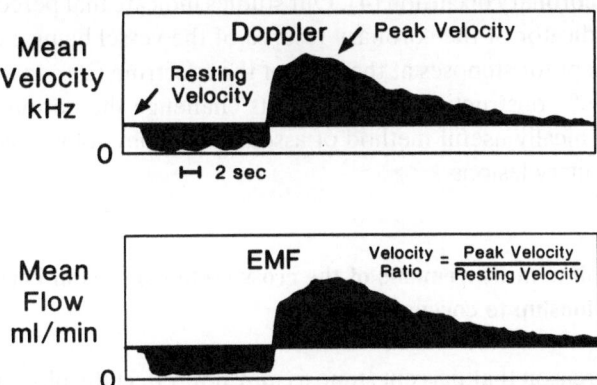

Mean Coronary Flow (ml/min) (timed venous outflow)

r = 0.975

Mean Coronary Velocity (volts)

Figure 1. Relationship between changes in blood flow (time venous collection from the coronary sinus) and changes in coronary blood flow velocity measured with the suction-Doppler in a dog. Flow was varied over a broad range by various pharmacological interventions. Changes in coronary blood flow velocity with the Doppler correlated closely with changes in coronary blood flow. (This figure was originally presented by Marcus *et al.* (4)).

Mean Velocity kHz

Doppler Peak Velocity

Resting Velocity

0

⊢⊣ 2 sec

Mean Flow ml/min

EMF

Velocity Ratio = Peak Velocity / Resting Velocity

0

Figure 2. Reactive hyperemic responses measured simultaneously in an anesthetized dog with the suction Doppler and an adjacent electromagnetic flow probe (EMF). The similarity of measured responses indicates that the reactive hyperemic response can be measured accurately with the suction Doppler. (Based on data originally presented by Marcus *et al.* (4)).

232

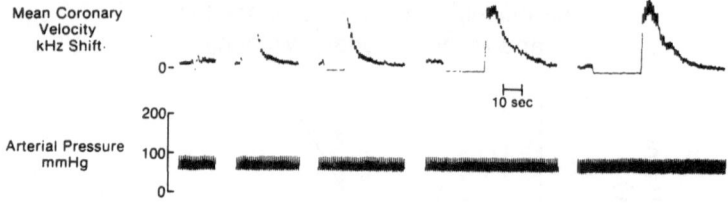

Figure 3. Coronary reactive hyperemic responses in a patient. The responses were obtained from a right ventricular branch of the right coronary artery. The coronary artery was angiographically normal and the right ventricle was also normal. Transient coronary occlusion did not alter arterial pressure or heart rate. In this patient the maximal reactive hyperemic response occurred following a 20-second coronary occlusion. (Data originally presented by Marcus *et al.* (4)).

Relationship between visual interpretation of the coronary arteriogram and coronary reserve

A large body of research (9–12) performed in normal dogs with localized mechanical coronary obstructive lesions of variable severity has shown in a convincing manner that there is an orderly relationship between coronary reserve and percent coronary stenosis (see Figure 4). It is unfortunate that cardiologists and cardiac surgeons have assumed that concepts derived from these elegant sophisticated animal experiments are applicable to the care of patients with coronary atherosclerosis.

At Iowa we have assessed coronary reserve in individual coronary vessels with our Doppler system and related these responses to percent coronary stenosis determined from visual interpretation of the patient's coronary arteriogram. Our index of coronary reserve was the peak-to-resting velocity ratio following release of a 20 second coronary occlusion (4). Our studies indicate that percent stenosis is a very poor indicator of the coronary reserve of the vessel being examined (see Figure 4). Except for stenoses at the ends of the spectrum (i.e., less than 10% or greater than 90% obstruction), these results challenge the notion that percent stenosis is a clinically useful method of assessing the physiologic significance of individual coronary lesions.

Studies of absolute measurements of the cross-sectional area of coronary lesions and their relationship to coronary reserve

One potential reason that percent stenosis may not reflect the physiologic significance of a coronary obstructive lesion is that the angiographically normal vascular segment adjacent to the lesion being assessed contains a variable degree of diffuse atherosclerosis. This concept is illustrated in Figure 5. If diffuse atherosclerosis of variable severity was the primary reason that percent stenosis was a poor index of

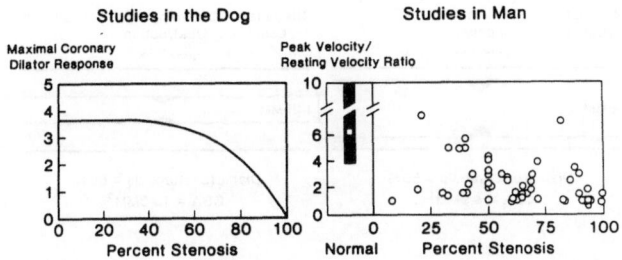

Figure 4. Relationship between maximal coronary blood flow or blood flow velocity and percent stenosis in an experimental study and in a clinical study. To achieve coronary blood flow velocity in the clinical study the coronary vessel being examined was occluded for 20 seconds and then the occlusion was released. Maximal coronary blood flow was expressed as a ratio of peak velocity following release of the occlusion and resting velocity. The percent stenosis of the vessel being examined was measured with calipers from the angiographic projection that showed the lesion to be most severe. The range of normal responses in humans is shown by the black bar in the figure on the right. Each open circle represents a study in one patient. Although there was an orderly relationship between percent stenosis and maximal coronary blood flow in the experimental study (left), this was not the case in the clinical study. (The clinical data is based on studies originally presented by White *et al.* (2)).

coronary reserve, one might postulate that measurements of absolute cross-sectional area would be a better predictor of coronary reserve. Measurements of absolute cross-sectional area of a lesion are not influenced by the presence or absence of angiographically undetected coronary atherosclerosis in other vascular segments in the vessel being examined.

The data presented in Figure 6 indicate that in patients with isolated single obstructive lesions in the proximal left anterior descending coronary artery measurements of absolute cross-sectional area provide a better separation of normal and abnormal coronary reserve than measurements of percent stenosis in the same patients. Furthermore, in the same patients, the cross-sectional area of the proximal vascular segment of the left anterior descending coronary artery that was angiographically normal was quite variable and correlated with the coronary reserve of the vessel (see Figure 7). These observations taken together provide strong support for the notion that diffuse atherosclerosis undetected by visual interpretation of the coronary arteriograms severely limits the usefulness of percent stenosis as an index of the physiologic significance of individual coronary obstructive lesions.

Although measurements of absolute cross-sectional area of a coronary lesion are useful under circumscribed conditions (i.e., isolated proximal lesions of the left anterior descending coronary artery) this approach has several limitations. First, normal values for multiple segments in the coronary tree have not been defined and there is reason to presume that such normal dimensions would be markedly influenced by the patient's coronary branching pattern, cardiac size and gender. Second, the absolute cross-sectional area of a lesion does not account for other geometric features of a stenosis such as lenght, exit angle and entrance

234

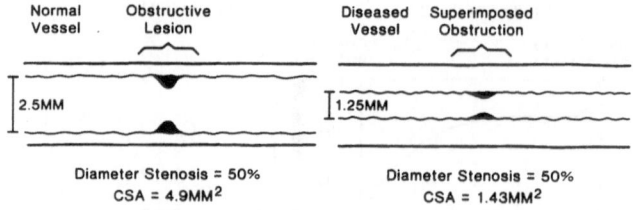

Diameter Stenosis = 50%
CSA = 4.9MM²

Diameter Stenosis = 50%
CSA = 1.43MM²

Figure 5. Effects of a 50% diameter stenosis in a normal vessel (left) and a vessel with diffuse obstructive disease (right). In the normal vessel, the obstructive lesion decreases the cross-sectional area (CSA) of the vessel at its narrowest point to 4.9 millimeters squared. In the diseased vessel, the obstructive lesion decreased the CSA at the narrowest point to 1.43 millimeters squared. Pathological studies indicate that coronary disease is often a diffuse process which involves the entire length of the coronary artery. As a consequence, percent stenosis is an inadequate approach to assessing the severity of coronary obstructive disease in patients with coronary atherosclerosis. (This figure was originally presented by Harrison *et al.* (3)).

angle that influence the hydraulic effects of any obstructive lesion (9–12). Third, because of the complex geometry of the coronary vasculature and vessel overlap, it is not practical or even possible to obtain adequate or orthogonal views of all coronary segments. Such high quality orthogonal angiograms would be needed to calculate absolute dimensions in multiple vascular segments in the coronary tree.

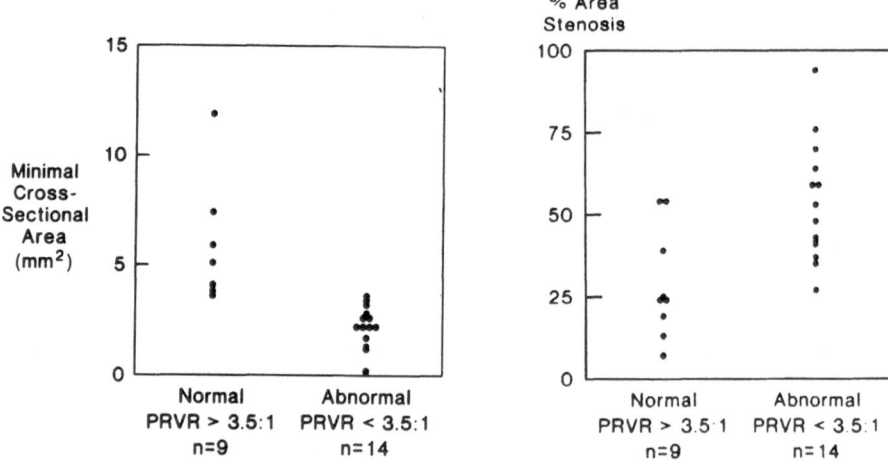

Figure 6. Effectiveness of minimal cross-sectional area (left) and percent area stenosis (right) in separating patients with normal and abnormal hyperemic responses. In our experience a peak-to-resting velocity ratio (PRVR) of 3.5:1 following the release of a 20 second occlusion is the lower limit of normal. Separation of abnormal and normal reactive hyperemic responses was best accomplished when minimal cross-sectional area was used as a criteria. (Based on data originally presented by Harrison *et al.* (3)).

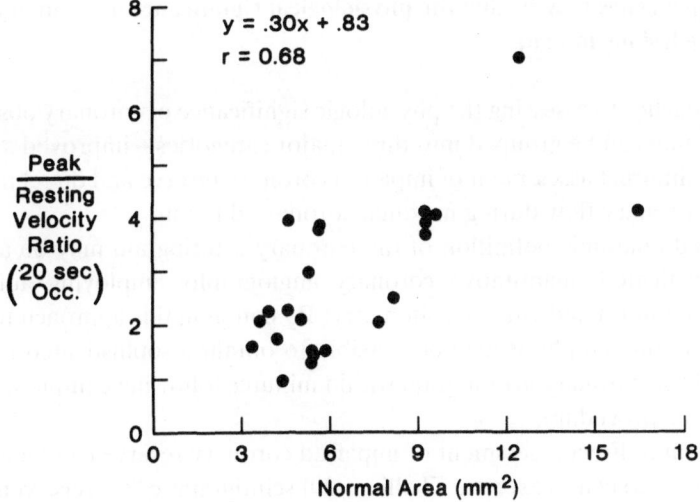

Figure 7. Relationship between peak-to-resting velocity ratio following a 20-second coronary occlusion and the cross-sectional area of a normal segment of a left anterior descending artery with a proximal stenosis. Note the wide range of normal areas in the apparently normal segment of the left anterior descending coronary artery. Also, there was a reasonable correlation (r = 0.68) between the peak-to-resting velocity ratio and the cross-sectional area of the normal portion of the left anterior descending coronary artery. The wide range of normal areas of the proximal left anterior descending coronary artery is best explained by the presence of a variable degree of diffuse atherosclerosis. (This figure was originally presented by Harrison *et al.* (3)).

Additional evidence of diffuse coronary atherosclerosis in man

Our studies of absolute coronary dimensions described above support the concept that diffuse coronary atherosclerosis can confound the interpretation of the coronary arteriogram. It is important to emphasize that this concept is also supported by other investigations utilizing totally different technologies. For example, pathological studies have emphasized that coronary atherosclerosis in man is a diffuse disease with superimposed local obstructions of greater severity as opposed to a localized disease process that occurs in an otherwise normal vessel (13). High-frequency echocardiography is a new technique that allows one to determine the thickness of the coronary wall as well as the cross-sectional area of the lumen. Studies utilizing high-frequency echocardiography at open-heart surgery have demonstrated that diffuse coronary atherosclerosis is ubiquitous in patients with angiographic evidence of localized coronary obstructive disease (14).

In view of the above, it is untenable to assume that a measurement of percent stenosis on an angiogram in a vessel with diffuse atherosclerosis of variable severity will ever provide a clinically useful estimate of the physiologic significance of a coronary obstructive lesion.

Future approaches to assessing the physiological significance of coronary obstructive lesions in man

New approaches to assessing the physiologic significance of coronary obstructive lesions in man can be grouped into three major categories – improved anatomic definition, indirect assessment of impaired coronary reserve and direct measurements of coronary flow during maximal coronary dilation.

Improved anatomic definition of the coronary arteriogram may be achieved with sophisticated quantitative coronary angiography employing automated border recognition and videodensitometry. By coupling this approach to digital subtraction angiography it may be possible to obtain a sophisticated anatomic analysis of the coronary arteriogram within minutes following completion of the angiographic procedure.

Functional indirect assessment of impaired coronary reserve can be achieved with techniques such as exercise Thallium-201 scintigrams or exercise ventricular function employing various modalities for examining cardiac geometry including nuclear angiograms, echocardiograms, digital subtraction angiography, nuclear magnetic resonance and cine computed tomography. With any of these systems the indirect assessment of coronary reserve will require measurements of relative myocardial perfusion or ventricular function during some type of pharmacologic or physiologic stress to the coronary circulation.

Direct assessment of coronary reserve is currently being pursued with a variety of approaches of measuring regional myocardial perfusion including digital subtraction angiography with contrast induced hyperemia (15), positron emission tomography utilizing rubidium 82 (16) and cine computed tomography utilizing contrast clearance (17). Also, the recent development of an intracoronary Doppler catheter is a very promising approach to assessing the physiologic significance of individual coronary obstructions in man (18).

In summary, this review emphasizes the limitations of utilizing percent coronary stenosis to estimate the physiologic significance of individual coronary obstructions in man. Since this time-honored standard has severe limitations the development of other more sophisticated approaches of assessing the physiologic significance of individual coronary obstructions in man should be strongly encouraged.

Acknowledgement

These studies have been supported in part by an Ischemic SCOR Grant HL 32295

References

1. Zir LM, Miller SW, Dinsmore RE, Gilbert JP, Harthorne JW: Interobserver variability in coronary angiography. Circulation 53, 1976: 627–632.
2. White CW, Wright CB, Doty DB, Hiratzka LF, Eastham CL, Harrison DG, Marcus ML: Does visual interpretation of the coronary arteriogram predict the physiologic significance of a coronary stenosis? N Eng J Med 310, 1984: 819–824.
3. Harrison DG, White CW, Hiratzka LF, Doty DB, Barnes DH, Eastham CL, Marcus ML: The value of lesion cross-sectional area determined by quantitative coronary angiography in assessing the physiologic significance of proximal left anterior descending coronary arterial stenoses. Circulation 69, 1984: 1111–1114.
4. Marcus M, Wright C, Doty D, Eastham C, Laughlin D, Krumm P, Fastenow C, Brody M: Measurements of coronary velocity and reactive hyperemia in the coronary circulation of humans. Circulation Research 49, 1981: 877–891.
5. Eastham C, Doty D, Wright C, Marcus M: Effects of age on coronary reserve in man. Circulation 62 (Suppl. III) 1980: III–64.
6. Marcus ML: The coronary circulation in health and disease. Chapter 3: Metabolic regulation of coronary blood flow. McGraw-Hill Book Company, New York, 1983.
7. Dole WP, Montville WJ, Bishop VS: Dependency of myocardial reactive hyperemia on coronary artery pressure in the dog. Am J of Phys 240(5), 1981: H709–H715.
8. Marcus ML, Doty DB, Hiratzka LF, Wright CB, Easthem CE: Decreased coronary reserve – A mechanism for angina pectoris in patients with aortic stenosis and normal coronary arteries. N Engl J Med 307, 1982: 1362–1367.
9. Gould KL, Lipscomb K, Hamilton GW: Physiologic basis for assessing critical coronary stenosis. Instantaneous flow response and regional distribution during coronary hyperemia as measures of coronary flow reserve. Am J Cardiol 33, 1974: 87–94.
10. Gould KL, Lipscomb K: Effects of coronary stenoses on coronary flow reserve and resistance. Am J Cardiol 34, 1974: 48–55.
11. Gould KL, Lipscomb K, Calvert C: Compensatory changes of the distal coronary vascular bed during progressive coronary constriction. Circulation 51, 1975: 1085–1094.
12. Gould KL: Pressure-flow characteristics of coronary stenoses in unsedated dogs at rest and during coronary vasodilation. Circ Res 43, 1978: 245–253.
13. Arnett EN, Isner JM, Redwood DR, Kent DM, Baker WP, Ackerstein H, Roberts WC: Coronary artery narrowing in coronary heart disease. Comparison of cineangiographic and necropsy findings. Ann Int Med 91, 1979: 350–356.
14. McPherson DD, Hiratzka LF, Brandt B; Lamberth WC, Kieso RA, Hite PR, Marcus ML, Kerber RE: Intraoperative characterization by high-frequency echo of lumen to wall ratios in coronary arteries. Clin Res, 32, 1984: 734 A; Circulation 70 (Supp II), 1984: II–394 (Abstract).
15. Vogel R, LeFree M, Bates E, O'Neill W, Foster R, Kirlin P, Smith D, Pitt B: Application of digital techniques to selective coronary arteriography. Use of myocardial contrast appearance time to measure coronary flow reserve. Am Heart J 107, 1984: 153–164.
16. Mullani NA, Goldstein RA, Gould KL, Marani SK, Fisher DJ, O'Brien HA, Loberg MD: Myocardial persfusion with Rubidium-82. I. Measurement of extraction fraction and flow with external detectors. J Nucl Med 24, 1983: 898–906.
17. Rumberger JA, Feiring AJ, Lipton MJ, Higgins CB, Marcus ML: Measurement of myocardial perfusion by ultrafast CT. JACC 5, 1985: 500 (Abstract).
18. Wilson RF, Hartley CJ, Laughlin DE, Marcus ML, White CW: Transluminal subselective measurement of coronary blood flow velocity and coronary vasodilator reserve in man. Am J Cardiol 3, 1984: 529.

Effects of coronary artery stenosis, aortic insufficiency and aortic stenosis on coronary blood flow in the dog

C. Richard Conti, R.L. Feldman, W.W. Nichols,
R.G. MacDonald and C.J. Pepine.

Summary

Physiologic experiments measuring coronary blood flow in an animal model were performed. Coronary narrowings were created in anesthetized open chest dogs using a calibrated snare or plastic occluder. Results of these experiments indicated that (1) short narrowings of 40–60% do not decrease resting coronary blood flow but slightly decrease hyperemic coronary blood flow; (2) increasing the length of the 40–60% narrowing from 1–5 mm further decreases the hyperemic coronary blood flow response; (3) increase in the length of the 40–60% narrowing to 10 mm decreases resting coronary blood flow and obliterates reactive hyperemic coronary blood flow; (4) sequential narrowings of 40–60% diameter stenosis decreased reactive hyperemic coronary blood flow greater than single narrowings of the same total length. In other experiments, acute aortic insufficiency was created. It was found that coronary flow reserve during reactive hyperemia in dogs with or without coronary narrowings is decreased during aortic insufficiency compared to dogs with competent aortic valves. The decrease in coronary flow reserve was more pronounced as the magnitude of aortic insufficiency increased.

In other experiments, dogs with acute aortic stenosis, and nonobstructed coronary arteries, mean coronary blood flow increased during the aortic stenosis, but coronary flow reserve during reactive hyperemia decreased. When the coronary artery was stenosed, aortic stenosis has an even more important hemodynamic influence on the coronary circulation.

Introduction

The primary goal of coronary angiography is to identify coronary artery disease sufficient to produce myocardial ischemia. The clinician is faced with the question:'What is the physiologic significance of a coronary artery stenosis observed during angiography?'. In this paper, we present five separate experiments that relate to this question and point out some of the problems of assessing coronary angiograms by simply reporting percent stenosis, i.e., percent diameter narrowing of the vessel. In these experiments, coronary stenoses were created in anesthetized open chest dogs using a calibrated snare or milled plastic occluder (1).

Methods

General experimental model

The studies were made in healthy mongrel dogs (20 to 30 kg). After premedication with morphine (1 mg/kg body weight) and pentobarbital (25 mg/kg) anesthesia, followed by an overnight fast, the animals were intubated. Respiration was controlled with a Harvard pump to maintain arterial blood gases and pH within the physiologic range. Through a left thoracotomy in the fifth intercostal space, the anterior descending or circumflex branch of the left coronary artery was approached. With the heart supported by a pericardial cradle, one of these branches was isolated by dissection. Only vessels averaging 3 mm or more in diameter over a length of 2 to 3 cm in their proximal portion were used. An appropriately sized cuff-type Narco Biosystems electromagnetic flow probe was positioned proximally around the artery to measure coronary blood flow. Aortic pressure, used to assess proximal coronary arterial pressure, was measured through a saline-filled catheter placed in the ascending aorta after insertion through a femoral artery. Distal coronary pressure was measured through a no. 4 Teflon catheter placed in a distal coronary branch beyond the flow probe and occluders. The pressure gauges (Statham P23Db) were made equisensitive by simultaneous calibration with the same test pressure using a Paley manifold. Pressure and flow signals and the electrocardiogram were monitored and recorded on an Electronics for Medicine model DR8 multichannel oscilloscopic recorder and on Hewlett Packard model 3960 magnetic tape.

Coronary arterial narrowings

A snare was attached to a Starrett machinist's micrometer to create calibrated focal constrictions. The lenght of subsequently produced obstructions was controlled with occluders made from Lucite rods 5 mm in external diameter. From each piece, milled at a constant concentric internal diameter, a set of occluders was created by cutting various lengths ranging from 1 to 15 mm. This procedure ensured that within a set of occluders only the length varied. The occluders were positioned on the artery through a small tapering keyhole. Each stenosis (regardless of length) was applied for the same duration. Particular care was taken to avoid kinking and distortion; only when they were excluded by both inspection and subsequent angiography were the data accepted for final analysis.

Confirmation of the degree of coronary arterial narrowing

Two techniques were used to confirm that the occluders create precise narrowings of predicted caliber, smooth and regular throughout their length. Selective coronary cineangiography of the coronary narrowings produced with all the sets of occluders was performed in multiple projections and the diameters of the prestenotic and stenotic sections were measured with calipers. Postmortem polysulfide casts were also used to verify the degree of diameter reduction produced by the occluders, and the degree of diameter reduction was measured with calipers.

Data accumulation and analysis

Measurements were made from the mean flow and pressure signals averaged from at least 10 consecutive beats. Flow measurements were made at rest and during reactive hyperemia after a 10 second complete coronary occlusion. Percent repayment of flow debt was calculated as reactive hyperemic flow/flow debt × 100 by planimetric integration of the mean flow signal. Flow debt = control flow rate × duration of occlusion. Reactive hyperemic flow = integral of flow curve during reactive hyperemia – (control flow rate × duration of reactive hyperemia).

Coronary artery blood flow related to percent stenosis

A typical experiment in a single animal study is illustrated in Figure 1. Aortic and distal coronary pressure and coronary blood flow were measured at rest and following a 10-sec coronary artery occlusion. The upper left panel represents resting and reactive hyperemic coronary blood flow in a nonobstructed coronary artery. There is no pressure gradient from the aorta to the distal coronary artery. Following a 10-sec occlusion, there is a small pressure differential and a typical hyperemic response. The upper right panel illustrates the effect of a 60% diameter stenosis produced by a snare. There is no diminution of resting coronary blood flow and there is no resting pressure gradient. Following a 10-sec coronary occlusion, there is a decrease of the peak reactive hyperemic response and a clear-cut pressure differential from aorta to distal coronary artery. In the lower left panel, the effect of an 80% snare narrowing reveals no resting pressure difference across the stenosis and no decrease in resting coronary blood flow. Following a 10-sec occlusion, there is a marked decrease in peak reactive hyperemic response

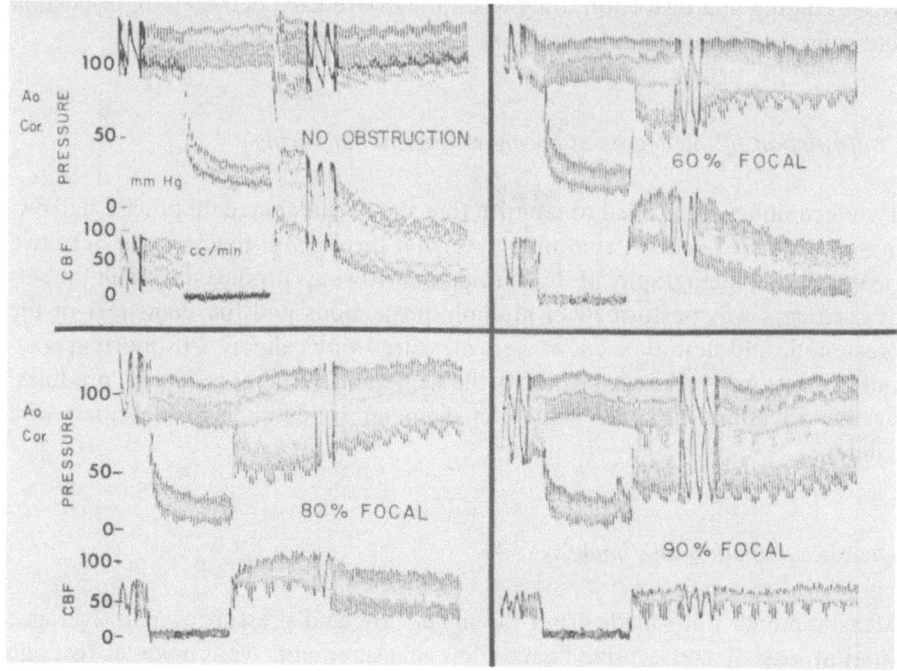

Figure 1. The effect of percent coronary artery stenosis on resting and reactive hyperemic distal coronary pressure and flow. Ao = Aortic, Cor = Coronary. CBF = coronary blood flow. See text.

and a large pressure difference across the stenosis which takes a long time to return to baseline. In the lower right panel, a 90% snare narrowing produces a marked decrease in resting coronary blood flow and a resting pressure difference across the stenosis. Following a 10-sec coronary artery occlusion, reactive hyperemia is essentially obliterated and the aorta coronary pressure gradient is increased. Recovery is markedly prolonged.

Coronary artery blood flow related to length of stenosis

Figure 2 is a representative experiment in a single dog to illustrate the physiologic effect of lengthening a 60% stenosis. The upper panel shows the effect of a 1 mm long 60% narrowing. There was no difference between this narrowing and the 60% snare occlusion shown in Figure 1. In the upper right panel, the length of this narrowing is increased to 5 mm which produces a striking increase in the resting pressure gradient across the stenosis and a slight decrease in resting coronary blood flow. The peak reactive hyperemic response is markedly decreased. In the lower left panel, increasing the length of the 60% narrowing to 10 mm decreases the resting coronary blood flow and eliminates the reactive hyperemic response.

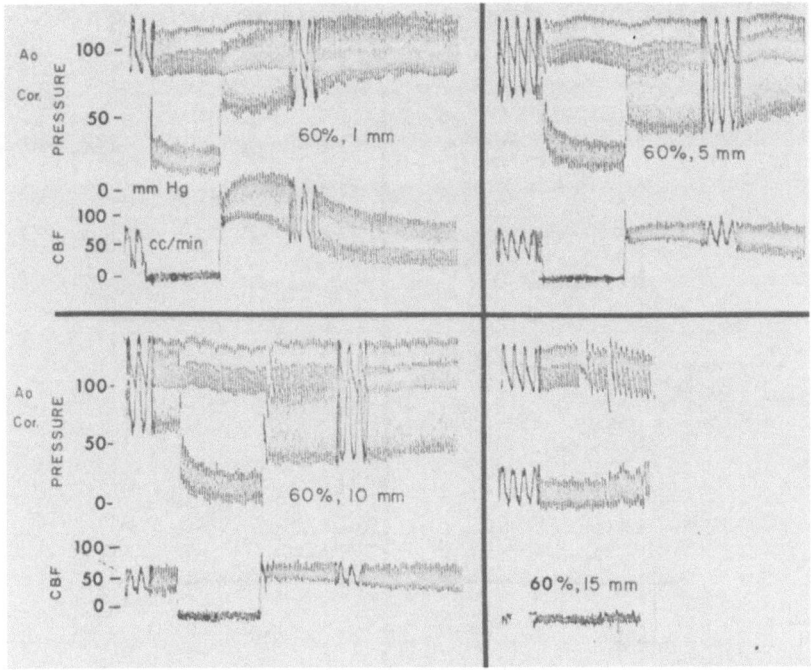

Figure 2. The effects of lengthening a 60% stenosis on resting and reactive hyperemic distal coronary artery pressure and flow. Ao = aortic, Cor = coronary. CBF = coronary blood flow. See text.

This was comparable to a 90% stenosis produced by the snare shown in Figure 1. In the lower right panel, the 60% narrowing 15 mm in length practically obliterates resting coronary blood flow and produces a large pressure gradient.

In a group of 8 dogs studied, a 90%, 1 mm long stenosis produced the greatest reduction in resting coronary blood flow, whereas a 70% narrowing had little effect. In the same animals it was apparent that as the length of the coronary artery narrowing increased, resting coronary blood flow decreased. Similar results were obtained during the reactive hyperemic response in these animals.

Coronary artery blood flow related to multiple stenoses in the same vessel

Experiments comparing the effects of single and multiple narrowings in the same coronary artery were performed in a fashion similar to the previous experiments (2). The effect of a 60% stenosis, 1, 2, and 3 mm in length was compared to a series of two and three 60% stenosis 1 mm in length. Two or three short narrowings (total length of 5 or 10 mm between lesions) resulted in larger decrements in flow and larger pressure gradients than with single narrowings of the same total length (2 or 3 mm). The hemodynamic responses observed with multiple 40% to 60%

244

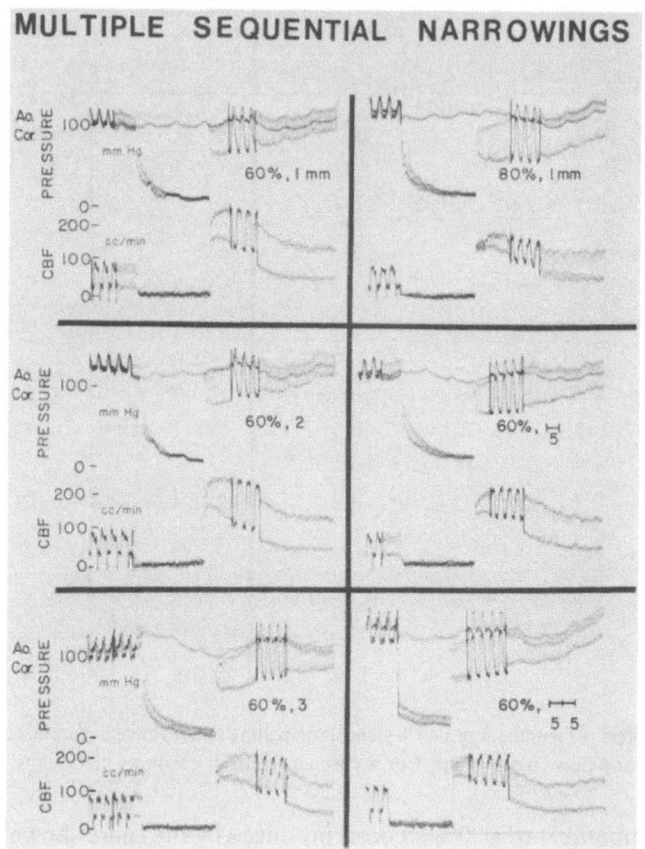

Figure 3. Six representative examples of coronary hemodynamic responses, comparing single 1 mm narrowings (panels 1 and 2), single 2 mm and 3 mm narrowings (panels 3 and 5), and multiple 1 mm narrowings (panels 4 and 6). Coronary blood flow (CBF), aortic (Ao) and coronary (Cor) pressures are shown. No decrease in resting coronary blood flow was observed; however, as degree of reduction in diameter increased, length increased (with reduction in diameter held constant at 60 percent), or number of narrowings increased, resting aorto-coronary pressure gradient increased slightly. Similarly, reactive hyperemic flow decreased as degree of narrowing increased, length of narrowing increased, or number of narrowings increased.

narrowings were comparable to effects previously observed with longer 40% to 60% narrowings and with short narrowings of approximately an 80% reduction in diameter (Figure 3). Thus, a series of narrowings has a greater effect on coronary flow and distal pressure than would be expected by simply adding effects of the narrowings studied individually.

What is the explanation for these observations? A stenosis has three sections, (1) a section of proximal contraction, (2) a section of expansion, and (3) a section of distal contraction. Viewed in this manner, the difference between a single narrowing and a series of narrowings, when the degree of reduction in diameter and the total length are constant, would be additional contractions and expansions of the multiple stenoses. Because the loss of energy in fluid flowing through a stenosis is greatest at the expansion, multiple narrowings might account for a larger loss of kinetic energy than single narrowings (3). Also, disruption of a normal pattern of laminar flow is believed to occur in the poststenotic region (3). If turbulent flow occurred at the entrance to a distal stenosis, an exaggeration of the loss in energy across this stenosis is also possible. Additionally, a series of stenoses could create new sites for wave reflection. If interaction occurred between incident and reflected waves, the responses of flow and pressure could be influenced. Considering these points, different distances between stenoses were evaluated but no significant hemodynamic differences over the 5 mm to 10 mm range studied was found. Therefore, these latter possible effects seem less important than the multiple sites for peak loss of energy.

These data indicate that coronary hemodynamics may be affected by moderate-degree (40% to 60%) stenoses of relatively modest length and by short stenoses in series. Thus, when multiple coronary arterial stenoses occur in one artery, a consideration of each as an isolated obstruction may not be appropriate.

Coronary artery blood flow related to aortic insufficiency and percent coronary artery stenosis

Coronary hemodynamic effects of controlled acute aortic insufficiency were studied in 40 open chest dogs with and without graded coronary diameter narrowing (4). An adjustable basket device was used to produce acute aortic insufficiency. This device was advanced to the aortic root through a standard catheter. When it exited the catheter it expanded and created acute aortic insufficiency. Three groups were created: (1) mild to moderate aortic insufficiency (regurgitant fraction <50%); (2) moderately severe aortic insufficiency (regurgitant fraction >50%); and (3) aortic insufficiency with mean aortic pressure restored to control levels. Figure 4 is a representative example of the coronary hemodynamic obtained in dogs with coronary stenosis with and without aortic insufficiency.

Mean coronary blood flow was similar to control values in dogs with mild to moderate aortic insufficiency but was higher in the other two groups. With coronary stenosis greater than 80%, coronary flow decreased with or without aortic insufficiency. Peak reactive hyperemic flow after release of a 10 second coronary occlusion also decreased during aortic insufficiency. The amount of decrease compared with control values was related to the magnitude of aortic insufficiency. This value with no coronary narrowing in the mild to moderate group was similar to peak reactive hyperemic flow with a 60% coronary narrowing during the control period. In the severe aortic insufficiency group peak reactive hyperemic flow was similar to that with an 80% coronary narrowing

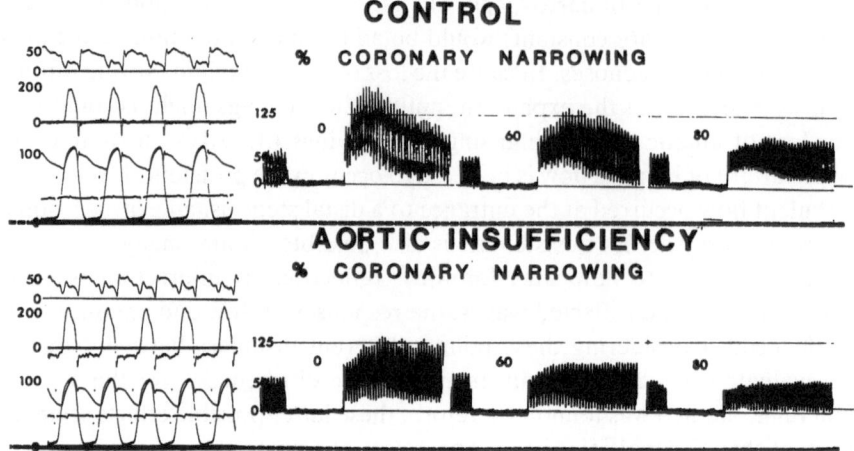

Figure 4. Representative example of coronary (ml/min) and aortic (ml/s) flows and aortic and left ventricular pressures (mmHg) during control and aortic insufficiency periods. During aortic insufficiency, the portion of coronary flow during systole increased as aortic diastolic pressure decreased and left ventricular diastolic pressure increased. Also during aortic insufficiency, reactive hyperemic flow with and without coronary narrowing decreased. AoF = aortic flow; AoP = aortic pressure; CF = coronary flow; VP = ventricular pressure.

during the control period. Restoring mean aortic pressure to control values did not restore peak reactive hyperemic flow to control values.

These data suggest that coronary flow reserve assessed with coronary stenoses during reactive hyperemia is decreased during aortic insufficiency. The decrease in coronary flow reserve was more pronounced as the magnitude of aortic insufficiency increased.

Coronary artery blood flow related to aortic stenosis and percent coronary artery stenosis

Coronary hemodynamic effects of controlled left ventricular outflow obstruction simulating aortic valve stenosis were studied in 20 open-chest dogs, with and without coronary artery stenosis (5). Aortic stenosis was created by balloon obstruction of the aortic root. The balloon catheter was introduced from the apex of the ventricle and advanced to the aortic valve. Aortic stenosis was regulated so that a mean left ventricular-aortic pressure gradient of 46 ± 20 mmHg (mean ± standard deviation) was created as both heart rate and stroke volume were unchanged. During aortic stenosis, mean aortic pressure and diastolic pressure time index/systolic pressure time index ratio decreased and end-diastolic left ventricular pressure increased.

Figure 5 is a representative experiment to illustrate the results. With no

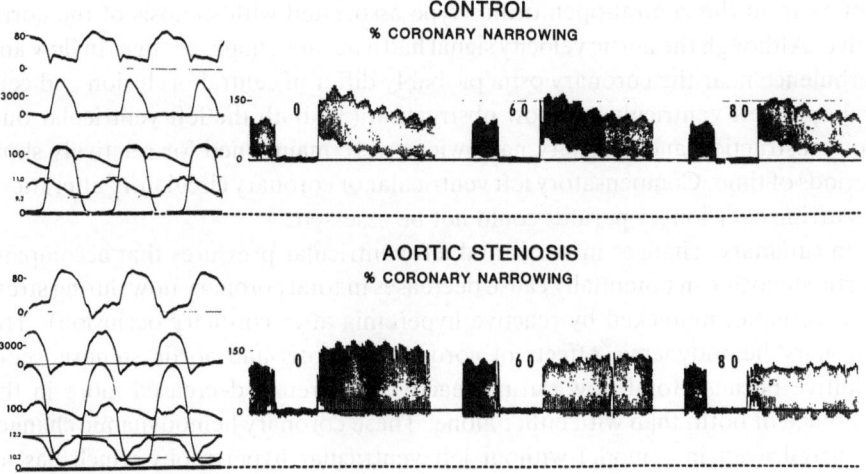

Figure 5. Left: at fast paper speed, coronary flow, aortic flow, and aortic and left ventricular pressure signals during control (top) and aortic stenosis (bottom). Right: at slow paper speed, phasic coronary flow signals before and during reactive hyperemia after a 10-second coronary occlusion for no coronary stenosis and for 60 and 80% coronary stenosis (control, top; aortic stenosis, bottom). Reactive hyperemic coronary flow values during aortic stenosis were similar to those during the control period with higher degrees of coronary narrowing. This example was chosen because mean aortic pressure was similar with and without aortic stenosis.

coronary narrowing, mean coronary flow increased during aortic stenosis (53 ± 23 to 62 ± 23 ml/min) as the percentage of diastolic flow increased (83 ± 6 to 89 ± 4, $p<0.05$). Peak reactive hyperemic flow decreased (168 ± 85 to 125 ± 73 ml/min, $p<0.05$). This value with no coronary narrowing was similar to peak hyperemic flow with 50% narrowing without aortic stenosis. With 80% coronary narrowing, mean coronary flow decreased with or without aortic stenosis.

These data suggest that although mean coronary flow is increased during aortic stenosis, coronary reserve as measured by a 10 second reactive hyperemic response is decreased. When a coronary artery is narrowed, aortic stenosis has an even more important hemodynamic influence on the coronary circulation.

Since these observation were made in an animal model of acute aortic stenosis, conclusions drawn may not apply to animals with chronic aortic stenosis or to patients with aortic stenosis. However although rare, acute aortic stenosis can occur in patients (for example, aortic valve thrombosis or aortic valve replacement with too small a valve in patients with previous aortic insufficiency). Several other factors deserve further comment: (1) these dogs did not have left ventricular hypertrophy. The presence of both left ventricular hypertrophy and changes in aortic and left ventricular pressure that occur during aortic stenosis would probably have additive effects on coronary hemodynamic function (2). The central-occlusion type of outflow tract obstruction caused by the balloon technique

248

differs from the central-open orifice type associated with stenosis of the aortic valve. Although the aortic velocity signal had a normal shape, changes in flow and turbulence near the coronary ostia probably differ in central-occlusion and central-open left ventricular outflow obstruction (3); both the left ventricular outflow obstruction and coronary narrowings were maintained for relatively short periods of time. Compensatory left ventricular or coronary circulatory alterations occurring over longer periods could not be assessed.

In summary, changes in aortic and left ventricular pressures that accompany aortic stenosis can potentially cause decreases in total coronary flow during stress (for example, mimicked by reactive hyperemia after coronary occlusion). The coronary hemodynamic effects of coronary stenosis and aortic stenosis seem additive because total flow during reactive hyperemia decreased more in the presence of both, than with either alone. These coronary hemodynamic changes occurred even in a model without left ventricular hypertrophy which has an additional effect on coronary flow.

Summary and conclusions

We can conclude from these experiments that: (1) short narrowings of 40–60% do not decrease resting coronary blood flow, but slightly decrease hyperemic coronary blood flow; (2) increasing the length of a 40–60% narrowing from 1 to 5 mm further decreases the hyperemic coronary blood flow response; (3) increasing the length of a 40–60% narrowing to 10 mm decreases resting coronary blood flow and obliterates reactive hyperemic coronary blood flow; (4) sequential narrowings of 40–60% decrease reactive hyperemic coronary blood flow greater than single narrowings of the same total length; (5) aortic valve disease (insufficiency or stenosis) will affect the coronary hemodynamic significance of a given coronary artery stenosis in a detrimental fashion.

Thus, it is hazardous for the cardiologist to make clinical decisions in patients based solely on the assessment of percent stenosis in the most severely affected vessel. The complex effects of percent stenosis, length of stenosis and the presence or absence of aortic valve disease on the physiology of coronary blood flow must always be considered by the clinician when evaluating angiograms for the physiologic significance of a stenosis.

Clinically, the physiologic significance of a stenosis observed at coronary angiography can best be evaluated by obtaining additional evidence of myocardial ischemia, e.g., stress testing with ECG monitoring, resting, and exercise isotope 'perfusion' studies or ventriculographic studies.

References

1. Feldman RL, Nichols WW, Pepine CJ, Conti CR: Hemodynamic significance of the length of a coronary arterial narrowing. Am J Cardiol 41, 1978: 865–871.
2. Feldman RL, Nichols WW, Pepine CJ, Conti CR: Hemodynamic effects of long and multiple coronary arterial narrowings. Chest 74, 1978: 280–285.
3. Streeter VL: Fluid Mechanics. McGraw-Hill Book Co, New York, 1971.
4. Feldman RL, Nichols WW, Conti CR, Pepine CJ: Influence of acute aortic insufficiency on the hemodynamic importance of a coronary artery narrowing. II. Various magnitudes of aortic insufficiency. JACC 1, 1983: 1281–1289.
5. Feldman RL, Nichols WW, Edgerton JR, Conti CR, Pepine CJ: Influence of aortic stenosis on the hemodynamic importance of coronary artery narrowing in dogs without left ventricular hypertrophy. Am J Cardiol 51, 1983: 865–871.

Pressure gradient, exercise thallium 201 scintigraphy, quantitative coronary cineangiography: in what sense are these measurements related?

Patrick W. Serruys, W. Wijns, R. Geuskens, P. de Feyter,
M. van den Brand and J.H.C. Reiber

Summary

During cardiac catheterization, the pressure-flow relationship across a coronary stenosis cannot be determined. On the other hand, the pressure distal to a coronary stenosis is measured routinely during the PTCA-procedure. The physiologic value of these measurements, even those obtained with the smallest catheters, must be questioned since the catheter impedes flow through the obstruction. In addition, it is well known that the mean pressure gradient is affected by phasis changes in flow velocity. In the present study, we attempted to assess the relationship between the pressure gradient measured during angioplasty, the angiographic severity of stenosis and the inducibility of regional perfusion defects during exercise Thallium-scintigraphy. As a first step, we decided to investigate the values and limitations of the transstenotic pressure gradient measured during PTCA by comparing the transstenotic gradient with the theoretical pressure drop calculated from the arterial dimensions and fluid-dynamic equations. Flow was measured in the great cardiac vein, (Q, ml/sec) in 13 patients, before (n = 10) and/or after (n = 10) angioplasty (PTCA) of a proximal LAD, not filled by collaterals. The mean transstenotic gradient (Grad, mmHg) measured with the balloon catheter was compared to the $\triangle P$ calculated from the occlusion area (occl A, mm^2). A 4-fold increase in the luminal area was associated with a 4-fold decrease in gradient (Grad). The occlusion A and the measured gradient were linearly correlated: Grad = 69–17. occl A; (r = 0.76). For the computed gradient $\triangle P$ the following relation was found: $\triangle P = 15.$ (occl A)$^{-2}$; (r = 0.87). Although, the present study clearly showed that the absolute values of the transstenotic pressure gradients obtained during angioplasty did not reflect accurately the flow resistances, we were still convinced that useful information could be derived from the gradient determination, at least in the setting of angioplasty. It is this concept that we tried to test in the second part of the study.

In other words, we studied the relationship between the stenotic diameter of a coronary artery and the pressure gradient across it on one hand and the extent of myocardial ischemia induced by exercise on the other. Thirty-one selected patients with stable exertional angina pectoris were studied; all were candidates for PTCA of an isolated proximal LAD-stenosis. The angiographic severity of stenosis was compared with the transstenotic pressure gradient measured with the dilatation catheter during angioplasty and with the results of exercise thallium-scintigraphy. A curvilinear relationship was found between the pressure gradient (normalized for the mean aortic pressure) and the residual minimal area of obstruction (after subtracting the cross-sectional area of the angioplasty catheter). The relationship was best fitted by the equation: normalized mean pressure gradient = a + b. log (obstruction area), (r = .74). The measurements of the percent area stenosis (cutoff 80%) and of the transstenotic pressure gradient (cutoff 0.30) obtained at rest correctly predicted the occurrence of thallium perfusion defects induced by exercise in 83% of the patients.

In summary, the functional significance of coronary stenoses can be evaluated in patients at rest by quantitative analysis of coronary dimensions and transstenotic pressure gradient measurements. In patients with single vessel disease of the left anterior descending coronary artery this allowed identification, while they were at rest, of those lesions responsible for thallium perfusion defects induced by exercise.

Introduction

During cardiac catheterization, the pressure-flow relationship across a coronary stenosis cannot be determined, although the feasibility of transluminal measurements of coronary blood flow velocity has been reported recently (1). On the other hand, the pressure distal to a coronary stenosis is measured routinely during the PTCA-procedure. The physiologic value of these measurements, even those obtained with the smallest catheters, must be questioned since the catheter impedes flow through the obstruction. In addition, it is well known that the mean pressure gradient is affected by phasic changes in flow velocity. In spite of these limitations, Vogel and his group have shown that the mean pressure gradient measured across the stenosis during angioplasty accurately predicts the coronary blood flow reserve measured by digital angiography (2).

In the present study, we attempted to assess the relationship between the pressure gradient measured during angioplasty, the angiographic severity of stenosis and the inducibility of regional perfusion defects during exercise Thallium-scintigraphy. As a first step, we decided to investigate the values and limitations of the transstenotic pressure gradient measured during PTCA by comparing the transstenotic gradient wih the theoretical pressure drop calculated from fluid-mechanic equations; the accuracy of the absolute value of the transstenotic gradients measured during PTCA must be questioned as the presence of the dilatation catheter further reduces the luminal area. Leiboff et al. (3) have shown in canine femoral arteries that the transstenotic gradient overestimated the 'true' gradient in a predictable manner, which is dependent on the ratio of the diameter of the angioplasty catheter to the stenosis diameter. In order to further characterize this relation in the coronary artery bed of humans, we compared the transstenotic gradient with the theoretical pressure drop calculated from fluid mechanic equations for steady flow of an incompressible fluid in rigid tubes. Therefore, the stenosis geometry was analyzed by quantitative coronary cineangiography and the mean myocardial blood flow was measured by the thermodilution technique in a selected group of patients with proximal left anterior descending coronary artery disease.

Part I: Values and limitations of transstenotic gradients measured during percutaneous coronary angioplasty

Patients and methods

Thirteen patients with exertional angina pectoris were studied; all were candidates for PTCA of an isolated proximal left anterior descending stenosis. The distal part of the vessel was not filled by collaterals, as judged from angiography.

The subjects gave informed consent and no complication resulted from the study. Details regarding the PTCA technique used in our laboratory have been described previously (4). The mean transstenotic pressure gradient was measured with the dilatation catheter and calculated on line after a data acquisition period of 20 seconds (5). The regional coronary blood flow measurement in the great cardiac vein, which must be known for the calculation of the theoretical gradient (see below), was obtained with a Baim catheter using the thermodilution technique (6). The position of the catheter was confirmed by dye injection before and after PTCA. Measurements were included only if selective sampling from the anterior vein was possible. Such selective great cardiac vein flows were available before PTCA in 3 patients, after PTCA in 3 patients, and before and after in 7 patients. Thus, 20 data points were available for comparison.

Quantitative coronary angiography

The quantitative analysis of selected coronary segments was carried out with the help of a computer-based Cardiovascular Angiography Analysis System (CAAS), which has been described in this book by Reiber et al., as well as extensively elsewhere (7–11). In short, the boundaries of a selected coronary segment were detected automatically from optically magnified and video digitized portions of a cineframe. Calibration of the diameter data of the vessels in absolute values (mm) was achieved by detecting the boundaries of a section of the contrast catheter and comparing the computed mean diameter in pixels with the known size in mm. Strictly speaking, this calibration factor is only applicable for coronary segments in the plane of the analyzed catheter segment parallel to the image intensifier input screen. The change in magnification for two objects located at different points along the X-ray beam axis is about 1.5% for each centimeter that separates the objects axially with the commonly used focus-image intensifier distances. In the present study, the axial distance between catheter and stenosis is short; hence the possible changes in the calibration factor would be negligible and no further corrections were used. In order to correct the contour positions of the arterial and catheter segments for the pincushion distortion, a correction vector was computed for each contour position based on a computer processed cineframe of a cm-grid placed against the input screen of the image intensifier (8).

The contour detection procedure requires the user to indicate a number of center positions with the writing tablet proximal and distal to the lesion such that the straight line segments connecting these points remain within the artery. The first centerline position was selected beyond the take-off of large daughter branches. The contours of the vessel are detected on the basis of the weighted sum of first and second difference functions applied to the digitized brightness information using minimal cost criteria.

From the detected contours, the diameter function, in absolute mm, is determined. From the minimal value of the diameter function determined by the computer and the mean diameter value at the reference position, the percentage area reduction, assuming circular cross-sections, is computed as:

$$\%\text{-A stenosis} = \{1 - (\text{minimal diameter/reference diameter})^2\} \times 100\%.$$

A representative analysis with the detected contours and the diameter function superimposed on the original video image is shown in Figure 1a. In arteries with a focal obstructive lesion and a clearly normal proximal arterial segment, the choice of the reference region is straightforward and simple. In cases where the proximal or distal part of the arterial segment shows combinations of stenotic and ectatic areas, the choice may be very difficult. Since the functional significance of a stenosis is related to the expected normal cross-sectional area of the vessel at the point of the obstruction, we have implemented two methods to define the reference: one is dependent on the user (user-defined reference), while the other technique is based on the computer estimation of the original arterial dimensions at the site of the obstruction (interpolated reference) (10, 11). For the latter method, the computed reference diameter function allows the vessel to taper. The resulting reference contours are shown in Figure 1b. The interpolated percentage diameter stenosis is then computed by comparing the minimal diameter value at the obstruction with the corresponding value of the reference diameter function at this position; as described earlier, the percentage area stenosis can be calculated as well.

The length of the stenotic segment was determined from the diameter function on the basis of curvature analysis of the D-function and expressed in mm.

The same angiographic projection was used before and after PTCA, except for 2 post-PTCA lesions where the mean value from two orthogonal projections was used. From an extensive validation study of the analysis procedure it has been shown that the variability (standard deviation of the differences) of repeated coronary acquisition and computer analysis is less than 0.22 mm for absolute arterial dimensions in a well-controlled study (11).

Theoretical pressure gradient

The theoretical pressure gradient was calculated according to the well-known formules described in the literature (12, 13):

$$\Delta P = Q \cdot (Rp + Q \cdot Rt),$$

where ΔP is the theoretical pressure drop (mmHg) over the stenosis, Q the mean coronary blood flow (ml/sec), Rp the Poisseuille resistance and Rt the turbulent resistance. These resistances have been defined as follows:

$$Rp = Cl \cdot \frac{(\text{length obstruction})}{(\text{obstruction area})^2} \left[\frac{\text{mmHg} \cdot \text{sec}}{\text{ml}}\right],$$

where $Cl = 8 \cdot \pi \cdot (\text{blood viscosity})$ with blood viscosity $= 0.03$ [g/cm · sec]

$$Rt = C2 \cdot \left(\frac{1}{\text{obstruction area}} - \frac{1}{\text{normal distal area}}\right)^2 \left[\frac{\text{mmHg} \cdot \text{sec}^2}{\text{ml}^2}\right],$$

where $C2 = \dfrac{\text{blood density}}{0.266}$ with blood density ≈ 1.0 [g/cm³]

In the formules given above the obstruction area calculated from the coronary cineangiograms must be corrected for by the cross-sectional area of the dilatation catheter; for this catheter area the value of 0.64 mm² was used.

Statistics

Comparisons between pre- and post-PTCA measurements were performed with the Student t-test for paired data.

Multiple regressions were performed between the obstruction area and either the measured or the theoretical gradient until the best fit was obtained. The individual data are tabulated in Table 1.

256

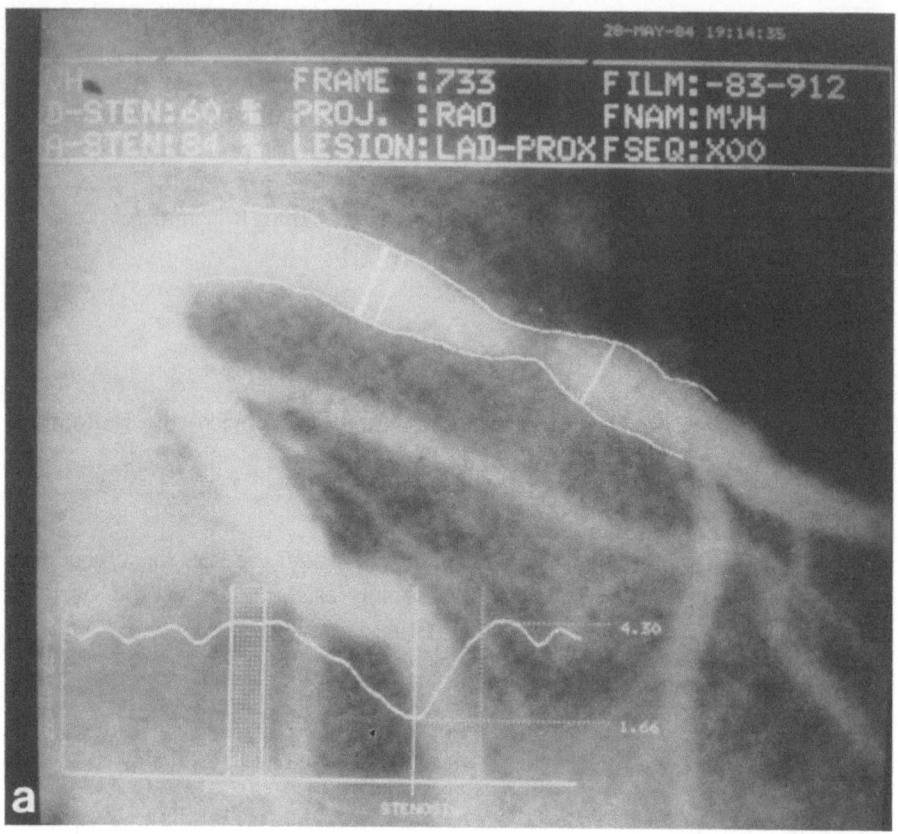

Figure 1. Detected contours superimposed on the original video image for a representative left anterior descending coronary artery stenosis. The diameter function is shown at the bottom. The calibrated diameter values in mm are plotted along the ordinate and the positions along the analyzed segment from the proximal to the distal part along the abscissa. 1a. The reference diameter (or area) was selected proximal to the stenosis. A percentage area stenosis of 84% resulted. 1b. The normal size of the artery over the obstruction has been estimated by the interpolated method. The resulting reference contours are shown and the difference in area between this boundary and the detected contours is a measure of the atherosclerotic plaque (shaded area). A percentage area stenosis of 83% resulted. 1c. Schematic representation of the coronary artery with the guiding catheter in the ostium (top left), the thermodilution catheter in the coronary sinus (bottom left) measuring the great cardiac vein flow (GCVF). The inset (top right) shows how the transstenotic pressure gradient was measured (between the white dots). The theoretical pressure drop was calculated from: 1) the reference diameter (or area) shown proximal to the stenosis for the sake of clarity; 2) the obstruction diameter (or area) and 3) the length of the stenosis.

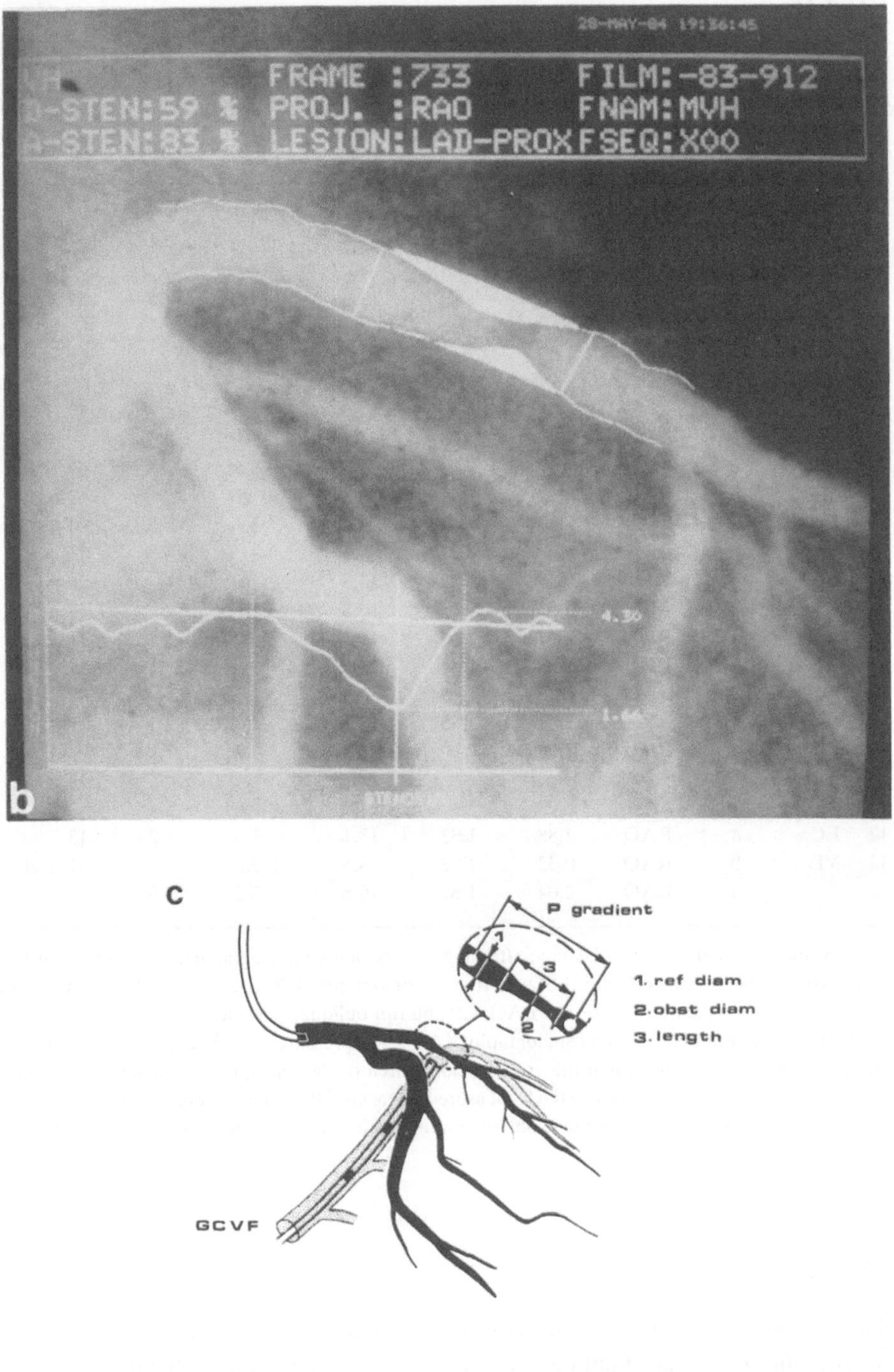

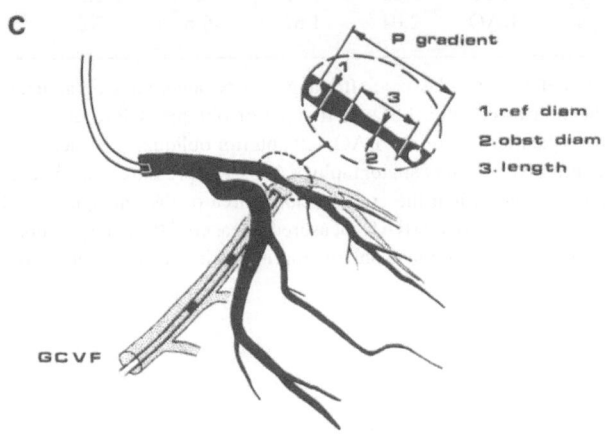

FRAME :733　　FILM:-83-912
D-STEN:59 %　PROJ. :RAO　　FNAM:MVH
A-STEN:83 %　LESION:LAD-PROX FSEQ:X00

4.30

1.44

b

c

P gradient

1. ref diam
2. obst diam
3. length

GCVF

Table 1. Measured versus calculated gradient.

No	Patient name		Angio view	Occlusion area mm²	GCV flow ml/s⁻¹	Sten length mm	ΔP calculated mmHg	(ΔP-CA) mmHg	GRAD measured mmHg
1	PO	b	RIO	0.96		7.0	18.9	–	
				2.13			80	occl	
		LSO	0.79		9.9	52.2	–		
2	VY	b	RAO	1.19	1.20	12.0	13.5	39.5	59
		a	CRA	2.43		7.3	1.9	3.9	
				1.52				5	
		a	RAO	4.26		11.9	0.8	1.2	
3	MA	b	RIO	1.52	1.40	7.9	5.5	18	59
		a	RIO	3.84	1.62	6.8	0.8	1.3	12
4	BO	b	LSO	1.47	1.02	7.5	3.5	12.3	69
5	ME	b	RAO	0.34	1.42	10.0	107.2	–	62 occl
6	BE	a	LSO	1.87	1.50	6.4	3.2	8.3	4
7	HE	b	CRA	0.48	1.27	8.8	8.2	–	71 occl
8	BA	b	RAO	0.57	1.23	14.3	55.6	–	56 occl
		b	RIO	0.53	1.23	10.8	51.9	–	52 occl
		a	RIO	2.97	1.50	11.3	1.0	2.8	11
9	GR	a	RIO	1.63	1.45	12.0	8.5	19.6	13
10	MA	b	RAO	2.38	1.68	6.9	2.3	5	48
		a	AP	3.41	1.85	10.5	0.9	2.1	17
11	PI	a	RIO	2.06		8.9	4.2	7.9	
					1.63				23
		a	LAO	3.08		4.1	0.8	1.4	
12	EC	a	RAO	2.88	1.33	13.1	1.5	3.2	13
13	VE	b	RAO	0.32	1.23	8.5	122.5	–	41 occl
		a	RAO	2.04	1.67	6.6	3.3	3.8	5

Abbreviations: b: before angioplasty; a: after angioplasty; angio: angiographic; GCV: great cardiac vein; RIO: right inferior oblique; LSO: Left superior oblique; CRA: cranio-caudal; RAO: right anterior oblique; AP: antero posterior; LAO: left anterior oblique; ΔP calculated: pressure gradient derived from quantitative coronary angiography; (ΔP–CA): pressure gradient derived from quantitative coronary angiography, when the cross sectional area of the angioplasty catheter (CA) is substrated from the obstruction area; GRAD measured: measured transstenotic pressure gradient; occl: when CA is greater than the luminal obstruction area, the vessel is considered to be completely occluded (occl).

Results

The median values and the ranges for the obstruction area, the measured gradient and the theoretical gradient before and after angioplasty are shown in Table 2. A fourfold increase in the luminal area was associated with a fourfold decrease in the measured gradient; however, the absolute values for the transstenotic gra-

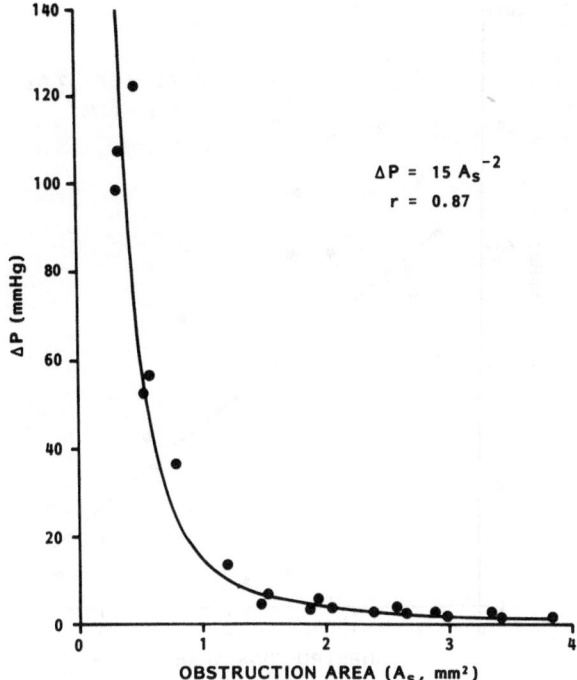

Figure 2. Curvelinear relationship between the obstruction area (A) and the theoretical pressure gradient ($\triangle P$). The relation is best fitted (r = 0.87) by the equation: $\triangle P = 15. A_s^{-2}$.

dient were consistently larger than the theoretical gradient. No changes in the reference area or the length of the stenosis were observed. The resting blood flow increased sligthly but not significantly from 1.3 to 1.6 ml/sec. The relation between the occlusion area and the theoretical pressure drop (Figure 2) was best fitted by the equation: $\triangle P = a \cdot$ (occlusion area)^b, where $\triangle P =$ theoretical gradient, a = 15 and b = −2 (r = 0.87). As expected from the laws of fluid dynamics, this relation is curvilinear and shows a steep increase in gradient once the critical value of 1 mm^2 for the occlusion area is reached. Figure 3 shows the

Table 2. Hemodynamic and angiographic measurements before and after PTCA.

	GCVQ ml/sec	Obstruction area (mm²)	$\triangle P$ mmHg	GRAD mmHg
Before	1.3 (1.0–2.1)	0.7 (0.3–2.4) *	44 (2–122) *	59 (41–80) *
After	1.6 (1.3–2.1)	2.8 (1.9–3.8)	2 (1–5)	13 (4–28)

The median value and the range are given; GCVQ = great cardiac vein flow; $\triangle P$ = theoretical or calculated pressure drop; GRAD = measured transstenotic gradient; * p<0.005.

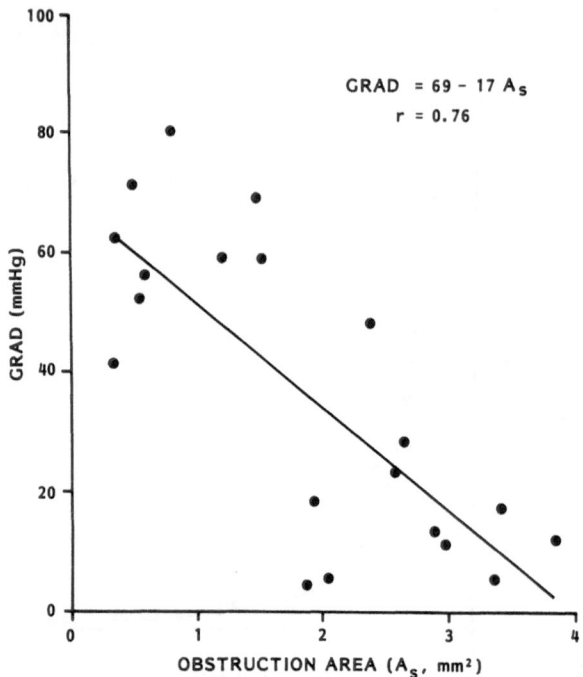

Figure 3. Linear relation between the obstruction area (A$_s$) and the transstenotically measured gradient (GRAD): GRAD = 69–17. A$_s$ (r = 0.76).

relation between the occlusion area and the measured transstenotic gradient, which was best fitted by the linear equation: GRAD = a − b. (occlusion area), where GRAD is the measured gradient, a = 69 and b = 17 (r = 0.76). According to this relation, the average gradient measured after PTCA, i.e. 13 mmHg, would correspond to a luminal area of 3.3 mm^2. The theoretical relation would predict with this area value, a pressure drop of 1.4 mmHg, at least within the observed range of flow. Thus, even when the lumen of the vessel is large as compared to the diameter of the angioplasty catheter, its presence leads to an overestimation of the 'true' gradient. In other words, these data show that the absolute value of the transstenotic pressure gradients obtained during angioplasty do not reflect accurately the flow resistances. As suggested by others (3, 14), this is related to the presence of the angioplasty catheter across the stenosis, further reducing its minimal luminal area. These findings are not surprising, but were until recently (15) never demonstrated in human coronary arteries. The data also show that calculation of theoretical pressure gradients on the basis of an hypothetical coronary blood flow could result in inaccurate numbers as the range of flows that we measured was rather large, even at rest (from 1.02 to 2.13 ml/sec.).

However, we were still convinced that useful information could be derived from the gradient determination, at least in the setting of angioplasty. And it is this concept that we tried to test in the second part of the study. In a second group of patients, we tried to evaluate during cardiac catherization what degree of narrowing of a major epicardial coronary artery will consistently lead to a definite transstenotic gradient at rest and to myocardial ischemia during exercise.

Part II: Quantitative angiography of the left anterior descending coronary artery: correlations with pressure gradient and results of exercise thallium scintigraphy

Patients and methods

Thirty-one consecutive patients with stable exertional angina pectoris were studied; all were candidates for percutaneous transluminal angioplasty of an isolated proximal left anterior descending stenosis. All subjects gave informed consent and no complications resulted from the study.

Quantitative coronary angiography

In this study, the coronary angiograms were obtained within five minutes after intracoronary injection of nifedipine (0.1 to 0.2 mg) in order to obtain a vaso-dilatation of the epicardial vessels and relief of a possible spasm (16, 17). Since the luminal cross section at the site of the coronary obstruction is frequently irregular in shape especially after angioplasty (18,19), the average obstruction area and percent area stenosis obtained from multiple views were used (mean of 1.7 views per segment). Since the presence of the dilatation catheter within the stenotic lumen further reduces lumen area, the difference between the luminal area measured from the coronary angiograms and the area of the balloon catheter (0.64 mm^2) was used as an approach to the actual residual lumen and related to the pressure gradient measurements. The mean pressure gradient across the stenotic lesion was measured with the dilatation catheter (mean diameter of 0.9 mm, Schneider 20–30 or 20–37) before and after angioplasty and calculated on line after a data acquisition period of 20 seconds (5).

Noninvasive testing

Exercise thallium-201 myocardial scintigraphy was performed before angioplasty in 7 patients, after angioplasty in 13 patients and before and after in 11 patients. Sequential imaging was performed according to a standard protocol immediately after a symptom limited exercise test and again 4 hours later. Scintigraphy was performed in the week before angiography (n = 18) and in the three weeks after successful angioplasty (n = 24). No patient had recurrence of angina pectoris during this time interval. During exercise, three orthogonal leads (X, Y, Z) were monitored and analyzed as previously described (20). The scintigraphic images were processed on a DEC gamma-11 system (21). Basically, circumferential profiles were computed in three projections (anterior, LAO 45, LAO 65) within the automatically detected contour of the left ventricle following interpolated background subtraction (22). The circumferential profiles, the processed images and the analog polaroid images were interpreted by three independent observers, who were unaware of the angiographic data. The myocardial uptake of thallium was scored in a total of 13 segments both for early and late exercise scintigrams in the following manner: 0 = no thallium uptake; 1 = severely abnormal; 2 = definitely abnormal; 3 = doubtfully abnormal; 4 = normal. These scores were summed per patient and the difference between late and early post-exercise sums was taken as a measure of the amount of redistribution. Using this approach, ischemia was considered to be present if at least two observers found that the redistribution score was two or more points higher than the early post-exercise one. Since only patients with single vessel disease were included, the left anterior descending artery stenosis was taken responsible for the regional defects observed in the anteroseptal, anterior, anterolateral as well as apical segments (23).

Statistical analysis

Simple regressions were used to attempt the best fit relation between the pressure gradient and the obstruction area. The Student test for paired data and linear least-squares regressions were used to compare the interpolated and user-defined percent area stenosis measurements. One-way analysis of variance followed by multiple comparisons was used to compare the angiographic measurements between three sub-groups of patients. Data are expressed as mean ± standard deviation.

Results

The absolute dimensions of the minimal obstruction areas are given in Table 3, ranked from the minimal obstruction area value of 0.15 mm^2 to the maximal value of 17.9 mm^2. The interpolated and user-defined percent area stenosis values are shown as well. The user-defined reference was taken proximal to the stenosis in all but 10 cases where it was taken distally due to the take-off of the left circumflex artery just before the stenosis. There was no significant difference between the interpolated and user-defined percent area stenosis: the difference between paired data was 1.7 ± 10 and the correlation coefficient was 0.91 (interpolated % Area st. = 0.95. (user % Area st.) + 4.8; SEE = 10). When the mean pressure gradient across the stenosis, normalized for the mean aortic pressure, was com-

Table 3. Individual data for quantitative angiography and exercise test results.

Patient		Obstr. area	D st. %	Area st. %		Measured Grad		Theor. ΔP		Exercise test		
				inter	user	Grad/ AoP	Grad	1	2	AP	ECG	TL201
1 HD	b	0.15	87	98	96	0.75	81	34	126	−	−	+
2 FA	b	0.30	85	98	94	0.49	39	16	42	+	+	−
3 HO	b	0.36	82	97	97	0.87	54	46	171	+	+	+
4 PL	b	0.45	79	96	84	0.46	38	12	32	+	+	+
5 EN	b	0.58	81	96	94	0.54	51	17	44	−	−	+
6 KS	b	0.58	71	92	91	0.55	51	13	46	−	−	−
7 BO	b	0.65	74	93	90	0.74	85	9	33	−	+	+
8 VD	b	0.80	69	90	(−)	0.38	27	4	16	−	BB	−
9 HN	b	0.88	68	89	89	0.63	65	6	17	−	+	+
10 EL	b	0.92	68	90	75	0.73	68	3	10	+	−	+
11 MS	b	0.98	54	80	85	0.67	63	5	19	−	−	+
12 HO	a	1.23	46	70	75	0.29	31	0	1	−	−	−
13 EM	a	1.58	47	72	55	0.16	20	1	2	−	+	−
14 KT	b	1.65	66	89	84	0.43	36	1	2	−	+	+
15 HE	b	1.74	70	91	89	0.65	73	1	3	+	+	+
16 SK	b	1.77	67	89	(−)	0.60	61	(−)	(−)	+	−	+
17 GI	b	2.06	66	88	90	0.39	35	4	12	+	BB	+
18 SR	b	2.09	65	88	87	0.72	72	4	15	−	+	+
19 DA	b	2.38	38	62	69	0.39	26	0	1	−	BB	+
20 RS	a	2.75	50	75	72	0.10	10	1	2	+	BB	−
21 MS	a	2.83	21	38	65	0.13	13	0	0	−	−	−
22 DA	a	2.95	19	34	50	0.18	15	0	2	+	−	−
23 HP	a	3.00	33	55	65	0.10	9	0	1	−	−	−
24 FN	a	3.11	31	54	64	0.13	13	0	0	−	+	−
25 HD	a	3.14	37	60	(−)	0.09	10	0	0	−	−	−
26 BE	a	3.14	10	44	32	0.06	4	0	0	−	−	−
27 WI	a	3.17	42	66	65	0.28	25	1	2	−	−	−
28 KL	b	3.33	41	65	65	0.15	13	4	9	−	−	+
29 MO	a	3.70	33	56	54	0.34	31	0	1	−	−	+
30 NS	a	3.94	38	61	30	0.16	13	0	0	−	−	−
31 BV	a	4.12	48	48	39	0.11	13	0	0	−	−	−
32 HT	a	4.16	41	66	48	0.16	14	0	0	−	+	−
33 FA	a	4.26	21	37	45	0.21	16	2	8	−	+	−
34 HN	a	4.34	40	65	56	0.04	5	0	0	−	−	−
35 KL	a	4.95	21	37	52	0.00	0	0	0	−	−	−
36 OW	a	5.68	25	44	43	0.16	15	0	0	−	−	−
37 SK	a	6.20	38	62	67	0.18	20	(−)	(−)	−	−	−
38 HE	a	7.07	40	64	53	0.21	24	0	0	−	−	+
39 SE	a	7.50	36	60	57	0.10	8	0	0	−	−	−
40 KN	a	8.29	3	6	14	0.21	26	0	0	−	+	−
41 KT	a	9.90	17	30	21	0.07	6	0	0	−	−	−
42 GI	a	17.87	3	6	6	0.06	5	0	0	−	−	−

Abbreviations: b = before angioplasty (PTCA); a = after PTCA; Obstr. Area = obstruction area in mm²; Area st. = percent area stenosis; inter = interpolated and user-defined reference; the measured mean pressure gradient (GRAD) is shown in absolute values (mmHg) as well as normalized for mean aortic pressure (AoP); theoretical gradients were calculated assuming constant coronary flows of 1 and 2 ml/sec, according to the frmula described by B.G. Brown et al. (12); (−) = missing data; AP = angina pectoris; ECG = ST depression ≥ 0.1 mV; TL201 = redistribution from exercise to rest scintigram; + = present; − = absent; BB = bundle branch block.

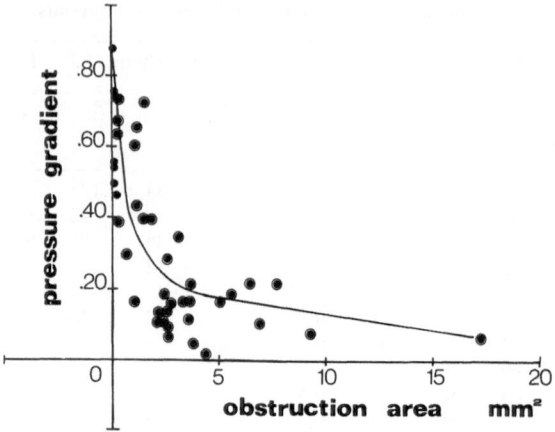

Figure 4. The relation between the mean pressure gradient normalized for the mean aortic pressure and the residual obstruction area in mm² (after subtraction of the area of the angioplasty catheter) is nonlinear; the best fit is obtained by the logarithmic function ($r = 0.74$). Filled symbols represent stenoses in which the angioplasty catheter totally obstructed the vessel.

pared to the residual obstruction area after subtracting the balloon area (Figure 4), a nonlinear relation was found which can be described by the equation:

$$\triangle P/AoP = a + b \cdot \log (\text{obstruction area}),$$

where $a = 0.35$ and $b = -0.12$ ($r = 0.74$).

It is shown that there is a steep increase in pressure gradient once a critical value of 1.5 mm² of the stenotic segment is reached. In seven cases, the angioplasty catheter almost totally obstructed the vessel. The computed cross-sectional area reduction is also related to the pressure gradient (Figure 5). Here, the steep increase in pressure gradient is observed once the critical reduction of 80% in cross-sectional area is reached.

During the exercise test, the maximal workload averaged $85 \pm 17\%$ of the predicted value. According to the results of the thallium scintigraphy, three types of responses are observed. In group I ($n = 25$), the scintigram is normal, with either normal or abnormal exercise ECG. In group II ($n = 7$), thallium scintigraphy is abnormal while the exercise test results are normal. In group III ($n = 10$), both thallium scintigraphy and exercise test results (angina and/or ST-segment changes) are abnormal. The percent area stenosis was 55 ± 23 in group I, 74 ± 17 in group II and 90 ± 4 in group III. The mean pressure gradient was: 0.18 ± 0.13 in group I, 0.44 ± 0.23 in group II and 0.62 ± 0.15 in group III. The pressure gradient measurements discriminated better between the groups than the area stenosis measurements (table IV). When combining both parameters, two groups of datapoints are delineated as shown in figure 5. Using cut-off values of 0.30 for

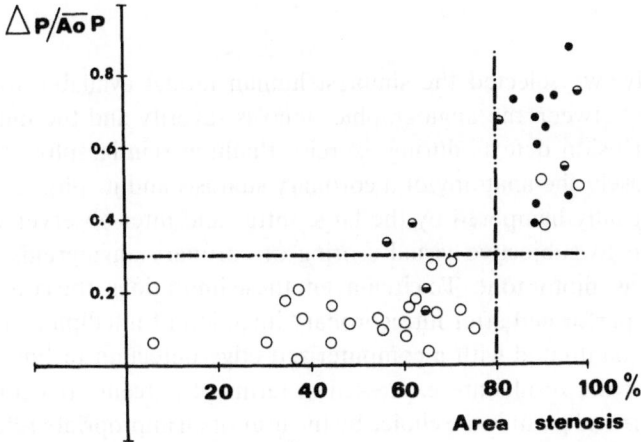

Figure 5. The relation between mean normalized pressure gradient, percentage area stenosis and the results of thallium scintigraphy is shown. Open circles represent patients with a normal scintigram (group I, n = 25), while half-filled circles represent patients with an abnormal thallium but normal exercise test (group II, n = 7). Filled circles represent patients with both abnormal thallium and exercise tests (group III, n = 10).

the pressure gradient and 80% for the cross-sectional area reduction, the result of the exercise thallium scintigram was correctly predicted from the angiographic data in 83% of the patients. An abnormal scintigraphy was observed in 13 of the 16 patients with a pressure gradient of at least 0.30 and a percent area stenosis equal to or greater than 80% (sensitivity of 81%). Two out of three patients with a normal thallium uptake and exercise test had important collaterals shown by angiography. Conversely, the thallium uptake is normal in 22 of the 24 patients with a pressure gradient less than 0.30 together with an area stenosis less than 80% (specificity 92%). Similar figures were found when the user-defined percent area was used instead of the interpolated method (sensitivity 85%, specificity 87%).

Table 4. Noninvasive test results and angiographic estimates of stenosis severity.

		n	% Area stenosis	Mean pressure gradient
Group I	(Tl−)	25	55 ± 23	0.18 ± 0.13
			n.s.	*
Group II	(Tl +/ET−)	7	74 ± 17	0.44 ± 0.23
			n.s.	n.s.
Group III	(Tl +/ET +)	10	90 ± 4	0.62 ± 0.15

Abbreviations as previously; n = number of patients; ET = exercise test result; + = abnormal; − = normal; n.s. = nonsignificant; symbols refer to p-values: * p<0.001; ** p<0.005

Discussion

In this study, we selected the simplest human model available to assess the relationship between the angiographic stenosis severity and the inducibility of regional perfusion defects during exercise thallium scintigraphy. Attempts to correlate closely the anatomy of a coronary stenosis and its physiologic significance are usually hampered by the large intra- and inter-observer variabilities (24, 25) due to subjective visual scoring of coronary angiograms and to the inconstant vasomotor tone. To circumvent these limitations, the coronary angiograms were performed after intracoronary injection of nifedipine and the cinefilms were quantitated with a computerized edge detection technique (10, 11). Since part of the results are expressed in terms of percent area (or diameter) stenosis, a critical point is the choice by the user of an appropriate reference area (or diameter). When a large vessel gives rise to a major daughter branch, the cross-sectional area of the main vessel distal to the branch point is significanty less than its area proximal to the branch point; hence, the choice of a proximal reference would not be appropriate. Conversely, the choice of an appropriate distal reference is often hampered by the presence of poststenotic ectasia and by anatomical tapering. Therefore, an alternative method was developed, similar to that used by Crawford et al. (26), which is based on the computer estimation of the 'original contour of the pre-atherosclerotic lumen', allowing the vessel to taper. The difference in area between the original lumen and the contours of the obstruction is a measure for the atherosclerotic plaque. Crawford et al. have demonstrated that such angiographic assessment of the atherosclerotic plaque by computer densitometry correlated with the cholesterol content of the corresponding human arterial specimen. Their approach includes both density and edge measurements; among these, the computer detected lumen with taper yielded the best correlation with the pathologic data (26). The data of Crawford et al. pertain to nonbranching segments of femoral arteries; they have not been confirmed for coronary arteries in which changes in lumen caliber occur predictably at branching points and not by taper (27). In the present as well as in earlier studies (18, 28), the user-defined and interpolated measurements were closely correlated. However, for the analysis of repeated angiograms (29, 30), the knowledge of the exact location of the reference, either proximal or distal to the stenosis, is not required when the interpolated method is used. For these theoretical and practical reasons, we favor the use of an automated definition of the reference area (or diameter) with the interpolated technique (19, 31).

From these data, obtained in a clinical setting, a curvilinear relation was found between the pressure drop across the stenosis and the minimal obstruction area as well as the percent cross-sectional area reduction. Both relations are similar to those calculated on theoretical grounds by Brown et al. (32), as well as to those experimentally derived from isolated human arteries (33) or dog experiments (34).

Such curvilinear relation is expected from the general equation of fluid dynamics showing that the pressure drop across a stenosis is influenced mainly by viscous losses in the stenotic segment and separation losses at the exit of the stenosis. For a given level of flow, the single most important determinant of stenosis resistance is its minimal cross-sectional area which appears as a second order term in both viscous and separation losses equations. In the animal laboratory, a coronary stenosis can be characterized precisely by simultaneous measurements of flow and stenosis gradient and related to the quantitative assessment of stenosis geometry. In such experimental setting, blood flow velocity and pressure drop across the stenosis are correlated in an exponential fashion (35). Recently, coronary blood flow velocity measurements were obtained in patients during heart surgery and related to the computer based analysis of their coronary angiograms (36, 37). It was shown that the minimal cross-sectional area was the best predictor of the physiological significance of a coronary stenosis. During cardiac catheterization, the pressure-flow relation across a coronary stenosis cannot be determined, although the feasibility of transluminal measurements of coronary blood flow velocity has been reported recently (1). However, the pressure distal to a coronary stenosis is measured routinely during the transluminal angioplasty procedure. This has stimulated the development of very small catheters for the in vivo investigation of the functional significance of pressure gradient measurements (38). The physiological value of these measurements, even those obtained with the smallest catheters, must be questioned since the catheter impedes flow through the obstruction. Experimental data obtained in dog femoral arteries suggest that the 'true' lesional gradient is overestimated in a predictable manner dependent on the ratio of the catheter diameter over the stenosis diameter (3). In addition, the mean pressure gradient is affected by phasic changes in flow velocity (35). The distal coronary pressure may be affected by collaterals and is entirely determined by collateral flow when the angioplasty catheter totally obstructs the vessel. In spite of these limitations, Vogel *et al.* (2) have shown that the mean pressure gradient measured across the stenosis during angioplasty predicted accurately the coronary flow reserve measured as the ratio of hyperemic over control myocardial contrast appearance times by digital angiography. In the present study, the gradient was related in a curvilinear way with the actual luminal area obtained by subtracting the area of the deflated balloon catheter from the minimal obstruction area as assessed by quantitative angiography. The major finding of this study was that the combination of pressure drop measurements across the stenosis with quantitative assessment of the luminal narrowing predicted the occurrence of exercise thallium perfusion abnormalities better than the measurements of the stenosis alone. Using the cut-off values of 0.30 for the pressure gradient and 80% for the percent cross-sectional area reduction, the result of the exercise thallium scintigram was correctly predicted from the angiographic data in all but six patients. In four of them, thallium perfusion abnormalities occurred without signs of ischemia in the presence of a noncritical cross-sectional area stenosis of about 60%. These discrepancies are not surprising since many other factors such as blood density, viscosity, stenosis length and divergence angle were not accounted for (32, 33). Two patients had normal scintigrams and exercise tests while ischemia was expected from the angiographics measurements. This can be due to the presence of coronary collaterals as shown by angiography, since previous work suggests that these could prevent the occurrence of thallium perfusion defects during exercise (39, 40).

In summary, the functional significance of a coronary stenosis can be evaluated at rest by quantitative analysis of coronary dimensions and transstenotic pressure gradient measurements. In patients with single left anterior descending coronary artery disease this allowed identification, at rest, of those lesions responsible or not for thallium perfusion defects induced by exercise.

References

1. Wilson RF, Hartley CJ, Laughlin DE, Marcus ML, White CW:Transluminal subselective measurement of coronary blood flow velocity and coronary vasodilator reserve in man. J Am Coll Cardiol 3, 1984: 529 (Abstract).
2. Vogel RA, Colfer HT, O'Neill WW, Walton JA, Aueron FM, Bates ER, Kirlin PC, LeFree MT, Pitt B: Correlations of arteriographically measured coronary cross-sectional area and coronary flow reserve with translesional gradient. J Am Coll Cardiol 1, 1983: 672 (Abstract).
3. Leiboff R, Bren G, Katz R, Korkegi R, Ross A: Determinants of transstenotic gradients observed during angioplasty: an experimental model. Am J Cardiol 52, 1983: 1311–1317.
4. Serruys PW, Brand M van den, Brower RW, Hugenholtz PG: Regional cardioplegia and cardioprotection during transluminal angioplasty, which role for nifedipine? Eur Heart J 4 (Suppl C), 1983: 115–121.
5. Brower RW, Meester GT, Zeelenberg C, Hugenholtz PG: Automatic data processing in the cardiac catheterization laboratory. Comp Progr in Biomed 7, 1977: 99–110.
6. Baim DS, Rothman MT, Harrison DC: Improved catheter for regional sinus flow and metabolic studies. Am J Cardiol 46, 1980: 997–1000.
7. Reiber JHC, Gerbrands JJ, Booman F, Troost GJ, Boer A den, Slager CJ, Schuurbiers JHC: Objective characterization of coronary obstructions from monoplane cineangiograms and three-dimensional reconstruction of an arterial segment from orthogonal views. In: Application of Computers in Medicine. MD Schwartz (Ed.). IEEE Cat. No. TH0095–0, 1982: 93–100.
8. Kooijman CJ, Reiber JHC, Gerbrands JJ, Schuurbiers JHC, Slager CJ, Boer A den, Serruys PW: Computer-aided quantitation of the severity of coronary obstructions from single view cineangiograms. First IEEE Comp. Soc. Int. Symp on Medical Imaging and Image Interpretation. IEEE Cat. No. 82 CH1804–4, 1982: 59–64.
9. Reiber JHC, Slager CJ, Schuurbiers JCH, Boer A den, Gerbrands JJ, Troost GJ, Scholts B, Kooijman CJ, Serruys PW: Transfer functions of the X-ray cine-video chain applied to digital processing of coronary cineangiograms. In: Digital Imaging in Cardiovascular Radiology. PH Heintzen, R Brennecke (Eds.) Georg Thieme Verlag Stuttgart, 1983: 89–104.
10. Reiber JHC, Kooijman CJ, Slager CJ, Gerbrands JJ, Schuurbiers JCH, Boer A den, Wijns W, Serruys PW, Hugenholtz PG: Coronary artery dimensions from cineangiograms; methodology and validation of a computer-assisted analysis procedure. IEEE Trans Med Imaging, MI–3, 1984: 131–141.

11. Reiber JHC, Serruys PW, Kooijman CJ, Wijns W, Slager CJ, Gerbrands JJ, Schuurbiers JCH, Boer A den, Hugenholtz PG: Assessment of short-, medium- and long-term variations in arterial dimensions from computer-assisted quantitation of coronary cineangiograms. Circulation 71, 1985: 280–288.

12. Brown BG, Bolson E, Frimer M, Dodge HT: Quantitative coronary arteriography. Estimation of dimensions, hemodynamic resistance, and atheroma mass of coronary artery lesions using the arteriogram and digital computation. Circulation 55, 1977: 329–337.

13. Gould KL, Kelly KO, Bolson EL: Experimental validation of quantitative coronary arteriography for determining pressure-flow characteristics of coronary stenosis. Circulation 66, 1982: 930–937.

14. Ganz P, Harrington DP, Gasper J, Barry WH: Phasic pressure gradients across coronary and renal artery stenoses in humans. Am Heart J 106, 1983: 1399–1406.

15. Sigward U, Grbic M, Goy JJ, Essinger A: High fidelity pressure gradients across coronary artery stenoses before and after transluminal angioplasty (PTCA). JACC 5, 1985: 521 (Abstract).

16. Serruys PW, Hooghoudt TEH, Reiber JHC, Slager C, Brower RW, Hugenholtz PG: Influence of intracoronary nifedipine on left ventricular function, coronary vasomotility, and myocardial oxygen consumption. Br Heart J 49, 1983: 427–441.

17. Amende I, Simon R, Hood WP, Hetzer R, Lichtlen PR: Intracoronary nifedipine in human beings: magnitude and time course of changes in left ventricular contraction/relaxation and coronary sinus blood flow. J Am Coll Cardiol 6, 1983: 1141–1145.

18. Serruys PW, Booman F, Troost GJ, Reiber JHC, Gerbrands JJ, Brand M van den, Cherrier F, Hugenholtz PG: Computerized quantitative coronary angiography applied to percutaneous transluminal coronary angioplasty; advantages and limitations. In: Transluminal Coronary Angioplasty and Intracoronary Thrombolysis. Coronary Heart Disease IV, M Kaltenbach, A Gruentzig, K Rentrop, WD Bussman. (Eds.) Springer Verlag, Berlin, Heidelberg, New York, 1982: 110–124.

19. Serruys PW, Reiber JHC, Wijns W, Kooijman CJ, Brand M van den, Katen HJ ten, Hugenholtz PG: Assessment of percutaneous transluminal coronary angioplasty by quantitative coronary angiography: Diameter vs densitometric area measurements. Am J Cardiol, 54, 1984: 482–488.

20. Simoons ML, Hugenholtz PG: Estimation of the probability of exercise-induced ischemia by quantitative ECG analysis. Circulation 56, 1977: 552–559.

21. Reiber JHC, Lie SP, Simoons ML, Wijns W, Gerbrands JJ: Computer quantitation location, extent and type of thallium-201 myocardial perfusion abnormalities. In: First IEEE Comp. Society Int. Symp. on Medical Imaging and Image Interpretation. IEEE Cat. No. 82 CH1804-4, 1982: 123–128.

22. Watson DD, Beller GA, Berger BC, Teates CD: Notes on the quantitation of sequential TL-201 images. Softwhere 6, 1979: 4–5, 10.

23. Rigo P, Bailey IK, Griffith LSC, Pitt B, Burow RD, Wagner Jr HN, Becker LC. Value and limitations of segmental analysis of stress thallium myocardial imaging for localization of coronary artery disease. Circulation 61, 1980: 973–981.

24. Detre KM, Wright E, Murphy ML, Takaro T: Observer agreement in evaluating coronary angiograms. Circulation 52, 1975: 979–986.

25. Zir LM, Miller SW, Dinsmore RE, Gilbert JP, Harthorne JW: Interobserver variability in coronary angiography. Circulation 53, 1976: 627–632.

26. Crawford DW, Brooks SH, Selzer RH, Brandt R, Beckenbach ES, Blankenhorn DH. Computer densitometry for angiographic assessment of arterial cholesterol content and gross pathology in human atherosclerosis. J Lab Clin Med 89, 1977: 378–392.

27. Hutchins GM, Miner MM, Boitnott JK: Vessel caliber and branch-angle of human coronary artery branch-points. Circ Res 38, 1976: 572–576.

28. Cherrier F, Booman F, Serruys PW, Cuillière M, Danchin N, Reiber JHC: L'angiographie coronaire quantitative. Application à l'évaluation des angioplasties transluminales coronaires. Arch Mal Coeur 74, 1981: 1377–1387.

29. Wijns W, Serruys PW, Brand M van den, Suryapranata H, Kooijman CJ, Reiber JHC, Hugen-holtz PG: Progression to complete coronary obstruction without myocardial infarction in patients who are candidates for percutaneous transluminal angioplasty: a 90-days angiographic follow-up. In: Prognosis of Coronary Heart Disease, Progression of Coronary Atherosclerosis, H. Ros-kamm (Ed.). Springer-Verlag, Berlin, Heidelberg, New York, Tokyo, 1983: 190–195.

30. Serruys PW, Lablanche JM, Reiber JHC, Bertrand ME, Hugenholtz PG: Contribution of dynamic vascular wall thickening to luminal narrowing during coronary arterial vasomotion. Z Kardiol 72, 1983: 116–123.

31. Serruys PW, Wijns W, Brand M van den, Ribeiro V, Fioretti P, Simoons ML, Kooijman CJ, Reiber JHC, Hugenholtz PG: Is transluminal coronary angioplasty mandatory after successful thrombolysis? Br. Heart J 50, 1983: 257–265.

32. Brown BG, Bolson EL, Dodge HT: Arteriographic assessment of coronary atherosclerosis. Review of current methods, their limitations, and clinical applications. Arteriosclerosis 2, 1982: 2–15.

33. Logan SE: On the fluid mechanics of human coronary artery stenosis. IEEE Trans. on Biom Eng BME-22, 1975: 327–334.

34. Mates RE, Gupta RL, Bell AC, Klocke FJ: Fluid dynamics of coronary artery stenosis. Circ Res 42, 1978: 152–162.

35. Gould KL: Pressure-flow characteristics of coronary stenoses in unsedated dogs at rest and during coronary vasodilation. Circ Res 43, 1978: 245–253.

36. Harrison DG, White CW, Hiratzka LF, Doty DB, Barnes DH, Eastham CL, Marcus ML: The value of lesion cross-sectional area determined by quantitative coronary angiography in assessing the physiologic significance of proximal left anterior descending coronary arterial stenoses. Circulation 69, 1984: 1111–1119.

37. Marcus M, Wright C, Doty D, Eastham C, Laughlin D, Krumm P, Fastenow C, Brody M: Measurements of coronary velocity and reactive hyperemia in the coronary circulation of hu-mans. Circ Res 49, 1981: 877–891.

38. Ganz P, Gaspar G, Barry BH: Phasic coronary stenosis pressure gradients in man; correlations with arteriography. Circulation 68, 1983: III-164 (Abstract).

39. Eng C, Patterson RE, Horowitz SF, Halgash DA, Pichard AD, Midwall J, Herman MV, Gorlin R: Coronary collateral function during exercise. Circulation 66, 1982: 309–316.

40. Rigo P, Becker LC, Griffith LSC, Alderson PO, Bailey IK, Pitt B, Burow RD, Wagner Jr HN: Influence of coronary collateral vessels on the results of thallium-201 myocardial stress imaging. Am J Cardiol 44, 1979: 452-458.

Index of subjects